Families & Chronic Illness

Lorraine M. Wright, RN, PhD
Director, Family Nursing Unit
Professor, Faculty of Nursing
University of Calgary
Calgary, Alberta, Canada

Maureen Leahey, RN, PhD
Team Director, Mental Health Services
Holy Cross Hospital
Adjunct Associate Professor
Faculty of Nursing, University of Calgary
Calgary, Alberta, Canada

Springhouse Corporation
Springhouse, Pennsylvania

Publisher: Keith Lassner
Senior Acquisitions Editor: Susan L. Taddei
Art Director: John Hubbard
Editorial Services Manager: David Moreau
Senior Production Manager: Deborah C. Meiris

Special thanks to Carol Robertson, Bernadette Glenn, and Jean Robinson, who assisted in the preparation of this volume.

CHAPTER 1
The author wishes to thank Fred Bozett, Jane Kirschling, Naomi Ballard, and Joanne Hall at the Oregon Health Sciences University for their early review of this manuscript. Merlene Lorenz-Cobb, Linda Waer, Barbara Edwards, and Dee Ceresero provided secretarial assistance. The author also gratefully acknowledges the faculty from the Department of Family Nursing at the Oregon Health Sciences University in Portland, Oregon, for allowing me to abstract ideas from the Philosophy, Conceptual Framework, and Objectives of the Department of Family Nursing and to share a working model that is in process.

CHAPTER 2
This chapter has appeared in *Family Systems Medicine* 2(3):245-62, 1984. New York: Brunner/Mazel, Inc. Reprinted with permission.

CHAPTER 3
Excerpts from this chapter have appeared in *Family Systems Medicine* 3(1):60-69, 1985. New York: Brunner/Mazel, Inc. Reprinted with permission.

CHAPTER 19
The author wishes to thank Dr. Mary Allen, Associate Professor, and Ms. Chloe Hammons, Assistant Professor, College of Nursing, University of Oklahoma, for their critical review of previous drafts of this chapter. Acknowledgment is also extended to Ms. Loretta Leach for her assistance in manuscript preparation.

Library of Congress Cataloging-in-Publication Data
Families and chronic illness.

(Family nursing series)
Includes bibliographies and index.
1. Chronic diseases—Nursing. 2. Chronically ill—Family relationships. I. Wright, Lorraine M., 1943- . II. Leahey, Maureen, 1944- III. Series.
[DNLM: 1. Chronic Disease—psychology—nurses' instruction. 2. Family—nurses' instruction. WY 152 F198]
RT120.C45F36 1987 616'.04 87-10196
ISBN 0-87434-091-8

To my brother and sister-in-law, Bob and Carol, and my favorite kids, Doran, Ryan, and Marcy, for valuing family life.

Lorraine M. Wright

To my brother and sisters, Don, Pat, and Barbara, and their families for encouraging the youngest child.

Maureen Leahey

ABOUT THE EDITORS

LORRAINE M. WRIGHT, RN, PhD, is Director, Family Nursing Unit, and Professor, Faculty of Nursing, University of Calgary. Dr. Wright's clinical and research interests include family somatics and systemic therapy; training and supervision of family clinical nurse specialists and family therapists; and split-opinion interventions. She maintains a part-time private practice in systemic marital and family therapy and is also a family therapy consultant. Dr. Wright is on the Board of the Alberta Foundation for Nursing Research and is a Member of the Research Committee of the American Association for Marriage and Family Therapy. She also serves on the editorial board of Contemporary Family Therapy—An International Journal.

MAUREEN LEAHEY, RN, PhD, is a nurse/family therapist specializing in work with children/adolescents and families with health problems. Dr. Leahey is a chartered psychologist. She is a Team Director and Director of the Family Therapy Institute, Mental Health Services, Holy Cross Hospital; Adjunct Assistant Professor, Department of Psychiatry, Faculty of Medicine; and Adjunct Associate Professor, Faculty of Nursing, University of Calgary. Dr. Leahey maintains a part-time private practice in strategic marital and family therapy and is a consultant. She is a Member of the Commission on Accreditation of the American Association for Marriage and Family Therapy.

Both editors have taught family nursing and family therapy to nursing and medical students, psychologists, social workers, and residents in family practice, pediatrics, and psychiatry. They have presented papers at national and international conferences in the United States, Canada, Israel, and Europe and have published their work in several journals. They are the co-authors of *Nurses and Families: A Guide to Family Assessment and Intervention* (Philadelphia: F.A. Davis Co., 1984).

CONTENTS

SECTION I: OVERVIEW OF FAMILIES AND CHRONIC ILLNESS

SECTION II: ASSESSING FAMILIES WITH CHRONIC ILLNESS

SECTION III: INTERVENING WITH FAMILIES WITH CHRONIC ILLNESS

PREFACE

Family Nursing Series

Although nurses have always interacted with the families of their patients, today's nurses are not only being encouraged but are also seeking ways to actively help families with health problems.

The Family Nursing Series, which consists of three volumes, focuses on clinically important family health issues. Titles include *Families and Life-Threatening Illness, Families and Chronic Illness,* and *Families and Psychosocial Problems.* Each volume provides an overview of family nursing with assessment and intervention sections on various health problems. Families at various stages of the developmental life cycle (for example, families with young children, families with adolescents, middle-aged families, and aging families) as well as various family forms (for example, single-parent, step-parent, and gay and lesbian families) are presented. Each chapter combines theory, research, and clinical examples to offer practical *how-tos* for assessment and intervention. Additionally, each chapter is organized according to the nursing process with direct access to information about assessment, planning, intervention, and evaluation.

Written for nursing students as well as practicing nurses, the Family Nursing Series provides current clinical information in a practical format. Essential theory is always presented in the context of clinical material, with the emphasis on sound family assessment and intervention. Descriptive case studies illustrate normal and dysfunctional families coping with health issues. Family Nursing Series contributors are authoritative clinicians and educators from a variety of distinguished nursing centers across North America.

Families and Chronic Illness

This volume offers an in-depth clinical guide to assessment and intervention with families with chronic illness. It offers specific, clear instruction on *how to* assess and intervene effectively.

The first section provides the conceptual base for working with families. To interview families and accurately identify their strengths and problems, a nurse must first have a sound conceptual framework. The chapters in this section deal with different aspects of family nursing and chronic illness. Reciprocity issues between the family and chronic illness are considered, as well as the nurse's assumptions about the family's ways to cope with the chronic illness. Intercultural issues are dealt with in a chapter on ethnicity.

The second section tells *how to* assess families with specific chronic illnesses, such as cystic fibrosis, Crohn's disease, chronic pain, and renal disease. Each chapter offers specific questions to use when assessing families.

The third section goes into depth about the issues involved in intervening with families with specific chronic illness. It considers various family forms, such as gay families and single-parent families. It focuses on families in various health care settings, for example, hospitals, community health clinics, outpatient clinics, and patient and caretakers' homes. Each chapter in this section is organized according to the nursing process and includes detailed case studies of families at all stages of the developmental life cycle. Intervention chapters focus on families of infants with Down syndrome, families of school-aged children with hypertension, families of adolescents with diabetes, and aging families and Alzheimer's disease. Other chapters in this section focus on current health problems, such as adolescent obesity, premenstrual syndrome, and cardiac surgery.

The major difference between this book and other books on families and chronic illness is that its primary emphasis is the application of family assessment and intervention models to deal with *specific* chronic illnesses in *specific* clinical settings with families in *specific* family developmental stages.

ACKNOWLEDGMENTS

We are grateful to our many colleagues and friends who have helped in countless ways to make the Family Nursing Series a reality. They stood by us through the moments of exhilaration and exasperation over the two and a half years of this project.

In particular, we are indebted to:

Susan Taddei, Senior Acquisitions Editor at Springhouse Corporation, who first thought of the idea of the series and inspired us to undertake it.

Bernadette Glenn and the staff at Springhouse Corporation for their helpfulness in overseeing the technical aspects of the Family Nursing Series.

The 76 authors who contributed 65 chapters in the Family Nursing Series and who have shared their expertise and vision of family nursing.

The secretaries who have graciously assisted us: Lynda Gourlie, Louise Hamilton, Ilona Schiedrowski, and Evy Stadey.

Douglas Leahey, who had confidence in our ability throughout the project. He encouraged and supported us in numerous ways, not least of which was transporting chapters to the courier.

Fabie Duhamel, who patiently listened to the many tales of the various stages of the Family Nursing Series and provided steady support. She was also a very willing, efficient "courier" who transported chapters between us.

Laura Crealy, who graciously took in all our packages from Federal Express.

In the process of editing these books, we have remained friends as well as colleagues and have discovered new dimensions to our friendship. We learned to hone our negotiating skills, oscillate in inspiring and supporting each other, and enjoy punctuating our progress through mini-celebrations.

M.L.
L.M.W.

GENOGRAM KEY

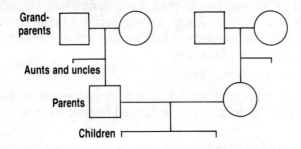

Grand-parents

Aunts and uncles

Parents

Children

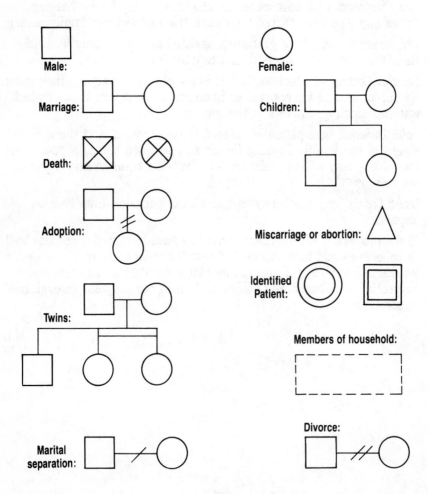

Male:

Female:

Marriage:

Children:

Death:

Adoption:

Miscarriage or abortion:

Identified Patient:

Twins:

Members of household:

Marital separation:

Divorce:

SECTION I

Overview of Families and Chronic Illness

1 Family nursing and chronic illness

Shirley M.H. Hanson, RN, PhD, FAAN
Professor
Department of Family Nursing
School of Nursing
Oregon Health Sciences University
Portland, Oregon

OVERVIEW

Nurses have cared for the chronically ill patient throughout their profession's history. Only recently, however, has family nursing and the role of nursing in chronic illness become more clearly delineated. This chapter provides a picture of family nursing and chronic illness in the United States. First, family nursing as a specialty is addressed, including both its historical development and present status. Issues in family nursing and a beginning conceptual framework are elucidated. Next, family nursing theory is discussed. A summary description of some of the nursing models is followed by the recommendation of an eclectic approach toward applying theory to practice.

The chapter's subsequent section addresses chronic illness and family nursing practice. Chronic illness is defined and a statistical picture given. Practice models, family tasks, and nursing implications illustrate nursing practice. Education for family and chronic care nursing are discussed next. The chapter concludes with a summary of the status of family research as well as the issues and concerns that family nurse researchers should consider when studying families with chronic illness.

The author trusts that this overall view of theory, practice, education, and research will give practicing nurses, nurse educators, researchers, and students a representative picture of the status of contemporary family nursing for chronic illness.

FAMILY NURSING AS A SPECIALTY

Evolution of Family Nursing

The concept of family nursing has been around for centuries. Long before the development of modern nursing, women were regarded as the primary healers (Ehrenreich and English, 1973). From the Dark Ages through the American colonial period, the home and family were society's basic units and women's work in particular centered around the family's survival and maintenance needs. Early "nurses" cared for entire sick populations including not only individuals, but also groups (families) and communities (Ham and Chamings, 1983). As formal caretaker groups such as the Knights Hospitalers arose, however, the focus of "professional" nursing shifted to individuals rather than families.

Florence Nightingale founded modern nursing in the mid-1800s—the beginning of the industrial revolution, a period when men moved to the factories and women stayed home. Nightingale's era also marked the beginnings of the traditional health care hierarchy, with the women nurturing children and patients (nursing) and the men thinking or healing (medicine).

Nightingale was an advocate of family life but also saw the family as an agency of repression. In 1852, at 32, she wrote:

> The family? It is too narrow a field for the development of an immortal spirit, be that spirit male or female. The family uses people not for what they are, not for what they are intended to be, but for what it wants them for—for its own uses...This system dooms some minds to incurable infancy, others to silent misery. (Nightingale, 1979, p. 37)

In spite of her personal sense of family constraint, Florence Nightingale firmly believed in the cradle-to-grave supportiveness of institutions (Hiestand, 1982). She forged her hygiene and health care views with women and children in mind, and encouraged better health by providing midwifery and nursing services in the home. She established the first Training School of Midwives in 1862 (Hiestand, 1982) and advocated nurse midwifery and nursing as a calling and career for educated women.

Nightingale also contributed much to the training of early public health (district or social) nurses. Her book, *Training Nurses for the Sick Poor*, discussed how home nurses could instruct families in hygiene and child care in the home environment (Nightingale, 1949). Recognizing the importance of family participation in maintaining or reviving members' health, she believed women were responsible for their family's health. For those who could not provide this vital health promotion and nursing to their own families, home nurses could substitute. Therefore, the early role of Nightingale–trained social or district nurses (and health missioners) was to promote in-home health and hygiene and provide families with the knowledge and skills to carry out these functions. Thus are public health nurses frequently viewed as the prototypical family nurses as well as the originators of maternal/child nursing.

Early nursing practice was divided between "sick" (hospital based) and "health" (home based) care from 1875–1933; American hospitals were staffed by student nurses, while trained professional nurses served in the homes. Visiting nurse associations were established in 1877, sending nurses into the homes of the sick poor who could not afford hospitals.

The Nightingale era in America ended with Lillian Wald's founding of modern public health and school nursing. Initially, public health nurses cared for the sick poor in New York's slums. This early concept of public health evolved into community health, which focused more on instructive and preventive care. Both fields, however, retained the traditional focus on the family as a care unit. Individual care in the family context was a recurrent theme throughout early American nursing, but particularly in community health.

America's industrial revolution ended this era of nursing, however. According to Ham and Chamings (1983), industrial management engineer Frederick Taylor followed Wald as the major shaper of United States nursing by introducing task orientation to individualized labor. This approach to work diverted nurses from the holistic family focus to that of performing tasks for individuals. Not long after, Max Weber developed the idea of hierarchical patterns of sub– and superordinates; this also hastened family compartmentalization. This complex of social and philosophical influences created a climate in which people's identities were dissected, with the ill person being seen as, for instance, a diseased gallbladder or a case of diabetes. The nursing ideal of holism gave way to reductionism in the face of inductive scientific methods. The family, initially the focus of nursing practice, fell from prominence, reemerging only in recent years.

Present Status of Family Nursing

Very few nursing specialties survived the transition from family–centeredness to fractionalization, let alone the transition back to the family focus that exists today. A few did survive, however, and family nursing today owes its background largely to four specialty areas.

Community health nursing. Public or community health probably has the strongest heritage of any nursing specialty, and it has retained its strong family focus. As early as 1910, one of Columbia University's first nursing baccalaureate programs incorporated family concepts into its community health curriculum. The family as client remains a strong focus within this specialty today.

Maternal/child nursing. Maternity and pediatric nursing also have strong family traditions; indeed, the promotion of mothers' and infants' health was one of nursing's earliest missions. Nurses in this specialty often view the family more as the context for individual care, however, than as the primary unit. Unlike community health, these specialties bridge inpatient and outpatient areas. There is a current movement to integrate (in health care facilities as well as in nursing schools) and rename the maternal and child specialties. Many departments have changed their names from Maternal/Child to Parent/Child, and moved from a medical to a nursing (pediatrics to childrearing) orientation, or have shifted their conceptual bases from individual to family.

Mental health nursing. Mental health or psychiatric nursing is another specialty with a claim on the family. Although the tradition of family nursing within psychiatric nursing is not as long as that of community health or maternal/child nursing, some within the mental health field have adopted a definite family orientation to practice. Seminal work in family-focused therapy was done in the 1930s, followed by 50 years of both theoretical and therapeutic development. All have made an impressive contribution to what is now called family nursing.

Family nurse practice. The family nurse practitioner (FNP) movement is the most recent nursing specialty to affect family nursing. This specialty developed in the 1960s, devoting its practice to the primary care of entire families. FNP roles include health promotion and protection— emphasizing wellness as well as illness. These nurses interact with and offer continuous coordinated health care to the family as a group (Ford, 1979, p. 98). Some nurses dismiss FNP programs as physician-extension rather than family nursing. Others believe the movement has placed nursing at the forefront of American health care, since primary care is the entry point into the health care system. When asked to define the family nurse, many health consumers conjure up the family nurse practitioner model.

Family nursing, then, is both old and new, and has always been an integral part of American nursing. It is simultaneously innovative and conservative. Because it is defined differently by different groups within nursing, it is not articulated well enough yet to give solid direction for prototype program development.

The status of the family nurse remains unclear. Family nurse practitioners, community-health, parent-child, and psychiatric/mental health nurses all stake their own territorial claims, not wanting to share their specialities' family component. Therefore, family content remains diluted throughout nursing curricula and practice.

Issues in Family Nursing

Leavitt (1982) says that, if family nursing is to progress as a specialty, it must overcome a number of obstacles. First, it must assemble and evaluate the vast amount of relevant information in the social science literature, and bring it together in a way meaningful for nursing practice.

Second, family theory and research methodologies must be included in most nursing curricula, a step that should come naturally as more nurses prepare in family studies and as more family content is incorporated into nursing curricula.

Third, comprehensive family assessment intervention and measurement tools must be developed. Some nurses have developed their own such instruments, but these do not always fit within existing social science conceptual/theoretical frameworks. In other words, there is a gap between knowledge of family theory, therapy, and nursing; nursing has not yet delineated what part of family theory/therapy is most pertinent to its needs.

Fourth, counterproductive attitudes must be overcome. Many people believe that family studies information is intuitive or good common sense; they find it hard to believe that there is a credible and scientific knowledge base about something as familiar as their own families of origin. Also, many people and cultures believe that the way their family functions and interacts is the right or best way, a "familio centrism" that inhibits alternative conceptualization.

Fifth, historical ties between nursing and medicine (Knafl, 1978) must be reevaluated. Nursing has tended to follow the medical model, emphasizing *individual* disease, diagnosis and treatment, and a problem-centered approach. In other words, nursing has tended to focus on individuals and pathology. Only recently has the profession explored health prevention, health promotion, and family health.

Other issues must also be addressed if family nursing is to develop completely. Health care takes place largely during the day, when families usually cannot receive care as a unit. Although some traditional practices are changing, the health care delivery system still precludes collective family participation.

Health insurance is also oriented to individual care; it focuses on individual illness and recovery rather than on healthy individuals or the family unit. Third-party payment plays an important role in guiding and directing the available health care model.

Like health insurance systems, the traditional and mechanized way of medical record-keeping also hinders family-oriented care. Since nursing has yet to master family assessment, family data remains difficult to record. A system of family nursing diagnosis is also needed.

Finally, while many nurses advocate family–focused care, most still deliver individualized care, just as they learned in the hospital setting. Although the family as the unit of nursing care seems logical, it remains elusive, more an ideal than a real focus. In both inpatient and outpatient settings, family nursing is more in the stage of *becoming* than of *being* family–centered. In short, family nursing as a distinct field remains in its infancy.

Toward a Conceptual Framework for Family Nursing

The concept of family nursing described in this section was developed by the faculty of the Department of Family Nursing, School of Nursing, the Oregon Health Sciences University. To begin, certain terms associated with family nursing—family, family nursing, and family health—must be defined. *Family* is defined broadly as "a social system comprised of two or more persons who coexist within the context of some expectations of reciprocal affection, mutual responsibility and temporal duration" (Department of Family Nursing, 1984), in order to transcend relationships based on blood or marriage. This definition includes traditional nuclear families (husband working, wife at home with children); dual earner families (both parents working); single and stepparent families; married, cohabitating, or homosexual couples; and any other group characterized by commitment, mutual decision making, and shared goals. This definitional breadth is important since people usually define "family" for themselves, and act on valued relationships even when they do not arise from blood ties, marriage, legal adoption, or common residence.

Family nursing focuses on the family not only as client but also as a framework for professional education, a focus for nursing research, and a unifying component for theory development.

Family nurses are commonly involved with families experiencing a situational or developmental transition(s) in their family life cycle. These transitions may be voluntary or involuntary, planned or spontaneous. Most often, they emanate from an individual family member or from society and the outside environment. In order to accomplish their goals, family nurses may intervene on behalf of individuals (subsystem), the family as a unit (system), or the larger community (suprasystem). Family nursing interventions include:

- The promotion, maintenance, and restoration of individual and family health;
- The enhancement of family resources; and
- The procurement of such outside-the-family resources as community, social, and health services.

In most chronic illness, the affected individual is the first to seek health care, but the assistance must come from within the family context. Illness affects the family as a whole, and the family affects the individual's response to his illness. By using this system perspective, the nurse will recognize individuals and families as interacting, dynamic wholes.

Family health is defined as a dynamic, relative state of well-being. Five dimensions—the biological, psychological, sociological, spiritual, and cultural—all combine into the holistic human system. The purpose of family nursing is to promote, maintain, and restore family health; it is concerned with the interactions between the family and society and among the family and individual family members.

One yardstick of family health status is the group's ability to rally when challenged. When the family's resources cannot meet the challenges at hand, stress occurs and the family requires outside intervention.

Family, family nursing, and family health cannot be understood in isolation from the larger environmental context. This external landscape includes the biological, physical, psychological, political, economical, spiritual, and cultural environments. Again, general systems theory helps explain the links between society and families, nursing, and family health, as well as how nursing, families, and family health affect the direction of American society (see Figure 1.1). All belong to an interdependent, interacting system.

Figure 1.1 Model for Family Nursing

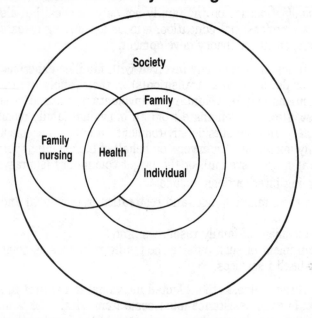

Source: "Statement of Philosophy and Conceptual Framework," Unpublished manuscript.
Portland, Ore.: Oregon Health Sciences University, School of Nursing, Department of Family
Nursing, 1984.

FAMILY NURSING THEORY

Since the early 1950s, social scientists and nursing theorists have tried to organize the accumulated conceptual knowledge of family and nursing. Existing theoretical writings have been continually refined, but no one theory, conceptual framework, or model from within or outside of nursing claims to be the single correct approach to analyzing family nursing in chronic illness. Each approach provides its own unique explanation of nursing and family phenomena. The growth of knowledge about family care emphasizes the need to identify key supporting concepts.

In 1983, Santora reported that two–thirds of all baccalaureate nursing programs followed one of three conceptual frameworks: the adaptation model, the general systems theory, or the developmental framework. Conceptual frameworks allow nursing scientists to analyze family behavior in an organized manner and to understand the predictable family interaction patterns that occur under certain circumstances (Dimond and Jones, 1983). Some of these conceptual frameworks have evolved from the social sciences, others from nursing. Those conceptual frameworks directed specifically toward nursing:
• Provide a basic structure for nursing education.
• Allow systematic classification of nursing knowledge, skills, and values.
• Provide a system for ordering facts that organizes data according to systemic function.
• Illustrate essential content relationships.

Family Social Science Models

Theoretical approaches to family analysis have changed over time. Hill and colleagues (1957) first identified at least seven theoretical approaches to the analysis of family development. Later, Hill and Hansen (1960), Christensen (1964), and Nye and Berardo (1981) reduced this number to five major strategies. The significant elements of these frameworks differed in their underlying assumptions about the nature of man, the family, and society. More recently, Burr and colleagues (1979) in a landmark work further elaborated these theories and boosted the family subfield into the mainstream of sociological theory (Dimond and Jones, 1983). In today's social sciences, theoretical writings about the family are usually categorized under three frameworks: structural-functional, interactional, and developmental. (For an in-depth discussion of the frameworks, the reader is encouraged to consult additional sources.)

Nursing Models

The 1960s brought systematization to nursing practice and nursing scholars began articulating the profession's philosophy and goals. Originally, these theorists focused on individuals (Abdellah et al., 1961; Wiedenback, 1964), but then recognized individuals as part of a social system (Smith, 1968; Becknell and Smith, 1975). Travelbee (1971) was the first to define nursing as an interpersonal process wherein the nurse helps the individual or group prevent or cope with illness and suffering, and if necessary, to find meaning in those experiences. Travelbee (1971) was an early proponent of formally including the family in the client system.

Imogene King (1981) followed a similar pattern. Her theoretical nursing framework incorporated individuals into groups; by 1981, she broadened the framework to include families/groups. Orem's (1980) self-care model viewed the family as a provider capable of delivering effective basic health service after careful instruction from professional caretakers.

The adaptation model (Roy, 1970) is one of the most useful in chronic care nursing. Although it did not include the family originally, this model has proven applicable to family and community issues (Riehl and Roy, 1980). In the adaptation model, nursing is rooted in a concern for man as a total being along a health-illness continuum, with assessment and intervention directed toward helping the patient and family to adapt. Characteristic nursing interventions include selection of strategies designed to promote adaptation, thereby saving the nurse's energy for healing.

These nursing theories and models will undoubtedly change with testing and application, but future trends appear supportive of family nursing.

Eclectic Approach

Each of the existing conceptual frameworks, whether originating within or outside of nursing, offers a distinct approach to nursing families in chronic illness. Focusing as they do on one aspect of family life, they yield certain insights but also overlook others of equal value. Utilizing only one framework inevitably discounts the multiple facets of family life. In practice, the nurse's choice of framework will depend on the questions being asked and the nursing care required.

Eclecticism may be the most efficient family nursing approach to chronic illness. Developmental theory (Duvall, 1977), for example, may help clarify family members' functions, roles, and tasks over time. As the family life cycle progresses, activities change and relationships among family members and between larger social institutions will alter. This theory may provide the structure by which long-term changes can be described and understood. It allows a more sweeping view of family development, helping to put issues into historical perspective.

The interactional framework (Hill and Hansen, 1960; Mead, 1934), on the other hand, examines family members' immediate behaviors and transactions. This framework illuminates family role enaction and associated family perceptions. Role theory is often part of the larger interactional framework; it can provide information on the norms which guide family members' interpretations of explicit and implicit messages regarding expected behavior. Families help individual role assumption and help members progress from one developmental phase to another.

In reality, many theoretical concepts overlap. For example, structural–functional elements can be applied to general systems theory, and the interactional framework can incorporate concepts from role theory and symbolic interaction. Nursing models derive from some of the broader family social science structures. For example, Roy's adaptation model has adapted some ideas from general systems and interactional theories.

No one framework encompasses every element in family nursing in chronic illness. Wright and Leahey (1984) may well have articulated the best eclectic family nursing approach to date. They call their model the Calgary Family Assessment Model (CFAM). It consists of three major frameworks (structural, developmental, and functional) and is based on a systems/cybernetics/ communication theory foundation. Friedman (1981) has also developed an eclectic assessment model, incorporating several structural–functional and interactional frameworks from family social science.

In the next decade, it remains for nursing scholars to bring the more conventional social science theories closer to nursing theories/models. This would connect family nursing to the broader disciplines of family social science; it would also help explicate conceptual frameworks that could be used for family nursing with chronically ill persons.

CHRONIC ILLNESS AND FAMILY NURSING PRACTICE

Chronic Illness

Chronic illness is the greatest health problem in the United States (Mayo, 1956; Anderson and Bauwens, 1981). An umbrella term encompassing many long-lasting diseases, chronic illness usually implies some degree of disability. Nursing practice has long been identified with the care and comfort of persons with chronic illness.

A number of formal definitions of chronic illness exist; that developed in 1956 by the Commission on Chronic Illness (Mayo, 1956, p. 9) is still in use:

> All impairments or deviations from normal which have one or more of the following characteristics: are permanent, leave residual disability, are caused by non–reversible pathological alteration, require special training of the patient for rehabilitation, may be expected to require a long period of supervision, observation, or care.

The terms chronic illness and chronicity are often used interchangeably to describe numerous pathological conditions occurring over long periods of time. Archbold and Perdue (Perdue et al., 1981) argue that not all chronic conditions are intrinsically pathological and that the word "chronicity" should replace "chronic disease" (Perdue et al., 1981, p. 3):

> Chronicity comprises all the vexing, weakening or troubling stressors of long duration associated with biological, cultural, economic, political or psychosocial imbalances which human systems possess and which influence all aspects of the system's relationship with any other system.

This latter definition covers a broad range of varied clinical phenomena, from heart conditions and hypertension to learning disabilities, mental health difficulties, arthritis, racism, and economic deprivation.

This chapter defines chronic illness as any impairment interfering with individual ability to function fully in the environment. In this sense, chronic illnesses are generally characterized by relatively stable periods, often interrupted by acute episodes requiring medical attention or hospitalization. Prognosis varies from normal life to unpredictable, early death. Chronic conditions are rarely cured, but are managed through individual and family effort (Thomas, 1984).

Statistics. Accurate statistics on the chronic illness incidence and prevalence in the United States are difficult to obtain. Incidence refers to the number of new cases and prevalence refers to the total number of cases of a particular disease—that is, new plus old cases. Assessing the prevalence of chronic health problems is difficult since chronic illness may be a slow, insidious process with mild or unnoticed beginnings. A survey carried out in the United States substantiated the prevalence of long-term illness as the *major* health problem, indicating that approximately 50% of the civilian population (23.3 million people) had one or more chronic conditions (U.S. Department of Health, Education and Welfare, 1971b; Strauss and Glaser, 1975; Epiopoulos, 1981).

The survey cited the following incidences (in percentage of the general population) of major chronic illnesses: heart conditions, 16.4%;

arthritis and rheumatism, 14.8%; impairment of back and spine, 8.2%; mental and nervous conditions, 7.8%; impairment of lower extremities and hips, 6.1%; visual impairments, 5.6%; and hypertension without cardiac involvement, 5.4%. People of different ages were found to suffer from different chronic conditions. Children under age 17 and young adults aged 17 to 44 are more likely than other age groups to develop complete or partial paralysis of the lower extremities and hips. Those over 45 are more likely to have arthritis, rheumatism, and heart conditions.

The leading health problems in the U.S. today are heart disease, stroke, and cancer, all of which largely affect adults. Arteriosclerosis and related conditions occur in one of every four adults and are the greatest cause of chronic illness and death. The incidence of cancer is rising, striking one of every four people; it has become the number two cause of mortality. Arthritis, the leading reason for immobility, affects one of every ten individuals.

The prevalence of chronic illness is also increasing, for a number of reasons. First, the elimination of infectious and parasitic disease through vaccination, immunization, and improved sanitation has helped enlarge the elderly population; where infection used to kill young people in great numbers, individuals are now living longer and dying from chronic illness. Indeed, chronic health problems are now the major obstacle to further increases in the life span from its current 73 years.

The aging population. Although chronic illness is not exclusively a problem of the elderly, they are more prone to such conditions. Middle-aged and older people are affected by the majority of disabilities, and chronic conditions account for a large proportion of overall health expenditures. In 1981, the leading chronic conditions afflicting Americans aged 65 and over were arthritis and hypertension. (Figure 1.2 shows the prevalence of chronic conditions among persons aged 45 to 64 and 65 plus.) Many elderly people are hospitalized for chronic digestive, circulatory, and neoplastic conditions rather than illnesses leading to death (American Association of Retired Persons, 1984). Circulatory problems, arthritis, and respiratory ailments prompt most visits to physicians in this population. Heart disease, cancer, and stroke account for more than 75% of all deaths among the elderly; before they reach that catastrophic stage they are also responsible for 20% of all doctor visits, 40% of hospitalization, and almost 50% of all days spent in bed. Arthritis and rheumatism, two of the leading chronic conditions, account for only 2% of hospital days but 16% of days spent in bed.

The future. The graying of the United States population and resultant increase in chronic illness is one of the most significant demographic trends of the twentieth and twenty-first centuries. Figure 1.3 tracks this

Figure 1.2   Prevalence of Top Chronic Conditions (in persons 45-64 years and 65 +)

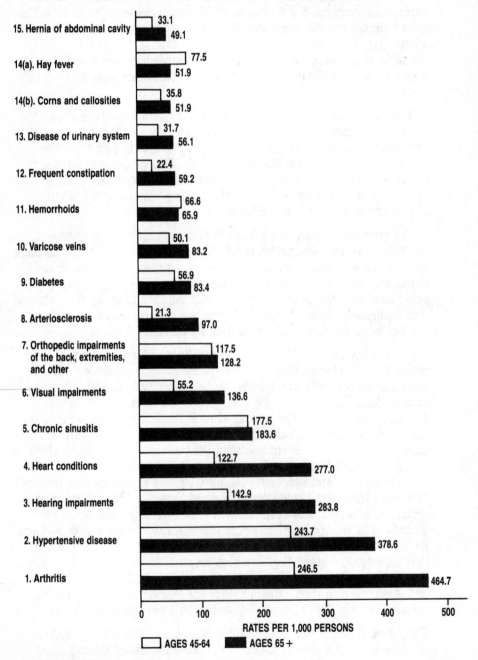

Source: *Aging America: Trends and Projections*. Washington, D.C.: American Association of Retired Persons, 1984.

Figure 1.3   Actual and Projected Population by Age (55 and older) 1900-2050

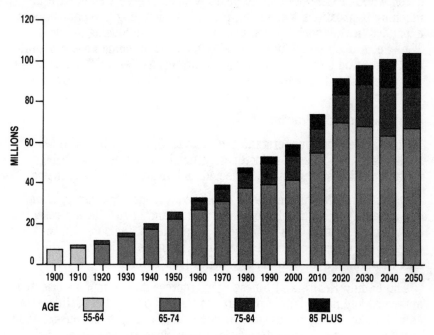

AGE
55-64   65-74   75-84   85 PLUS

Source: *Aging America: Trends and Projections.* Washington, D.C.: American Association of Retired Persons, 1984.

trend from 1900 and extrapolates it through the year 2050. In 1982, more than one in five Americans was 55 years or over; currently, the 75-plus group is the fastest growing segment of the population. By 2050, one of every three persons will be over 55 years of age and one out of four will be over 65.

The elderly constitute 11% of the total population, but account for approximately 30% of all health care expenditures. Half of those over 65 have one or more chronic conditions that limit their activity. By 2050, some 31.8 million people will suffer some degree of health-related activity limitation. Eight of the 10 major causes of death among the elderly are chronic degenerative diseases. Eighty percent of all older persons have at least one chronic illness. Of these, 46% have some limitation and 40% are limited in *major* activities of daily living. Because male life expectancy is less than female, these health problems, like most of the social and economic problems of the elderly, predominately affect women. Too, the elderly nonwhite population is growing faster than the elderly white population. The aged see their physicians and spend time in the hospital twice as much as do their younger counterparts (CNA, 1985).

All regions of the world are currently witnessing an increase in the absolute and relative size of their older populations. By 2025, one in seven world citizens will be 60 years or older. These trends have far-reaching implications for nursing practice since aging populations need expanded health, social, income maintenance, and housing services. The effects of chronic illness on independent functioning have a significant impact on service demand and future needs. By 2025, twice as many health and long-term care services will be needed as are now available.

Frameworks for Practice

Family nurses must understand the practical interface between family health care and illness; unfortunately, much of the material being written on this subject is disconnected and lacks any logical schema.

Doherty and McCubbin (1985) published a model, the *Family Health and Illness Cycle*, that helps organize family and health theory, research, and practice. Within this framework, there are *six* temporal phases of the family's efforts to reduce illness risk, manage initial onset, and adapt to illness and, if necessary, death (see Table 1.1).

The Family Health and Illness Cycle represents a symptom–oriented approach, keying on family preparation for and prevention of illness as well as on family definitions, reactions, and coping techniques. Family nursing assessment and intervention takes place at each phase of the cycle; thus the model represents a way of organizing nursing knowledge and skills. The relationship between the model's components, and thus to nursing practice, is illustrated in Figure 1.4.

Many family nurses question the relative importance of their work with individual patients and with family units. When, for instance, should members of the health care team (nurses and other professionals) assemble the whole family unit? Doherty (1985) developed a continuum addressing this issue (see Figure 1.5); although explicated for use in family medicine, it has nursing implications. Doherty recommends that the family of a chronically ill patient always be included in health care planning. He emphasizes that health care professionals in such cases need a knowledge base of family systems and skills in working with families and groups. Nurses who work primarily with the chronically ill need foundations in family theory, general systems theory, and group process.

Family Tasks

Strauss and Glaser (1975) discussed some of the tasks that families of chronically ill patients must perform. Each task has nursing implications. First, there is (medical) crisis prevention and management, especially in those chronic diseases characterized by potentially fatal crises.

Table 1.1   Phases of the Family Health and Illness Cycle

Phase	Characteristic(s)
Family health promotion/risk reduction	• Emphasizes identification and shaping of health-promoting environmental, social, psychological, and interpersonal factors within or surrounding the family.
Family vulnerability/illness onset	• Life events precipitating illness or rendering the family vulnerable.
Family illness appraisal	• Family attempts to assign meaning to illness.
Family acute response	• Immediate emotional and interactional aftermath of illness; family appraisal of the experience.
Family and health care system	• Family seeks outside help or decides to handle problem(s) internally.
Adaptation to illness	• Long-term impact of illness; family role in rehabilitation and recovery.

Source: Doherty, W.J., and McCubbin, H.I. "Families and Health Care: An Emerging Area of Theory, Research, and Clinical Intervention," *Family Relations* 34(1):5–11, 1985.

Cardiac conditions are one example, but severe diabetes and epilepsy are equally threatening. Family members must learn to organize their lives for crisis management, a process that should begin by asking key questions:

• How probable is a crisis?
• Could a crisis be fatal?
• What are the crisis' signs and symptoms?
• Can crisis be avoided?
• What should the family do in case of crisis?
• How can the nurse help prevent and/or assist during crisis?

The second major family task is regimen management. What kind of health routine has been established for the individual? How must family members adjust in order to accommodate it? Do patient and family comply with their regimens? What are the consequences of noncompliance? What part does nursing play in the regimen?

Symptom control is the third major family task; it is closely linked to regimen adherence. Patient and family must rely on their own judgment, wisdom, and ingenuity to control symptoms. Though the nurse

Figure 1.4   Family Health and Illness Cycle

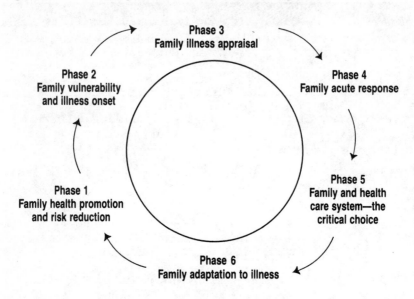

Source: Doherty, W.J., and McCubbin, H.I. "Families and Health Care: An Emerging Area of
Theory, Research, and Clinical Intervention," *Family Relations* 34(1):5–11, 1985.

might tell them what to expect when symptoms are not controlled, the
individuals must ultimately be sensitive to their own physiologic idio-
syncrasies. The nurse's role here is to educate clients about signs,
symptoms, and appropriate responses.

Fourth, families must adjust to the temporal and role disruption
which usually accompany chronic disease. Often the chronically ill find
themselves with too much time on their hands. People forced to quit
their jobs or abandon leisure activities often face boredom and depression. At the same time, chronic illness can impose added responsibility
on healthy family members, who must assume the roles and functions
previously performed by the patient.

Families must also learn to handle the disease course, or trajectory,
the fifth task. Some chronic disease trajectories plunge straight down,
some deteriorate slowly, while others vacillate back and forth. Families
adjust more easily to a predictable trajectory.

Overcoming social isolation is the sixth major family task. The patient's reduced energy, impaired bodily functioning, disfigurement, time-
consuming medical regimen, and possible desire to hide the disease
and its management can all disrupt or disintegrate social relationships.
This is especially true for aging families in which the patient's spouse
becomes the caretaker and has no respite. In chronic illness, the family

Figure 1.5   Assembling the Family in Health Care

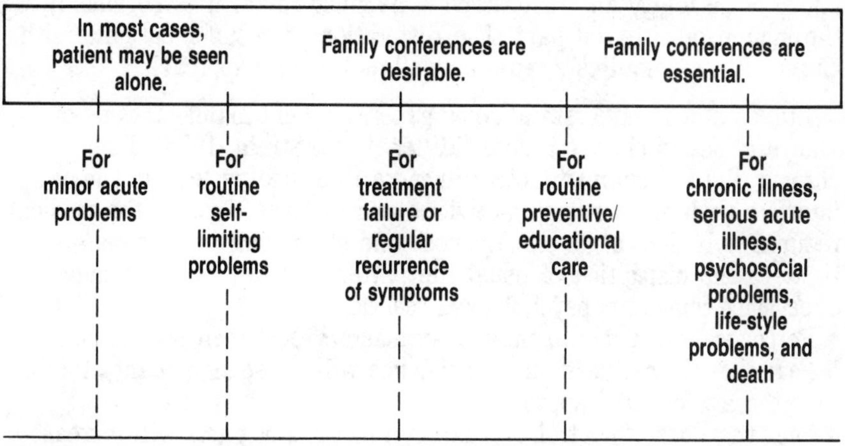

In most cases, patient may be seen alone.		Family conferences are desirable.		Family conferences are essential.
For minor acute problems	For routine self-limiting problems	For treatment failure or regular recurrence of symptoms	For routine preventive/ educational care	For chronic illness, serious acute illness, psychosocial problems, life-style problems, and death

Source: Doherty, W.J. "Family Interventions in Health Care," *Family Relations* 34(1):129–37, 1985.

must maintain as normal an existence as possible despite the disease. This normalcy depends on establishing social arrangements, managing symptoms and regimen, and storing useful knowledge and skills.

The final family task in chronic illness is to find the necessary funding for treatment and daily needs in the face of partial or complete loss of income. Health care is especially costly when it extends over a number of years. Chronic illness can easily drain a family's financial resources.

Both families and patients must develop strategies for performing all these tasks. The most effective techniques involve organization, family cooperation, and evaluation of consequences.

Nursing Implications

Virtually every practicing nurse in the United States works with patients having some form of chronic disability. Virtually all health care facilities have patients presenting with one or more chronic conditions.

Nursing management of chronic illness can begin at any point in the health care system from entry to discharge (Craig and Edwards, 1983). Chronic illness nursing is really rehabilitation nursing, if rehabilitation is defined as individual and family restoration to the fullest possible physical, mental, social, vocational, and economic capacity (Stryker, 1977).

Nurses working with the chronically ill must realize that rehabilitation begins when patients first suffer acute disease, trauma, or early symptoms of a progressive debilitating condition (Stryker, 1977). The two basic rehabilitative aims in chronic illness are prevention of further injury or disability and restoration of as much function as possible in the injured or diseased part. The restoration process for patients with chronic illness requires a team as well as a family approach.

Nurses should understand some general patient manifestations of and reactions to chronic illness (Miller, 1983; Strain, 1974). First, chronic illness impairs function in more than one system and may interfere with many normal activities and routines. Second, the medical regimen is limited in its effectiveness and often contributes substantially to the disruption of usual life patterns. Third, patients may experience numerous psychological reactions:

• Perceived threat due to the loss of mastery over their own bodies.
• Fear that their illness and dependence will cause significant others to withdraw love and approval.
• Fear that loss of control over bodily functions or parts will increase dependence on others.
• Anxiety about separation from supportive, protective loved ones and environments.
• Fear of pain.
• Fear of strangers who must provide intimate care.

Clients' reactions to chronic illness may vary with age, cultural values, race, and ethnicity (Anderson and Bauwens, 1981). Even when diseases are not age–specific, different age groups react differently to the experience. (For additional information, refer to Chapter 4, Ethnicity and families with chronic illness.) Too, each person's cultural background and personality affects reactions to illness, pain, and impairment; each culture, for instance, has beliefs and values about health and illness and how people should respond. Race and ethnicity also affect the occurrence of and response to chronic health problems. Certainly some chronic problems are more prevalent among specific races; the occurrence of hypertension and diabetes in nonwhite populations is one example.

Several of the nursing goals in chronic care are aimed not at curing the client but at controlling his health problems and his anxiety over the threat of full-blown incapacitation (Miller, 1983). The nurse should help chronically ill clients and families accept the changes precipitated by the disease, and thus preserve everyone's physical and psychological integrity. Improving function, if possible, might be a realistic goal, but the nurse must recognize that, in some cases, a standstill or even slow regression might imply progress.

The nurse can improve function by teaching an individual with disabling arthritis how to use special utensils and self–care devices.

She might work to prevent secondary complications by supervising diabetic self–care or by teaching COPD patients to eat properly, perform breathing exercises, and identify sputum changes. Yet another nursing goal, delaying deterioration and disability, might be achieved by helping a family maintain maximum orientation and self–care for an Alzheimer's victim.

Adaptation, however, is the ultimate family nursing goal in chronic illness. Families of the chronically ill incur many biological, psychological, and sociological losses, and there are no clear–cut norms of behavior for anyone involved (Craig and Edwards, 1983). Nurses can help families adjust to this situation; if necessary, they may also have to help patient and family achieve the ultimate goal: death with peace, comfort, and dignity.

FAMILY NURSING EDUCATION AND CHRONIC ILLNESS

Information about the preparation of nurses for family–centered practice in either acute or chronic illness is scarce. Some scattered material, mostly in clinical journals, addresses nursing roles in a variety of specific chronic conditions, such as diabetes. This chapter offers general comments about nursing education and curriculum and their need to prepare nurses for family care in chronic illness.

There is no standardized nursing curriculum. The National League for Nursing (NLN) accreditation process sets institutional standards but does not specify curriculum. However, most nurse education programs appear to revolve philosophically, conceptually, and substantially around four general concepts: people, health, nursing, and environment, and their interrelationships (Bozett & Fields, 1984).

The identification of key concepts in nursing education gained acceptance largely due to the NLN's requirement of a guiding framework for curriculum decisions. Santora (1983) recently surveyed schools of nursing in the United States for their major curricular concepts. The nine most commonly cited were: man, nursing, nursing process, health, illness, family, community, social systems, and environment. (Note that the four concepts reported earlier have been expanded to nine concepts, and that illness and the family are now included.) Santora noted that these concepts were often isolated from any conceptual framework or other broad intellectual schema. In other words, faculty believed it important to include information about the family and illness (chronic and acute) in their curriculum, but they did not present these concepts systematically or explore the connections between them.

The quality or quantity of family concepts in nursing curricula vary with the school or level of preparation. At the undergraduate level, family concepts may be taught only in such prerequisite courses as sociology, psychology, human growth and development, or anthropology. No systematic requirement ensures that every undergraduate student entering the nursing segment of the curriculum understands family dynamics and their nursing implications. Some schools, however, appear to have integrated family content throughout their curricula. For example, students learning to assess maternity patients also learn the importance of the family context to prenatal nursing care. This delivery of family content is most often included in pediatrics, community health, or mental health nursing courses. Placement of family content may be serendipitous, reflecting the instructor's preferences, or it may be logical and sequential. Some undergraduate programs are so committed to family concepts that they develop specific courses for it. In these programs, all nursing students are required to learn family concepts and apply them to the clinical settings encountered throughout the rest of the program. Although the actual state of family nursing instruction is unknown, institutions with a strong undergraduate family focus still constitute a minority.

The status of family-related concepts in graduate education is equally elusive. Traditional master's degree preparation concentrates on developing a clinical nursing specialty (maternal/child, mental health, medical–surgical, or community health) and/or on role preparation (teaching, administration, clinical practice, or research). Advanced family concepts are more often offered at the graduate level or are obtained through social science courses supplemental to the nursing program. It seems likely that many students graduating with master's degrees in maternal/child, mental health, family practitioner, or community health nursing have had some exposure to family concepts. Some master's programs even offer a family nurse clinical specialist track, but the role of these graduates remains unclear and their numbers are small.

In recent years, several schools have taken the concept of family more seriously; a few now include Departments of Family Nursing. How many schools have done this is unknown, but the Oregon Health Sciences University in Portland and the University of California in San Francisco are two leading examples. Structured family nursing programs require more than a simple amalgamation of existing traditional maternity, pediatrics, and geriatrics course material with the addition of new family concepts; they require the evolution of an entirely new philosophy and conceptual framework.

The status of doctoral education in family nursing is unknown. Although the numbers of doctoral programs have substantially increased, there is no accrediting body like the National League for Nursing to keep track of curricula. Nurses seeking doctoral preparation can pursue a PhD, ND, DNSc, or doctorate in a related field. At that level, professional and research programs may include enough family concepts to allow a family major, but it is more likely that doctoral candidates design much of their own program. More and more nurses are doing advanced family work through family studies, family social sciences, family sociology, and similar programs in other schools. The family knowledge base is just starting to filter back into the nursing literature and curriculum.

The educational preparation of nurses for chronic care is as desultory as that for family work. Much nursing education, particularly at the undergraduate and master's levels, concentrates on acute care; even chronic conditions are viewed in terms of acute exacerbations. Many students are mesmerized by intensive care or emergency nursing and the advanced pathophysiologic and technical knowledge required to care for such patients. Basic supply and demand compels many schools to spend a disproportionate amount of both theoretical and practicum time in acute settings. Courses devoted specifically to chronic care are practically nonexistent. Where chronic illness does exist in the curriculum, the focus is on nursing care during acute manifestations, as might occur in the hospital setting.

Some graduate schools offer majors in chronic care, but most nursing majors are in such clinical specialties as neurological or cardiovascular nursing. Students of geriatrics or rehabilitation are most likely to complete advanced work in chronic illness.

Aydelotte (1983) projects a marked increase over time in the demand for nurses skilled in gerontology and chronic care. Both population and health care trends indicate that nurses will eventually assume major responsibility for chronic illness management. Those employed in hospital and ambulatory/home settings will require advanced skills and scientific knowledge to help individuals and their families adapt to the changes associated with chronic disease; therefore family and chronic illness nursing education remain important mandates for the future.

FAMILY NURSING RESEARCH AND CHRONIC ILLNESS

The closing part of this chapter will explore some of the problems in conducting family nursing research and what the questions and methods pertaining to chronic illness might be.

Family nursing research is in its infancy. Family scientists from many disciplines, including nursing, are still trying to discern basic conceptual and methodological issues; in recent years, some nursing scholars have turned to the family as an analytic unit and tried to relate their material to the larger theoretical and conceptual frameworks of nursing and family social science.

Feetham (1985) has summarized the status of family nursing research and identified future issues and directions. She contends that
nursing researchers do not use the theoretical concepts commonly used
in mainstream family studies, and that authors of the major nursing
models have only begun to include the family in their own conceptuali-
zations. She concludes that nurse researchers can contribute meaning-
fully to knowledge about the family and family health. Nurses should
build on knowledge and research from other disciplines to develop
nursing models and examine the family as a unit of analysis. By understanding how families help each other, how they cope, and how they
grow, nurses can learn much about family health promotion and protection. Nurse researchers should direct their attention to defining family
health and determining the predictors of family well-being and
strengths.

Like family nursing, chronic care remains relatively unexplored by
nurse researchers. However, numerous nursing authors have proposed
and outlined future explorations of the subject.

Two sociologists at the University of California in San Francisco,
Strauss and Glaser (1975), characterized present research on chronic
illness as piecemeal, categorical, and overly focused on the biomedical
aspects of isolated diseases. Future research on chronic illness should
therefore consider several arguments. First, in order to treat any chronically ill person's medical problems, one must supplement medical
knowledge with psychological and social knowledge. That expanded
knowledge base should include not only how families handle chronic
disease and the associated medical regimens, but how these diseases,
regimens, and symptoms affect individual and collective lives.

The second argument against a strictly disease-oriented research
approach is that chronically ill persons often display associated psychological problems. Although each disease or group of diseases gives
rise to different issues, an understanding of the common rather than
the unique problems can be of considerable value in improving patients'
lives. These common problems are complex; they and their nursing
implications deserve further study.

In short, chronic care nurses need information about patients' and
families' psychological problems. How might families coping with a
particular chronic illness better manage their lives? How can nurses
help resolve problems arising in the wake of chronic illness and
treatment—problems like social stigma, isolation, family disruption,
marital discord, and domestic role transformation? How can the nurse
help prevent crises within the family or the community?

Dimond and Jones (1983) discussed nursing and chronicity over its
life span, and identified two major methodological issues: a need for

descriptive longitudinal designs, and use of cohort studies. Chronic illness, Dimond and Jones argue, should be studied as it occurs—over time. Longitudinal designs that study the stages of chronic illness help the nurse plan effective intervention strategies. Investigators interested in interventions and their effects on coping should obtain premorbid information if possible as well as follow-up assessments after treatment (Watson and Kendall, 1983).

Second, cohort studies would allow investigators to select a specific disease and describe how it is experienced by three different age groups. They could gather data simultaneously from several groups and compare across cohorts. This approach, combined with longitudinal design, would provide a rich comparison of age groups over time.

Watson and Kendall (1983) also addressed a few pertinent methodological and research issues, but focused specifically on coping. They believed that chronic disease patient populations are often mistakenly viewed as single and homogeneous. Patients seen at single sites might not constitute a representative sample, so multiple site sampling may be desirable. Researchers should employ predictive analyses as well as simple mean comparisons. Correlating patient characteristics at disease onset with later coping levels would facilitate early intervention for both patients and families. Also, alternative interventions could be developed for patients not likely to be helped by current treatment programs.

Much of the research on the psychological characteristics of chronic disease patients is based upon subjective data. More objective information must be gathered and appropriate control group comparisons used. Outcome studies require comparison groups that control for time passage and placebo effects. Patients with different disease entities could be compared.

Chronic illness and coping are multidimensional concepts, not assessable through a single measure; multimethod, multivariate studies would yield much more useful information—although investigators must be careful not to overtax subjects with too many instruments (Watson and Kendall, 1983).

Finally, Litman (1973) summarized existing empirical work and made some suggestions for further inquiry. He advocated greater application and integration of family theory in health care research. Family theorists should no longer ignore health care research; neither should health care researchers continue to ignore family theory. Family health behavior should be connected to general family theory in order to be generalizable, that is, to illuminate how coping with illness compares to coping with other kinds of family crisis.

One needs also to consider how the family life cycle might dictate health and nursing care. For instance, did nursing interventions vary with the different family behaviors characteristic of specific family stages? And how were nursing and age related in chronic care?

Nursing needs more valid and reliable instruments to measure family health, illness, and functioning. To date, researchers have found it difficult to devise broadly applicable family measurement instruments yielding generalizable information. Even if such instruments were developed, many methodological and analytical issues would remain. For instance, should family data collected from individuals in a family unit be analyzed separately or collectively?

Intergenerational health and health care studies are also needed. Cross-sectional and one-generational studies do not address changing family health dynamics.

Comprehensive health data on the general public is also lacking. While accurate statistics are available on how people die, little is known about actual public health status. Such information could help identify "high risk" families and establish health norms.

As yet, little is understood about illness' impact on the family unit. For example, why are some families strengthened by a health crisis while others disintegrate? Do families with acute illness cope differently from families with chronic disorders? How do roles change as a result of various kinds of illnesses and do such changes affect interactions and relationships? How does long-term chronic illness alter relationships between the patient and kin and among the nuclear and extended family? Where does the social support system enter into illness and recovery? Who are the actors in this social support system and how and why do they differ?

More needs to be learned about the effects of chronic illness on families of varying life styles and structures, and how those effects vary with the patient's role. What if the victim is a child, breadwinner, or grandparent? Do single-parent families respond differently from stepfamilies or nuclear families? Does family response vary with diagnosis, rate of onset, medical regimen, and attitudes toward illness?

More and more people suffer from some kind of chronic disorder. Except during acute episodes, when they are hospitalized or placed in long-term care facilities, most remain at home. What is the home caretaker's role? How is family life altered, and what price is paid for the increasing reliance on home care of the chronically disabled?

Many research questions could be asked in regard to family nursing and chronic illness, far more questions than have been answered by previous work. Just as family nurses have an important role to perform in care provision, nursing education, and advancement of family nursing theory, they must take the lead in research to help solve many of the problems facing families with chronic illness.

CONCLUSIONS

This chapter provided a general picture of family nursing and chronic illness. A history of family nursing as well as its present status and future issues were discussed. Existing nursing models were summarized and the need to integrate these models with mainstream family social science was pointed out. Family nursing practice, education, and research were also reviewed.

Several conclusions can be drawn. Family nursing has both old and new elements, but it is still an emergent specialty. The idea of viewing the family as a unit of care and of analysis still requires much study. Since the world population is inevitably aging, and the incidence of chronic illness is thereby increasing, nurses must learn more about chronic conditions, their short- and long-term effects on the family unit, and family responses to chronically ill members. Combining the concepts of family nursing care and chronic illness in this chapter has been a challenge, since little has been written about either one. It is hoped this chapter will serve as a foundation for future work on nursing families with chronic illness.

REFERENCES

Abdellah, F.G., et al. *Patient–Centered Approaches to Nursing.* New York: Macmillan Publishing Co., 1961.

American Association of Retired Persons. *Aging America: Trends and Projections.* Washington, D.C.: American Association of Retired Persons, 1984.

Anderson, S.V., and Bauwens, E.E., eds. *Chronic Health Problems: Concepts and Application.* St. Louis: C.V. Mosby Co., 1981.

Anderson, T.P. "Educational Frame of Reference: An Additional Model for Rehabilitation Medicine," *Archives of Physical Medicine and Rehabilitation* 59(5):203–06, 1978.

Archbold, P., and Perdue, B. "Chronicity: A Systems Approach," Unpublished manuscript. New Brunswick, N.J.: Rutgers University, 1976.

Auger, J.R. *Behavioral Systems and Nursing.* Englewood Cliffs, N.J.: Prentice–Hall, 1976.

Aydelotte, M.K. "The Future Health Care Delivery System in the United States," in *The Nursing Profession. A Time to Speak.* Edited by Chaska, N. New York: McGraw–Hill Book Co., 1983.

Beavers, W.R. "Hierarchical Issues in a Systems Approach to Illness and Health," *Family Systems Medicine* 1(1):47–55, 1983.

Becknell, E.P., and Smith, D.M. *Systems of Nursing Practice.* Philadelphia: F.A. Davis Co., 1975.

Blum, R.W. *Chronic Illness and Disabilities in Childhood and Adolescence.* New York: Grune & Stratton, 1984.

Bozett, F.W., and Fields, M.R. *The Role of the Nurse in Providing Family Health Care.* Oklahoma City: University of Oklahoma, College of Nursing, 1984.

Broderick, C.B. "Beyond the Five Conceptual Frameworks," *Journal of Marriage and the Family* 33:139–59, 1977.

Burr, W.R., et al., eds. *Contemporary Theories about the Family.* New York: Free Press, 1979.

California Nurses' Association. *The Preparation, Utilization and Regulation of Nursing Personnel.* San Francisco: California Nurses' Association, 1985.

Christensen, H., ed. *Handbook of Marriage and the Family.* Chicago: Rand McNally, 1964.

Clements, I.W., and Roberts, F.B., eds. *Family Health: A Theoretical Approach to Nursing Care.* New York: John Wiley & Sons, 1983.

Cohen, R., and Lazarus, R.S. "Coping with the Stresses of Illness," in *Health Psychology.* Edited by Stone, G.C., and Alder, N.E. San Francisco: Jossey-Bass, 1979.

Craig, H.M., and Edwards, J.E. "Adaptation in Chronic Illness: An Eclectic Model for Nurses," *Journal of Advanced Nursing* 8:397–404, 1983.

Department of Family Nursing. "Statement of Philosophy and Conceptual Framework," Unpublished manuscript. Portland, Ore.: Oregon Health Sciences University, School of Nursing, 1984.

Dimond, M., and Jones, S.L. *Chronic Illness Across the Life Span.* East Norwalk, Conn.: Appleton–Century–Crofts, 1983.

Doherty, W.J. "Family Interventions in Health Care," *Family Relations* 34:129–37, 1985.

Doherty, W.J., and McCubbin, H.I. "Families and Health Care: An Emerging Area of Theory, Research, and Clinical Intervention," *Family Relations* 34(1):5–11, 1985.

Duvall, E.M. *Marriage and Family Development.* Philadelphia: J.B. Lippincott Co., 1977.

Ehrenreich, B., and English, D. *Witches, Midwives, and Nurses: A History of Women Healers.* Old Westbury, N.Y.: The Feminist Press, 1973.

Epiopoulos, C. "Chronic Care and the Elderly: Impact on the Client, the Family, and the Nurse," *Topics in Clinical Nursing* 3(1):71–83, 1981.

Eshleman, J.R. *The Family: An Introduction.* Boston: Allyn & Bacon, 1974.

Fawcett, J. "The Family as a Living Open System: An Emerging Conceptual Framework for Nursing," *International Nursing Review* 22:113–16, 1975.

Feetham, S.L. "Family Research: Issues and Directions for Nursing," in *Annual Review of Nursing Research,* vol. 2. Edited by Werley, H.H., and Fitzpatrick, J.J. New York: Springer Publishing Co., 1985.

Feldman, D.J. "Chronic Disabling Illness: A Holistic View," *Journal of Chronic Disease* 27:287–91, 1974.

Ford, L.E. "The Development of Family Nursing," in *Family Health Care: General Perspectives,* vol. 1. Edited by Hymovich, D.P., and Barnard, M.U. New York: McGraw–Hill Book Co., 1979.

Friedman, M.M. *Family Nursing: Theory and Assessment.* East Norwalk, Conn.: Appleton–Century–Crofts, 1981.

Ham, L.M., and Chamings, P.A. "Family Nursing: Historical Perspectives," in *Family Health: A Theoretical Approach to Nursing Care.* Edited by Clements, I.W., and Roberts, F.B. New York: John Wiley & Sons, 1983.

Hiestand, W.C. "Nursing, the Family, and the 'New' Social History," *Advances in Nursing Science* 4(3):1–12, 1982.

Hill, R., and Hansen, D. "The Identification of Conceptual Frameworks Utilized in Family Studies," *Marriage and Family Living* 22:299–311, 1960.

Hill, R., et al. "An Inventory of Research in Marriage and Family Behavior: A Statement of Objectives and Progress," *Marriage and Family Living* 19:89–92, 1957.

Janosik, E.H., and Miller, J.R. "Theories of Family Development," in *Family Health Care: General Perspectives,* vol. 1. Edited by Hymovich, D.P., and Barnard, M.U. New York: McGraw–Hill Book Co., 1979.

Johnson, A.E. "The Behavioral System for Nursing," in *Conceptual Models for Nursing Practice.* Edited by Reihl, J.P., and Roy, S.C. East Norwalk, Conn.: Appleton–Century–Crofts, 1980.

Katz, S., et al. *Effects of Continued Care: A Study of Chronic Illness in the Home.* Washington, D.C.: U.S. Government Printing Office, 1972.

King, I. "How Does the Conceptual Framework Provide Structure for the Curriculum?" in *Curriculum Process for Developing or Revising Baccalaureate Nursing Programs.* New York: National League for Nursing, 1978.

King, I.M. *A Theory for Nursing: Systems, Concepts, Process.* New York: John Wiley & Sons, 1981.

Knafl, A. *Families Across the Life Cycle: Studies for Nursing.* Boston: Little, Brown & Co., 1978.

Leavitt, M.B. *Families at Risk: Primary Prevention in Nursing Practice.* Boston: Little, Brown & Co., 1982.

Lindemann, J.E. *Psychological and Behavioral Aspects of Physical Disability: A Manual for Health Practitioners.* New York: Plenum Press, 1981.

Litman, T.J. "The Family as a Basic Unit in Health and Medical Care: A Social-Behaviorial Overview," *Social Science and Medicine* 8:495–519, 1973.

Mace, D.R. "The Family Specialist, Past, Present and Future," *Family Coordinator* 21:291–94, 1971.

MacVicar, M.G., and Archbold, P. "A Framework for Family Assessment in Chronic Illness," *Nursing Forum* 15(2):180–94, 1976.

Mayo, L. "Problem and Challenge," in *Guides to Action on Chronic Illness.* New York: National Health Council, 1956.

Mead, G.H. *Mind, Self and Society.* Chicago: University of Chicago Press, 1934.

Miller, J.F., ed. *Coping with Chronic Illness: Overcoming Powerlessness.* Philadelphia: F.A. Davis Co., 1983.

Moulton, P.J. "Chronic Illness, Grief, and the Family," *Journal of Community Health Nursing* 1(2):75–88, 1984.

National League for Nursing: Nursing Data Book 1983–1984. New York: National League for Nursing, 1984.

Nightingale, F. "Sick Nursing and Health Nursing," in *Nursing of the Sick— 1893.* Edited by Hampton, et al. New York: McGraw–Hill Book Co., 1949.

Nightingale, F. *Cassandra.* Westbury, N.Y.: The Feminist Press, 1979.

Nye, F.I., and Berardo, F.M. *Emerging Conceptual Frameworks in Family Analysis.* New York: Praeger Pubs., 1981.

Orem, D.E. *Nursing Concepts of Practice.* New York: McGraw–Hill Book Co., 1980.

Perdue, B.J., et al., eds. *Chronic Care Nursing.* New York: Springer Publishing Co., 1981.

Phipps, L.B. "Theoretical Frameworks Applicable to Family Care," in *Family Focused Care.* Edited by Miller, J.R., and Janosik, E. New York: McGraw–Hill Book Co., 1980.

Preston, R.P. *The Dilemmas of Care: Social and Nursing Adaptations to the Deformed, the Disabled and the Aged.* New York: Elsevier, 1979.

Prince-Embury, S. "The Family Health Tree: A Form for Identifying Physical Symptom Patterns Within the Family," *The Journal of Family Practice* 18(1):75–81, 1984.

Reif, L. "Beyond Medical Intervention: Strategies for Managing Life in Face of Chronic Illness," in *Nurses in Practice: A Perspective on Work Environments.* Edited by Davis, M., et al. St. Louis: C.V. Mosby Co., 1975.

Riehl, J.P., and Roy, S.C. *Conceptual Models for Nursing Practice.* East Norwalk, Conn.: Appleton–Century–Crofts, 1980.

Roberts, F.B. "The Health Care Delivery System and Family Health," in *Family Health: A Theoretical Approach to Nursing Care.* Edited by Clements, I.W., and Roberts, F.B. New York: John Wiley & Sons, 1983.

Roberts, F.C. "The American Family," in *Family Health: A Theoretical Approach to Nursing Care*. Edited by Clements, I.W., and Roberts, F.B. New York: John Wiley & Sons, 1983.

Rogers, M.E. *An Introduction to the Theoretical Basis of Nursing*. Philadelphia: F.A. Davis Co., 1970.

Rogers, R.H. *Family Interaction and Transaction: The Developmental Approach*. Englewood Cliffs, N.J.: Prentice–Hall, 1973.

Rolland, J.S. "Toward a Psychosocial Typology of Chronic and Life-Threatening Illness," *Family Systems Medicine* 17:1–16, 1984.

Roy, S.C. "Adaptation: A Conceptual Framework for Nursing," *Nursing Outlook* 18:42–45, 1970.

Santora, D. "Conceptual Frameworks of Undergraduate and Graduate Nursing Programs," in *The Nursing Profession: A Time to Speak*. Edited by Chaska, N. New York: McGraw–Hill Book Co., 1983.

Schwenk, T.L., and Hughes, C.C. "The Family as Patient in Family Medicine. Rhetoric or Reality?" *Social Science and Medicine* 17:1–16, 1983.

Shapiro, J. "Family Reactions and Coping Strategies in Response to the Physically Ill or Handicapped Child: A Review," *Social Science and Medicine* 17(14):913–31, 1983.

Smith, D.M. "A Clinical Nursing Tool," *American Journal of Nursing* 68(1):2384–88, 1968.

Strain, J. "Psychological Reactions to Chronic Medical Illness," *Psychiatric Quarterly* 51:287, 1974.

Strauss, A.L., and Glaser, B.G. *Chronic Illness and the Quality of Life*. St. Louis: C.V. Mosby Co., 1975.

Stryker, R. *Rehabilitative Aspects of Acute and Chronic Nursing Care*. Philadelphia: W.B. Saunders Co., 1977.

Thomas, Robin B. "Nursing Assessment of Childhood Chronic Conditions," *Issues in Comprehensive Pediatric Nursing* 7:165–76, 1984.

Travelbee, J. *Interpersonal Aspects of Nursing*. Philadelphia: F.A. Davis Co., 1971.

Turk, D.C., and Kerns, R.D. *Health, Illness and Families: A Life-Span Perspective*. New York: John Wiley & Sons, 1985.

U.S. Department of Census. *Statistical Abstract of the United States: 1985*. Washington, D.C.: U.S. Government Printing Office, 1985.

U.S. Department of Health, Education and Welfare. *Chronic Conditions and Limitations of Activity and Mobility, U.S. July 1965–June 1967*. Washington, D.C.: U.S. Government Printing Office, 1971a.

U.S. Department of Health, Education and Welfare. *Vital and Health Statistics: Prevalence of Chronic Conditions of the Genitourinary, Nervous, Endocrine, Metabolic and Blood and Blood Forming Systems and Other Selected Chronic Conditions*. Washington, D.C.: U.S. Government Printing Office, 1971b.

Watson, D., and Kendall, P. "Methodological Issues in Research on Coping with Chronic Disease," in *Coping with Chronic Disease*. Edited by Burish, T.G., and Bradley, I.A. New York: Academic Press, 1983.

Wiedenbach, E. *Clinical Nursing: A Helping Art*. New York: Springer Publishing Co., 1964.

Wright, L., and Bell, J. "Nurses, Families and Illness: A New Combination," in *Treating Families with Special Needs*. Edited by Freeman, D., and Truce, B. Ottawa: The Canadian Association of Social Workers, 1981.

Wright, L., and Leahey, M. *Nurses and Families: A Guide to Family Assessment and Intervention*. Philadelphia: F.A. Davis Co., 1984.

2 Chronic illness and the family: An overview

John S. Rolland, M.D.
Assistant Clinical Professor
Department of Psychiatry
Yale University School of Medicine
New Haven, Connecticut

Medical Director
Center for Illness in Families
New Haven, Connecticut

OVERVIEW

Impediments to the advancement of clinical practice and psychosocial research in the area of chronic and life-threatening illness suggest the need for 1) a categorization scheme that organizes similarities and differences between diseases in a manner useful to psychosocial rather than biomedical inquiry, and 2) greater attention to how illnesses vary over their time course. To address these needs, a conceptual model is described that distinguishes types of illnesses and key phrases in their natural history. Possibilities are discussed for this model's research applications, and its potential as a basis for more comprehensive family assessment and treatment planning in a wide range of medical and mental health settings is presented.

This chapter will offer a conceptual base for theory building, clinical practice, and research investigation in the area of chronic and life-threatening illness. This proposed scheme organizes a wide range of chronic diseases according to key landmarks in their natural history. It furnishes a central reference point from which clinicians and researchers of many persuasions may forge their own trails.

PSYCHOSOCIAL FACTORS IN CHRONIC ILLNESS

Health professionals, patients, and their families generally agree that chronic or life-threatening illness exerts a powerful impact on individuals and their families. Indeed, a rapidly expanding group has begun to study the way social and psychological factors might affect the course of disease, and many clinicians and researchers have struggled to clarify the important variables involved. Weiner (1977), in his comprehensive and scholarly review, concluded that our knowledge of the psychosocial factors that modify disease course is still in its infancy. Recent reviews of the psychosocial modifiers of stress emphasize the fuzziness that exists in the definitions of various individual, small group, and environmental factors that might be important (Elliott and Eisdorfer, 1982; Kasl, 1982; Weiss et al., 1981). Divergent or conflicting research results, inconclusive findings, and variably successful clinical approaches are cited as manifestations of this problem.

More precise operational definitions of psychosocial concepts like "social networks," or better measurement techniques would be the best means to clarification, critics (Fox, 1982) in this field have said. This is valid criticism, but it obscures two essential aspects of the problem. First, insufficient attention has been given to the differences and similarities between one chronic illness and another. Second, there has been a glossing over of the differences in how a single chronic disease manifests itself over its time course. Chronic illnesses need to be conceptualized in a manner that organizes these similarities and differences over the disease course so that the type and degree of demands relevant to psychosocial research and clinical practice can be identified.

This discussion will focus on developing a typology of illness. Some possibilities will be briefly highlighted for using this typology with family systems theory in a synergistic, complementary manner to create an overall model. A future chapter will detail a systemic model for family assessment and treatment formulation of chronic illness cases using this typology.

All psychosocial inquiry, for clinicians and researchers alike, must focus on interaction. In the arena of chronic illness, one's concern is the interaction between a disease and an individual, family, or other biopsychosocial system. In order to think in a systemic manner about the interface of an illness and an individual or family, one must characterize the illness itself. A schema to conceptualize chronic diseases, which is relevant to that interactive purpose, is required. A common metalanguage that transforms or reclassifies biological language is needed to bridge the biological and psychosocial worlds.

Before proposing a solution, let us examine the problem more closely. The great variability of chronic illnesses over time has vexed those psychosocial investigators who have tried to extract practical findings of a generalizable nature. The difficulty originates when social scientists or psychotherapists accept a disease classification that is based on purely biological criteria. This nosology fits the world of anatomy, physiology, biochemistry, histology, microbiology, physical diagnosis, pharmacology, surgery, and so forth. From a traditional medical point of view, the diagnosis of a specific illness is of primary concern because it dictates subsequent treatment planning. Even in the field of primary prevention, which has considered risk factors for a broader constellation of illnesses, there remains a tendency to emphasize biological risks (smoking, obesity, diet). One can argue that the problem of psychosocial research in physical illness suffers as much from a blind acceptance of this unshakable model of medicine as from its own shortcomings. We hinder progress in clarifying the relationship of psychosocial factors to disease course if we limit ourselves to a biological framework that categorizes information solely to diagnose and treat illness from a biological perspective.

Historically, this illness orientation has guided investigations of the relationship between psychosocial factors and physical illness toward opposite ends of a continuum. Truths are sought either in each specific illness or in "illness" in general. Most investigators have examined a specific disease. For example, an intervention study with lung cancer patients might be designed to clarify the impact on the disease course of a specific intervention, such as family therapy. This kind of study may be important, but it can mislead researchers in two ways. Findings with one disease are often generalized to cover all illnesses indiscriminately. Or, findings are held to be not generalizable and researchers study each illness in a narrowly focused way.

Both extremes hamper the clinician. Without guidelines to balance unifying principles and useful distinctions, clinicians can become bewildered by the wide variety of chronic illnesses. To reduce anxiety, they may inappropriately apply a monolithic treatment approach to all chronic illnesses. Extensive experience with a single kind of illness that requires intensive focus on issues of separation and loss, like terminal cancer, may get transferred to a chronic illness, like stroke, where other issues such as role reallocation predominate.

The psychosocial importance of different time phases of an illness is not well enough understood. A major reason for this in research has been the relative predominance of cross-sectional, in contrast to longitudinal, studies. Some cross-sectional studies have been timed to clarify aspects of either the crisis, chronic, or terminal phases of a specific illness. More often, studies include cases that vary widely in the amount of time families have lived with chronic illness (Atcherberg et al., 1977; Blumberg, et al., 1954; Turk, 1964). Often, separate investigations of the same disease produce conflicting results. Debates ensue without either side recognizing the factor of time phase as an explanation for the different results. Likewise, clinicians often become involved in the care of an individual or family coping with a chronic illness at different points in the "illness life cycle." Clinicians rarely follow the interaction of a family illness process through the complete life history of a disease. As when we arrive for the second act of a play and are later told the rest of the story, we get an incomplete view of the drama.

A few studies have explored short-range psychosocial effects on disease course. One study noted a synchronicity of emotional and behavioral factors with joint tenderness ratings in individuals with rheumatoid arthritis (Moldofsky and Chester, 1970). Others have studied diabetic and asthmatic exacerbations (Baker et al., 1975; Bradley, 1979; Hamburg et al., 1980; Matus and Bush, 1979; Minuchin et al., 1978). Minuchin, in his classic study of children with brittle diabetes, used the accepted medical correlation between a rise in blood serum free fatty acid levels and the development of diabetic ketoacidosis. He demonstrated a sustained rise of serum levels when the children were led into an interview where the parents were discussing conflictual issues. However, these projects concerned microfluctuations rather than broader scale phases of an illness (crisis, chronic, end-stage, or terminal).

The importance of broad time phases of illness has surfaced periodically in the chronic illness literature. One example is the role of denial at different points of the disease course. Denial may enable the parents of a child with leukemia to perform necessary duties during the illness, but might lead to devastating consequences for them if maintained during the terminal phase (Chodoff et al., 1964; Wolff et al., 1964). Denial may be helpful for recovery on a coronary care unit after a myocardial infarction, but harmful if this translates into ignoring medical advice about diet, exercise, and work stress over the long-term recovery (Croog et al., 1971; Hackett et al., 1968).

There is an obvious need for a conceptual model that can guide both clinical practice and research, and that allows dynamic, open communications between these disciplines. The first section of this chapter proposes a typology of chronic or life-threatening illnesses. The illnesses are grouped according to biological characteristics that dictate different psychosocial demands for the ill individual and his family. The model will address the problems of illness variability and time phases on two separate dimensions: chronic physical illnesses grouped according to biological similarities and differences; and the prime developmental time phases in the natural evolution of chronic disease. These two dimensions, together, provide a matrix. Within this matrix we can compare data and generate hypotheses about psychosocial factors pertinent to the course of chronic illness. The model will illuminate the effects of disease on the patient, family, or social network, as well as the impact of the patient, family, or social network on the course of the illness.

TYPOLOGY OF ILLNESS

Any typology of illness is by nature arbitrary. A particular typology must select a limited number of variables from a universe of choices. The attributes chosen must neither be too few and too general, nor too many and unwieldy. The present typology has a particular goal: to create categories for a wide array of chronic illnesses. It is designed not for traditional medical treatment or prognosis, but to study the relationship between family or individual dynamics and chronic disease.

This typology conceptualizes four broad distinctions: onset, course, outcome, and degree of incapacitation of illness. These attributes have been chosen for several reasons. For many diseases, these attributes are considered the most significant at the interface of the illness and the individual or family. There is also a correspondence between each of the attributes: onset, course, and outcome, and a particular temporal phase of chronic disease. Although each variable is actually a continuum, it will be categorized by selection of key points along the continuum. In reality, much finer distinctions exist. Particular anchor points are chosen because they provide useful discriminating features.

Onset

Onset of illness can be divided into two categories: acute and gradual. This division is not meant to differentiate types of biological development, but instead, types of symptomatic presentation. Strokes and myocardial infarction are examples of illnesses with sudden clinical presentation, but arguably long periods of preliminary biological change. For illnesses with gradual onset, like rheumatoid arthritis or angina pectoris, diagnosis as a confirmation point can occur at any time after clinical symptoms have started.

A gradual crisis differs from a sudden crisis in the type of stressor it presents to a family or individual. The total amount of readjustment of family structure, roles, problem-solving, and affective coping might eventually be the same for both types of crisis, but for acute onset illnesses, like stroke, these readjustments are compressed into a short time frame. This will require the family to mobilize its crisis management skills much faster. Gradual onset diseases, like rheumatoid arthritis or Parkinson's disease, allow the family more time to adjust, though they may generate more anxiety before a diagnosis is made. For acute onset diseases, there is immediate strain on the family members to juggle their energy between protecting against further disintegration and trying to maximize mastery through restructuring or problem-solving (Adams and Lindemann, 1974).

Course

Chronic diseases take three courses: progressive, constant, or relapsing/
episodic. A progressive disease by this definition is one that is continually symptomatic and progresses in severity. The family is faced with
a perpetually symptomatic family member whose increasing degrees
of disability occur in a stepwise or progressive fashion. Periods of relief
from the demands of the illness tend to be minimal; continual adaptation and role change are implicit. Increasing strain on family caretakers
arises from exhaustion and the continual addition of new caretaking
tasks. Also, the family duties of the ill member may need to be re-
allocated as the disease becomes more incapacitating. Family flexibility
and the availability of outside resources become important.

It seems profitable to distinguish further between illnesses that
progress rapidly or slowly. The demands on the family with a rapidly
progressive illness such as nonresponsive lung cancer or leukemia differ
from the demands of slowly progressive illnesses like rheumatoid arthritis, chronic obstructive pulmonary disease (emphysema, chronic
bronchitis), or adult onset diabetes. The pace of adapting to ever new
demands of a rapidly progressive disease mounts as the time course
shortens. By contrast, a slowly progressive illness may place a higher
premium on stamina rather than adaptation.

In constant course illness, an initial event is followed by a period of
biological stability. Stroke, myocardial infarction, trauma with resulting
amputation, or spinal cord injury with paralysis, are examples of this.
Typically, after an initial period of recovery, the chronic phase is
characterized by a clear–cut deficit such as paraplegia, amputation,
speech loss, or a cognitive impairment. There may also be a residual
functional limitation, such as diminished physical stress tolerance or a
restriction of previous activities. Recurrences can occur, but the
individual or family faces a semipermanent change that is stable and
predictable over a considerable time span. The potential for family
exhaustion exists without the strain of new role demands over time.

The third kind of course is characterized as relapsing or episodic.
Illnesses like ulcerative colitis, asthma, peptic ulcer, migraine headaches, and multiple sclerosis are typical. Forms of cancer in remission,
such as resectable and chemotherapy-responsive kinds, might be included in this category. Its distinguishing feature is the alternation of
stable periods of varying length, characterized by a low level of absence
of symptoms, with periods of flareup or exacerbation. Often the family
can carry on a "normal" routine. However, the specter of a recurrence
hangs over their heads.

Relapsing illnesses demand a somewhat different sort of family adaptability. Relative to progressive or constant course illnesses, they may require the least ongoing caretaking or role reallocation. But the episodic nature of such an illness requires a flexibility that permits movement back and forth between two forms of family organization. In a sense, the family is on call to enact a crisis structure to handle exacerbations of the illness. Strain on the family system is caused by both the frequency of transitions between crisis and noncrisis, and the ongoing uncertainty of when a crisis will next occur. Also, the wide psychological discrepancy between periods of normalcy and illness is a particularly taxing feature unique to relapsing chronic diseases.

Outcome

The extent to which a chronic illness is a likely cause of death and the degree to which it can shorten one's life span is a critical distinguishing feature with profound psychosocial impact. On one end of the continuum are illnesses that do not typically affect the life span, such as lumbosacral disc disease, blindness, arthritis, spinal cord injury, or seizure disorders. At the other extreme are illnesses that are clearly progressive and usually fatal, such as metastatic cancer, acquired immune deficiency syndrome (AIDS), and Huntington's chorea. There is also an intermediate, more unpredictable category. This includes both illnesses which shorten the life span, such as cystic fibrosis, juvenile diabetes, and cardiovascular disease, and those with the possibility of sudden death, such as hemophilia, or recurrences of myocardial infarction or stroke.

All chronic illnesses potentially involve the loss of bodily control, self-identity, and intimate relationships (Sourkes, 1982). A life-threatening illness entails greater consequences—death and the permanent loss of relationships. The ill member fears that his life is ending before he has lived out his "life plan," and that he is alone in death. The family fears becoming survivors alone in the future. For both, an undercurrent of anticipatory grief and separation permeates all phases of adaptation. Families are often caught between a desire for intimacy and a pull to "let go" emotionally of the ill member. The future expectation of loss can make it difficult for a family to maintain a balanced perspective; a virtual torrent of affect can distract a family from the myriad practical tasks and problem-solving that maintain family integrity (Weiss, 1983). Also, the tendency to see the ill family member as practically "in the coffin" can set in motion maladaptive responses; there may be unwarranted role reallocation that divests the ill member of important responsibilities. The result can be the structural and emotional isolation of the ill person from ongoing family life. This kind of psychological alienation has been associated with poor medical outcome in life-threatening illness (Davies et al., 1973; Derogatis et al., 1979; Schmale and Iker, 1971; Simonton, 1980).

Illnesses that shorten life or cause sudden death imply less imminence of loss than metastatic cancer, so that issues of mortality are less predominant in day-to-day life. The probability of a fatal outcome in these cases is relatively uncertain. For that reason, this type of illness provides a fertile ground for idiosyncratic family interpretations. The "it could happen" nature of these illnesses creates a nidus for both overprotection by the family and powerful secondary gains for the ill member. This is particularly relevant to childhood illnesses such as hemophilia, juvenile diabetes, and asthma (Minuchin et al., 1978; Minuchin et al., 1975).

Incapacitation

Illnesses that cause incapacitation also belong in this typology. Incapacitation can result from impairment of cognition, sensation, movement, energy production, or disfigurement. Cognition includes: memory, integration of sensory input, judgment, insight, and language processes. Examples of illnesses affecting these areas are Alzheimer's disease and stroke with aphasia. Sensory limitations include blindness and deafness. Motor limitations are seen in such illnesses as stroke with paralysis, multiple sclerosis, and Parkinson's disease. Some illnesses, such as cardiovascular and pulmonary disease, impair the body's ability to produce raw energy. They may reduce peak performance or the ability to sustain motor, sensory, or cognitive efforts. Finally, some illnesses, such as leprosy, neurofibromatosis, or severe burns, are visibly disabling to the extent that sufficient social stigma impairs normal social interaction.

The different kinds of incapacitation imply sharp differences in the specific adjustments required of a family. For instance, the combined cognitive and motor deficits of a person with a stroke necessitate greater family role reallocation than would be required for a spinal cord–injured person who retains his cognitive faculties. Some chronic disease, such as hypertension, peptic ulcer, many endocrine disorders, or migraine headache, may cause only mild, temporary, intermittent incapacitation, or none at all. This highly significant factor moderates the quality and quantity of the stressors facing a family. For some illnesses, like stroke or spinal cord injury, incapacitation is worst at the time of onset and exerts its greatest influence then. Incapacitation at the beginning of an illness magnifies family coping issues related to onset, expected course, and outcome. For progressive diseases, like multiple sclerosis, rheumatoid arthritis, or dementia, disability looms as an increasing problem in later phases of the illness. This allows a family more time to prepare for anticipated changes. In particular, it provides an opportunity for the ill member to participate in disease-related family planning.

As a caveat, several studies cite the importance of the family's expectations of a disabled member. Expectations that the ill member will continue to have responsible roles and autonomy was associated with a better rehabilitation response and more successful long-term reintegration into the family (Bishop and Epstein, 1980; Cleveland, 1980; Hyman, 1975; Litman, 1974; Slater et al., 1970; Sussman and Slater, 1971; Swanson and Maruta, 1980). Bishop and Epstein (1980) envisioned that the family would have the greatest difficulty in deciding realistic role expectations in both mildly disabling illnesses, which were ambiguous in their demands, and the most severely incapacitating ones, because of the sheer amount of role change required.

Overall, the effect of incapacitation on a particular individual or family depends on both the type of incapacitation and the pre–illness roles occupied by the ill member. However, it may be the presence or absence of significant incapacitation that constitutes the principal dividing line relevant to a first attempt to build a model (Viney and Westbrook, 1981).

By combining the kinds of onset (acute versus gradual), course (progressive versus constant versus relapsing/episodic), outcome (fatal versus shortened life span versus nonfatal), and incapacitation (present versus absent) into a grid format, we generate a typology with 32 potential types of illness. It is clear that certain types of disease (i.e., constant course fatal illnesses) are so rare or non–existent that for practical purposes they can be eliminated. This grid is shown in Table 2.1. The number of potential categories can be reduced further by combining or eliminating particular factors. This would depend on the relative need for specificity in a particular situation.

The extent to which illnesses are predictable has not been formulated as a separate category in the typology. Rather, it seems more profitable to consider predictability as a kind of metacharacteristic that overlays and colors the other attributes of onset, course, outcome, and incapacitation. There are two distinct facets to the predictability of a chronic illness. Diseases can be uncertain as to the actual nature of the onset, course, outcome, or presence of incapacitation. And, they can vary to the rate at which changes occur. Some disease, like spinal cord injury, can be accurately typed at the point of diagnosis and have a highly predictable course. Other illnesses, such as stroke, myocardial infarction, hypertension, or lung cancer, are unpredictable as to course and outcome. The initial prediction of type may change if a relapse occurs. For instance, hypertension can be constant (stable) or progressive.

Table 2.1 Categorization of Chronic Illnesses by Psychosocial Type

	Incapacitating		Nonincapacitating	
	Acute	Gradual	Acute	Gradual

Fatal

	Acute	Gradual	Acute	Gradual
Progressive		• Lung cancer with CNS metastases • AIDS • Bone marrow failure • Amyotrophic lateral sclerosis	• Acute leukemia • Pancreatic cancer • Metastatic breast cancer • Malignant melanoma • Lung cancer • Liver cancer	• Cystic fibrosis
Relapsing			• Cancers in remission	

Possibly Fatal, Shortened Life Span

	Acute	Gradual	Acute	Gradual
Progressive		• Emphysema • Alzheimer's disease • Multi-infarct dementia • Multiple sclerosis (late) • Chronic alcoholism • Huntington's chorea • Scleroderma		• Juvenile diabetes • Malignant hypertension • Insulin-dependent adult-onset diabetes
Relapsing	• Angina	• Multiple sclerosis (early) • Episodic alcoholism	• Sickle cell disease • Hemophilia	• Systemic lupus erythematosis
Constant	• Stroke • Moderate/severe myocardial infarction	• PKU and other inborn errors of metabolism	• Mild myocardial infarction • Cardiac arrhythmia	• Hemodialysis-treated renal failure • Hodgkin's disease

(continued)

	Incapacitating		Nonincapacitating	
	Acute	Gradual	Acute	Gradual
Nonfatal				
Progressive		• Parkinson's disease • Rheumatoid arthritis • Osteoarthritis		• Non-insulin-dependent adult-onset diabetes
Relapsing	• Lumbosacral disk disease		• Kidney stones • Gout • Migraine • Seasonal allergy • Asthma • Epilepsy	• Peptic ulcer • Ulcerative colitis • Chronic bronchitis • Other inflammatory bowel diseases • Psoriasis
Constant	• Congenital malformations • Spinal cord injury • Acute blindness • Acute deafness • Survived severe trauma and burns • Posthypoxic syndrome	• Nonprogressive mental retardation • Cerebral palsy	• Benign arrhythmia • Congenital heart disease	• Malabsorption syndromes • Hyperthyroidism/hypothyroidism • Pernicious anemia • Controlled hypertension • Controlled glaucoma

If a second episode occurs, a stroke or myocardial infarction can be considered relapsing or progressive. Lung cancer, as an example of an acute onset/progressive/fatal illness, can become incapacitating if there is brain metastasis. Some cases of lung cancer progress at a rapid rate. Others advance slowly with a long remission, or not at all ("spontaneous cure"). Some illnesses, like rheumatoid arthritis or migraine headache, tend to have predictable long-range courses, but can be highly variable as to day-to-day flareups. This kind of uncertainty interferes more with day-to-day rather than with long-term planning. The typology of illness cannot predict these changes. In a particular case, if important changes occur during the course of the disease, an individual's situation can switch from one category to another. At present it is unclear how much of this individual variation can be explained by the effects of psychosocial factors, like family functioning, on disease course and outcome.

Several other important attributes that differentiate illnesses were excluded from this typology because they seemed of lesser importance or were relevant to only a subgroup of disorders. When appropriate, they should be considered in a thorough, systemically oriented evaluation. Genetically transmitted illnesses, because of their intergenerational nature, often foster blame, guilt, and strain at the marriage and family planning stage of the life cycle. The complexity, frequency, and efficacy of the treatment regimen, the amount of home versus hospital-based care required by the disease, and the frequency and intensity of symptoms vary widely across illnesses and have important implications for individual and family adaptation. Finally, the age of the patient at illness onset in relation to child, adult, and family stages of development is a critical factor beyond the scope of this paper.

TIME PHASES

To complete a matrix, the time phases of an illness need to be considered as a second dimension. Often one hears about "coping with cancer," "managing disability," or "dealing with life-threatening illness." These cliches can create a kind of tunnel vision that blinds one to the phases of an illness. Each phase has its own psychosocial tasks which require different strengths, attitudes, or changes from a family.

Depending on the need for detail, time lines of varying degrees of complexity can be outlined. To capture the core psychosocial themes in the natural history of chronic disease, three major phases can be described: crisis, chronic, and terminal. The relationship between a more detailed chronic disease time line and one grouped into broad time phases can be diagrammed as in Figure 2.1.

Figure 2.1 Time Line and Phases of Illness

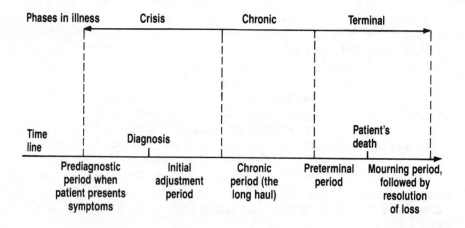

The crisis phase includes any symptomatic period before actual diagnosis when the individual or family senses that something is wrong, but doesn't know the exact nature and scope of the problem. It includes the initial period of readjustment after the problem has been diagnosed and initial treatment begun.

During this period, there are several key tasks for the ill member and his family. They must create a meaning for the illness event. They must grieve for the loss of the pre-illness family identity and accept the permanent change while maintaining a sense of continuity between their past and future. The family must pull together to undergo both short-term crisis reorganization and, in the face of uncertainty, develop a special system flexibility toward future goals.

The chronic phase usually consists of the time span between the initial diagnosis and readjustment period, and the third phase when issues of death and terminal illness predominate. It can be marked by constancy, progression, or episodic change. In this sense, its meaning cannot be grasped simply by knowing the biological behavior of an illness. Rather, it is a psychosocial construct, often referred to as "the long haul," and "day–to–day living with chronic illness" phase. Often the individual and family have come to grips psychologically and/or organizationally with the permanent changes presented by the illness and have devised an ongoing plan of action. At the extremes, this phase can last for decades in a stable, nonfatal chronic illness, or it may be virtually nonexistent in an acute, rapidly progressive, fatal disorder, in which the crisis phase is contiguous with the terminal or third phase. The ability of the family to maintain normal life under the "abnormal" presence of a chronic illness and heightened uncertainty is a key task of this period. It is a time of "living in limbo" with a fatal illness. For certain highly debilitating, not clearly fatal illnesses, such as a massive stroke or dementia, the family may be saddled with an exhausting and endless problem. Paradoxically, some families' only hope to resume a "normal" life cycle might be death of their ill member. This highlights another crucial task of this phase: the maintenance of maximal autonomy for all family members in the face of growing mutual dependency and caretaking.

The last phase is the terminal period. It includes the preterminal stage of an illness where death is inevitable and predominates family life. It encompasses the periods of mourning and resolution of loss, and it may include significant elements of crisis. Separation, death, grief, resolution of mourning, and resumption of "normal" family life beyond the loss are the issues that distinguish this phase, however.

Beyond their own significance, the three phases illuminate critical transition points that link each period. Apt descriptions in the adult development and family life cycle literature have clarified the importance of transition periods (Levinson, 1978; McGoldrick and Carter, 1980). It is the same for the transitions between developmental eras in the course of disease. This is a time for reevaluation of the previous family life structure in the face of new illness-related development demands. Unfinished business from the previous phase can complicate or block the transitions. Families or individuals can become frozen in an adaptive structure that has outlived its utility (Penn, 1983). For example, the act of pulling together in the crisis period can become maladaptive and stifling for all family members in the chronic phase. Enmeshed families, because of their rigid and fused nature, have particular difficulty negotiating this delicate transition.

The three time phases—crisis, chronic, and terminal—describe the natural evolution of illnesses. The point in the disease history at which an individual seeks a diagnosis and medical care can often determine variation between cases. Mechanic (1978) has written eloquently on this subject which he terms "illness behavior."

Variation in illness behavior is highly significant vis–à–vis early versus late detection of an illness. For an illness such as breast cancer it may mean the difference between a high expectancy of "cure" and an expectancy of death. For these two extremes of breast cancer both the prognosis and the character of the time phases of the illness would differ accordingly. Breast cancer detected in an early stage is potentially curable by local surgery. The possibility of a fatal outcome exists, but an optimistic view by the family is realistic. Breast cancer that is far advanced at diagnosis may be incurable. Pessimism or hopelessness would tend to prevail. In this situation the crisis and terminal phase are juxtaposed with an elimination of the relatively stable middle chronic period. These complexities are mentioned so that those using the model can account for differences between individuals. These factors will help the clinician use the model to think through an approach to a particular family. For the researcher, it may help explain discrepancies between previous studies of a particular disease, and guide refinements in design for future studies.

At this point, we can combine the typology and phases of illness to construct a matrix (see Table 2.2). This matrix permits the grouping and differentiation of illnesses according to important similarities or differences. It subdivides types of chronic illnesses into three time phases. This allows a more refined examination of a chronic illness. Although beyond the scope of this discussion, the inclusion of a family systems model as the third dimension might reveal the relative importance of various family patterns to specific types of illness at a particular phase of their natural history.

Table 2.2 Matrix of Illness Types and Time Phases

ONSET	COURSE	OUTCOME	INCAPACITATION
A = acute	P = progressive	F = fatal or	Yes = (+)
G = gradual	C = constant	shortened life	No = (−)
	R = relapsing	span	
		NF = nonfatal	

ILLNESS TYPE		PHASE	
	I	II	III
	CRISIS	CHRONIC	TERMINAL
A P F +			
A P F −			
A P NF +			
A P NF −			
A C F +			
A C F −			
A C NF +			
A C NF −			
A R F +			
A R F −			
A R NF+			
A R NF−			
G P F +			
G P F −			
G P NF +			
G P NF −			
G C F +			
G C F −			
G C NF +			
G C NF −			
G R F +			
G R F −			
G R NF+			
G R NF−			

CLINICAL IMPLICATIONS

There are several important applications for this model in clinical practice. The major contribution may be the provision of a framework for assessment and clinical intervention for a family facing a chronic or life-threatening illness. The same kind of categorical thinking that will aid the researcher will also aid the clinician.

By using the components of the typology of illness rather than traditional biological diagnosis, the clinician can think with greater clarity and focus. Attention to features of onset, course, outcome, and incapacitation provides markers that facilitate assessment. This will

focus the clinician's interviews with the family. For instance, acute
onset illnesses demand high levels of adaptability, problem-solving, role
reallocation, and balanced cohesion. A high degree of family enmesh-
ment, because of its interference with meeting these demands, would
flash a warning sign of family vulnerability to possible difficulties in
the crisis phase. Forethought on this issue would alert a clinician to the
need for a more appropriate assessment interview. At their core, the
components of the typology provide a means to grasp the character of a
chronic illness in psychosocial terms. They provide a meaningful bridge
for the clinician between the biological and psychosocial worlds.

The concept of time phases encourages a clinician to think longitudi-
nally. A long-range perspective enables the clinician to more fully
understand a chronic illness as an ongoing process with landmarks,
transition points, and changing demands. An illness time line delineates
psychosocial developmental tasks. Kaplan (1968) has emphasized the
importance of solving phase-related tasks within the time limits set by
the duration of each successive developmental phase of an illness. He
suggests that failure to resolve issues in this sequential manner can
jeopardize the coping process of the family. Therefore, attention to time
allows the clinician to assess a family's strengths and vulnerabilities
in relation to the present and future phases of the illness.

Taken together, the typology and time phases provide a context to
integrate other aspects of a comprehensive assessment. This would
include consideration of the developmental stages of the family unit and
individual members; the family history of dealing with crisis, illness,
and loss; the family's contingency crisis planning; the pre–illness roles
of the ill member; the meaning of the illness to the family; and the
family paradigm vis–à–vis locus of control. For instance, imagine that
an accident paralyzes the family breadwinner, a carpenter. The role
changes necessitated by this disability can coincide with the loss of the
family's financial base and the former breadwinner's main source of
status in the family. This convergence of role changes can overwhelm
even high-functioning families. In this case, if the family was also
at an important developmental transition, the problem would be complicated further. The only son, now 15, has dreams of going away to
college in two years. The specter of financial hardship and the perceived
need for "a man in the family" creates a serious dilemma of choice for
the son and the family. In this case there is a clash between developmental issues of separation, of individuation, and of the demands of the
chronic disability upon the family. The model will facilitate a systems-
oriented assessment of these intertwined issues.

The model also clarifies treatment planning. First, an awareness of
the components of family functioning most relevant to particular types

or phases of an illness can guide goal setting. Use of the time phases can improve short- and long-range treatment plans. One could hypothesize that because the clinician will feel more certain about the important issues and their timing, he will convey this to the family therapeutically. The act of sharing this information with the family and deciding upon specific goals will provide the family with a better sense of control and more realistic hope. This knowledge alerts the family to warning signs that might signal a need for family treatment. This permits families not accustomed to psychiatric care to call upon a family therapist at appropriate times for brief goal-oriented treatment.

Maladaptive patterns of coping usually start in the crisis phase (Caplan, 1964). To maximize prevention of these patterns, initial clinical intervention should target the crisis phase of a chronic illness. This is especially true for acute onset, incapacitating types of illnesses which present the greatest strain to a family.

Finally, the model enables clinicians to decide upon realistic extensions or restrictions of treatment approaches. For instance, with this typology, disparate diseases such as rheumatoid arthritis, multiple sclerosis, and Parkinson's disease would be considered similar. They are all gradual onset, progressive, nonfatal, and incapacitating illnesses. Thus clinicians can apply their clinical experience with rheumatoid arthritis to Parkinson's disease. On the other hand, a slow-growing brain tumor is similar to these diseases in onset, course, and incapacitation, but it is fatal. Clinicians could still use their experience with multiple sclerosis and Parkinson's disease if they alter it to take into account the family dynamics important in fatal illness.

RESEARCH IMPLICATIONS

The model has important implications for research. First, reexamination of previous studies using this model might dispel the confusion surrounding conflicting results or lack of statistical significance. Stratification by illness type and/or phase might bring significant associations to light.

Cognizance of the time phases is essential to study design. An investigator must be aware of the time phase—crisis, chronic, or terminal—that a case is in as it enters a study for assessment or intervention. Different results are likely if studies differ in their timing. The time phases can clarify a methodology for longitudinal studies. Multiple observations could be spaced at chronological intervals.

The typology should facilitate research designed to sort out the relative importance of psychosocial variables across a spectrum of diseases. Grouping illnesses by the parameters of this typology should help in this regard. According to the premises for this typology, illnesses appearing within the same category have the highest congruence of psychosocial demands on the family. In other words, pooling results from studies of Parkinson's disease, rheumatoid arthritis, chronic obstructive pulmonary disease, and multiple sclerosis (all gradual onset/progressive course/incapacitating/nonfatal) would allow significant generalizations for that cluster of diseases. Illnesses within a particular category will be roughly matched as to type of onset, course, outcome, and incapacita-tion. Since each of these variables exists as a continuum, the degree of homogeneity of study cases can be fine-tuned according to the desire of the investigator. Specific criteria for subdivisions are feasible for any of the typology's attributes.

Theoretically, the typology can isolate a "critical" aspect of chronic illness for more intensive study. For instance, one might ask, "What is the relative importance of family adaptability for chronic diseases with and without incapacitation?" A comparison could be made between two types of illnesses that vary on the presence or absence of incapaci-tation but are matched for the other typology attributes. So, lumbosacral disk disease (incapacitating/acute onset/relapsing/nonfatal) and peptic ulcer disease (nonincapacitating/acute or gradual onset/relapsing/nonfatal) could be used to investigate the relative importance of high versus low family adaptability in incapacitating versus nonincapacitating diseases.

Also, the model simplifies the design of studies intended to explore the interactional effects of the typology's components. As an extension of the hypothetical study just described, by using a 2 by 2 design one could investigate how fatal versus nonfatal outcome interacts with the presence or absence of incapacitation.

Overall, the typology and time phase matrix provides a framework to generate and test hypotheses about the relationship of different compo-nents of family or individual functioning to different phases of illness. If we operationalize the typology, the phases of illness, and the compo-nents of family functioning as three distinct variables, then three kinds of comparisons can be generated by holding any two variables constant. This would allow asking the following sorts of questions: Given illness type X in the crisis phase, how does high versus low family cohesion affect disease course? Given illness type X with high family cohesion, how is disease course affected in each of the three time phases? How does high family cohesion in the chronic phase affect the course of different types of illnesses?

The implications for research can be summarized. Use of the model for re-analysis of previous studies may lead to new insights. The model will significantly improve our ability to generate more succinct hypotheses. Definitions of independent and dependent variables will be clearer. Components of the typology of illness and time phase identify what needs to be controlled in a study design. Used in conjunction with a well-researched family systems model like the McMaster (Epstein et al., 1978; Epstein and Bishop, 1981; Epstein et al., 1983), Structural (Minuchin et al., 1978; Minuchin et al., 1975), Beavers-Timberlawn (Lewis et al., 1977), or Circumplex (Olson et al., 1979a; Olson et al., 1979b; Olson and McCubbin, 1981; Russell, 1979; Sprenkle and Olson, 1978), the typology should improve family systems medical research.

CONCLUSIONS

This chapter has described a conceptual model that clarifies and enhances the work of clinicians and researchers with chronic and life-threatening illness. Two problems were identified as major impediments to progress in this field. These difficulties suggest the need for a categorization scheme that organizes similarities and differences between diseases in a manner useful to psychosocial rather than medical inquiry, and greater attention to how illnesses vary over their time course.

A model was proposed to address these needs. The first dimension described a typology of illness with four components: onset, course, outcome, and presence or absence of incapacitation. The second dimension distinguished three phases of chronic illness: crisis, chronic, and terminal.

The typology of illness can facilitate a key goal of family systems medicine to integrate a number of sovereign territories into a truly coherent discipline (Bloch, 1983). When used in an interlocking way with typological models of the family or an illness-oriented family assessment, this categorization scheme provides the researcher and clinician with a clearer path. Clinically, it will help most when applied in the initial diagnostic phase of the illness, when the family and health care providers must grasp the myriad issues surrounding medical treatment and family system readjustment. A vision of this model's use for preventive screening of high risk families seen in a variety of medical settings, and as part of an overall evaluation for symptomatic families, will be discussed in a future paper.

REFERENCES

Adams, J.E., and Lindemann, E. "Coping with Long-Term Disability," in *Coping and Adaptation*. Edited by Coelho, G.V., et al. New York: Basic Books, 1974.

Atcherberg, J., et al. "Psychological Factors and Blood Chemistries as Disease Outcome Predictors for Cancer Patients," *Multivariate Experimental and Clinical Research* 3:107–22, 1977.

Baker, L., et al. "Psychosomatic Aspects of Juvenile Diabetes Mellitus: A Progress Report," in *Modern Problems in Pediatrics 12*. White Plains, N.Y.: S. Karger, 1975.

Bishop, D.S., and Epstein, N.B. "Family Problems and Disability," in *Behavior Problems and the Disabled: Assessment and Management*. Edited by Bishop, D.S. Baltimore: Williams & Wilkins Co., 1980.

Bloch, D.A. "Family Systems Medicine: The Field and the Journal," *Family Systems Medicine* 1:3–12, 1983.

Blumberg, E.M., et al. "A Possible Relationship Between Psychological Factors and Human Cancer," *Psychosomatic Medicine* 16:277–86, 1954.

Bradley, C. "Life Events and the Control of Diabetes Mellitus," *Journal of Psychosomatic Research* 23:159–62, 1979.

Burr, W.R. *Theory Construction and the Sociology of the Family*. New York: John Wiley & Sons, 1973.

Caplan, G. *Principles of Preventive Psychiatry*. New York: Basic Books, 1964.

Chodoff, P., et al. "Stress, Defenses and Coping Behavior: Observations in Parents of Children with Malignant Disease," *American Journal of Psychiatry* 120:743–49, 1964.

Cleveland, M. "Family Adaptation to Traumatic Spinal Cord Injury, Response to Crisis," *Family Relations* 29:558–65, 1980.

Croog, S.H., et al. "Denial Among Male Heart Patients: An Empirical Study," *Psychosomatic Medicine,* 33:385–97, 1971.

Davies, R.K., et al. "Organic Factors and Psychological Adjustment in Advanced Cancer Patients," *Psychosomatic Medicine* 35:464–71, 1973.

Derogatis, L.R., et al. "Psychological Coping Mechanisms and Survival Time in Metastatic Breast Cancer," *Journal of the American Medical Association* 242:1504–08, 1979.

Elliott, G.R., and Eisdorfer, C. *Stress and Human Health: Analysis and Implications of Research*. New York: Springer Publishing Co., 1982.

Epstein, N.B., and Bishop, D.S. "Problem-Centered Systems Therapy of the Family," in *Handbook of Family Therapy*. Edited by Gurman, A., and Kniskern, D. New York: Brunner-Mazel, 1981.

Epstein, N.B., et al. "McMaster Model of Family Functioning," *Journal of Marriage and Family Counselling* 4:19–31, 1978.

Epstein, N.B., et al. "The McMaster Family Assessment Device," *Journal of Marital and Family Therapy* 9(2):171–80, 1983.

Fox, B.H. "A Psychological Measure as a Predictor in Cancer," in *Psychological Aspects of Cancer*. Edited by Cohen, J., et al. New York: Raven Press, 1982.

Hackett, T.P., et al. "The Coronary-Care Unit: An Appraisal of Its Psychologic Hazards," *New England Journal of Medicine* 279:1365–70, 1968.

Hamburg, B.A., et al., eds. *Behavioral and Psychological Issues in Diabetes.* Washington, D.C.: U.S. Goverment Printing Office, 1980.

Hyman, M. "Social and Psychological Factors Affecting Disability among Ambulatory Patients," *Journal of Chronic Diseases* 28:99–216, 1975.

Kaplan, D.M. "Observations on Crisis Theory and Practice," *Social Casework* 49:151–55, 1968.

Kasl, S.V. "Social and Psychological Factors Affecting the Course of Disease: An Epidemiological Perspective," in *Handbook of Health, Health Care and the Health Profession.* Edited by Mechanic, D. New York: Free Press, 1982.

Levinson, D.J. *The Seasons of a Man's Life.* New York: Alfred A. Knopf, 1978.

Lewis, J.H., et al. *No Single Thread: Psychological Health in Family Systems* New York: Brunner-Mazel, 1977.

Litman, T.J. "The Family as a Basic Unit in Health and Medical Care: A Social Behavioral Overview," *Social Science and Medicine* 8:495–519, 1974.

Matus, I., and Bush, D. "Asthma Attack Frequency in a Pediatric Population," *Psychosomatic Medicine* 41:629–36, 1979.

McGoldrick, M., and Carter, E.A., eds. *The Family Life Cycle: A Framework for Family Therapy.* New York: Gardner Press, 1980.

Mechanic, D. *Medical Sociology,* 2nd ed. New York: Free Press, 1978.

Minuchin, S., et al. *Psychosomatic Families.* Cambridge, Mass.: Harvard University Press, 1978.

Minuchin, S., et al. "A Conceptual Model of Psychosomatic Illness in Children: Family Organization and Family Therapy," *Archives of General Psychiatry* 32:1031–38, 1975.

Moldofsky, H., and Chester, W.J. "Pain and Mood Patterns in Patients with Rheumatoid Arthritis: A Prospective Study," *Psychosomatic Medicine* 32:309–18, 1970.

Olson, D.H., and McCubbin, H.I. "Circumplex Model of Marital and Family Systems: Application to Family Stress and Crisis Intervention," in *Family Stress, Coping, and Social Support.* Edited by McCubbin, H.I. New York: Springer Publishing Co., 1981.

Olson, D.H., et al. "Circumplex Model of Marital and Family Systems I: Cohesion and Adaptability Dimensions, Family Types, and Clinical Applications," *Family Process* 18:3–28, 1979a.

Olson, D.H., et al. "Circumplex Model of Marital Family Systems II: Empirical Studies and Clinical Intervention," in *Advances in Family Intervention, Assessment and Theory.* Edited by Vincent, J. Greenwich, Conn.: JAI Press, 1979b.

Penn, P. "Coalitions and Binding Interactions in Families with Chronic Illness," *Family Systems Medicine* 1:16–25, 1983.

Russell, C.S. "Circumplex Model of Marital and Family Systems III: Empirical Evaluation with Families," *Family Process* 18:29–45, 1979.

Schmale, A.H., and Iker, H. "Hopelessness as a Predictor of Cervical Cancer," *Social Science and Medicine* 5:95–100, 1971.

Simonton, C.O., et al. "Psychological Intervention in the Treatment of Cancer," *Psychosomatics* 21:226–33, 1980.

Slater, S.B., et al. "Participation in Household Activities as a Prognostic Factor for Rehabilitation," *Archives of Physical Medicine and Rehabilitation* 51:605–11, 1970.

Sourkes, B.M. *The Deepening Shade: Psychological Aspects of Long–Term Illness.* Pittsburgh: University of Pittsburgh Press, 1982.

Sprenkle, D.H., and Olson, D.H. "Circumplex Model of Marital and Family Systems IV: Empirical Study of Clinic and Non–Clinic Couples," *Journal of Marital and Family Therapy* 4:59–74, 1978.

Sussman, M.B., and Slater, S.B. "Reappraisal of Urban Kin Networks: Empirical Evidence," *The Annals* 396:40, 1971.

Swanson, D.W., and Maruta, J. "The Family's Viewpoint of Chronic Pain," *Pain* 8:163–66, 1980.

Turk, J. "Impact of Cystic Fibrosis on Family Functioning," *Pediatrics* 34:67–71, 1964.

Viney, L.L., and Westbrook, M.T. "Psychosocial Reactions to Chronic Illness Related Disability as a Function of Its Severity and Type," *Journal of Psychosomatic Research* 25:513–23, 1981.

Weiner, H. *Psychobiology and Human Disease.* New York: Elsevier, 1977.

Weiss, H.M. Personal communication, 1983.

Weiss, S.M., et al., eds. *Perspectives on Behavioral Medicine.* New York: Academic Press, 1981.

Wolff, C.T., et al. "Relationship Between Psychological Defenses and Mean Urinary 17–Hydroxycorticosteroid Excretion Rate. I. A Predictive Study of Parents of Fatally Ill Children," *Psychosomatic Medicine* 26:576–91, 1964.

3 Families and chronic illness: Assumptions, assessment, and intervention

Maureen Leahey, RN, PhD
Team Director, Mental Health Services
Director, Family Therapy Institute
Holy Cross Hospital
Calgary, Alberta, Canada

Lorraine M. Wright, RN, PhD
Director, Family Nursing Unit
Professor, Faculty of Nursing
University of Calgary
Calgary, Alberta, Canada

OVERVIEW

This chapter presents certain basic assumptions about families with chronic illness. Guidelines for conducting a family assessment are outlined and examples of circular questions are given. Indications and contraindications for family intervention and concepts about the process of change are highlighted. General and specific interventions directed at the cognitive, affective, and behavioral levels of family functioning are described.

The family system influences the course of illness in a variety of ways. Thus, the family should be the context in which the challenges of coping with illness are resolved. Interventions target the whole family system since chronic illness cannot be treated solely by a physician or nurse. As Griffin (1980, p. 254) has written,

> Medical intervention is of paramount importance but even the implementation of medical treatment will eventually become the obligation of the family. After the medical program is outlined, it is the family who must see that procedures are followed sensibly, that medications are taken, and that diet and rehabilitation programs are observed. Family members quickly become experts on chronic illness suffered by one of them, and their daily observations usually provide reliable data for health professionals in attendance. Family

attitudes and actions are crucial in determining the course
of the illness and contribute to remission or exacerbation
of symptoms.

Working from the premise that *family* intervention is paramount, this
chapter presents basic assumptions about families with chronic illness.
Guidelines for conducting a family assessment and examples of circular
questions are given. Indications and contraindications for family intervention and concepts about the process of change are highlighted.
Specific family interviewing skills as well as particular types of interventions useful in work with families with chronic illness are addressed.

BASIC ASSUMPTIONS ABOUT FAMILIES WITH CHRONIC ILLNESS

Effective intervention with a family system is possible only after thorough family assessment. Nursing requires certain assumptions so that
nurses can maximize opportunities for systemic change.

Assumption #1: There are Predictable Points of Family Stress

If a chronic disease symptom conflicts with a normal developmental
milestone, stress is predictable. For example, families of children with
Crohn's disease often experience stress when growth failure conflicts
with the usual adolescent growth spurt; this can be particularly
stressful if younger siblings become taller than the ill child. Another
predictable stress point (Power and Orto, 1980) comes when a developmental milestone is not met or is delayed. A family may cope quite
well with a child's congenital disability until it prevents the child from
entering school at the usual time.

Assumption #2: Families Vary in Their Level of Tolerance for the Patient's Physical Condition

Families may tolerate some symptoms when they cannot accept others
(Blazer, 1984). It is important to assess a family's tolerance level and
not insist that family members cope with symptoms before they are
ready to. One family may deal well with chronic pain, by seeking appropriate assistance and perceiving the situation as a challenge. Another
family, however, may perceive chronic pain as an undue and unfair form
of suffering; members may become angry and despondent, affectively
blocking problem-solving efforts.

An adult child might successfully care for an elderly parent until
that parent becomes incontinent of feces and urine, at which point care
becomes intolerable. When the family's tolerance level is exceeded,
other arrangements, such as institutionalization, must be considered.

Assumption #3: Families Under Stress Tend to Hold to Previously Proved Patterns of Behavior, Whether or Not They are Effective Under Current Circumstances

Some families minimize or deny problems which can be useful (Power and Orto, 1980). If, however, a father has had a recent stroke and requires extensive care, then the normal pattern of minimalization may not be effective. Family members will not fully appreciate or admit the amount of effort and time that will be required for his care.

Assumption #4: Families Usually Go Through a Grief-Loss Process Following the Diagnosis of a Disabling Condition

A chronic illness diagnosis represents a major family loss and adjustment that goes beyond the suffering of the patient, and produces different reactions. For example, a patient may openly mourn the loss of eyesight or memory. Family members, on the other hand, may be unable to openly express their feelings about the loss of the valued "normal" relative. Family members sometimes feel guilty for complaining about this change in their situation in light of the change the patient experiences.

Health professionals should not intervene prematurely in this grief process or insist that all family members cope with it in similar ways. In terms of intervention, nurses must not insist upon "required grieving" or impose on family members' specific grief techniques.

Assumption #5: Families Play a Significant Role in Encouraging or Discouraging Chronically Ill Members to Participate in Particular Therapies

Families can increase or hasten the rehabilitation process if they actively support and encourage prescribed therapies.

Assumption #6: Families React to Particular "Illness Behaviors"

Chronically ill patients often become dependent on other family members. However, family reactions to such expressions of dependency and helplessness vary. Some relatives become angry and fail to recognize the patient's real needs, while other members may overcompensate and foster dependence. Therefore, before intervening a nurse must first assess family reactions to displayed illness behaviors.

Assumption #7: Many Families Have Difficulty Adjusting to a Chronic Physical Illness Because of Incorrect or Inadequate Disease-Related Information

Families need up-to-date information regarding their member's illness, although such information may produce guilt or shame in family members, or add to existing anxiety. Health care professionals should recognize that some families cannot comprehend the information given to them at first. Therefore, a nurse should assess not only family members' needs for information, but also their ability to comprehend and process it. The latter is critical if the family already has accurate information but persists in maladaptive behavior, despite intervention efforts.

Assumption #8: In Chronic Illness, Families Must Adjust to Changed Expectations of Each Other

Many of the changes in physical functioning brought on by chronic illness may subtly change expectations for family members. These changes often go unacknowledged and may contribute to family disruption. For example, a young mother confined to a wheelchair with multiple sclerosis often cannot adequately discipline her preschool children. All family members may realize this but never discuss it openly and may, therefore, retain unrealistic expectations.

Assumption #9: A Family's Perception of the Illness Event is the Greatest Influence Upon Ability to Cope

"Besides adjusting its structure in order to cope, a family also develops explanations of illness in order to bring some measure of certainty to the unknown, the unexplainable and the unjust" (Phipps and Desplat, 1984, p. 301). Some families perceive illness as a threat; others perceive it as a challenge; and still others see it as an enemy or test. Nurses must understand the family's perception of the illness before they attempt to intervene. Often, the most important goal of health care intervention is to change family members' perceptions of and thoughts about the illness event. In chronic illness the nurse's primary objective is to help the family adjust and adapt to the situation, not necessarily to accept it.

FAMILY ASSESSMENT

Family assessment is the evaluation of a family system. Although families are composed of individuals, a family assessment should focus less on the individual and more on the relationships and behaviors among *all* the individuals in the unit; thus, the family is viewed as a system of interacting members.

The nurse who conducts a family assessment assumes that individuals are best understood within their immediate social context. The nurse conceives of the individual as defining and being defined by that context (Sluzki, 1974). Relationships with family members and other meaningful members of the social environment are thus very important factors in family assessment.

If the nurse thinks "relationship" rather than "individual" then individual family members' behavior will be seen not in isolation, but in context. In interviewing family members as a group, the nurse can observe how they spontaneously interact and influence each other. Furthermore, the nurse can ask questions about the impact that family members have on one another. Although many variables of family functioning (e.g., roles and control) may also be assessed, the evaluation of relationships must remain the thrust of family assessment.

Family Assessment Models

The nurse may choose between family assessment frameworks. The model referred to in this chapter is the Calgary Family Assessment Model (CFAM) (Wright and Leahey, 1984), a multidimensional framework consisting of three major categories (structural, developmental, and functional). CFAM is based on a systems/cybernetics/communication theory foundation. This chapter will be devoted to the practical application of this model in family interviews.

HOW TO CONDUCT A FAMILY INTERVIEW

Before conducting a family interview, the nurse must have a clear conceptual framework. This will be influenced by her basic assumptions about families and chronic illness. The following guidelines are designed for family nurse interviewers and are an extension of the beginning family interviewing skills described by Wright and Leahey (1984). They are based on the theoretical foundation of a strategic/systemic approach to family interviewing (Haley, 1977; Watzlawick et al., 1974; Selvini-Palazzoli et al., 1980), and encourage a problem-solving, goal-oriented, time-limited approach to family interviewing.

Pre-Interview Guidelines

Developing hypotheses. Prior to meeting the family for the first time, the nurse should develop a basic hypothesis—a hunch or explanation about the family and the presenting problem in its relational context. Tomm (1984) defines hypothesis as a supposition generated to guide executive activity during the interview. Such assumptions orient the nurse's questioning and offer meaning to family behaviors. In short, hypotheses provide order for the interviewing process.

In dealing with families facing chronic illness, the nurse can generate hypotheses based on information gathered during hospital admission, visiting hours, or from the other staff. This information may consist of opinions, behavioral observations, or analogic (nonverbal) data. Fleuridas et al. (1986) suggest that hypotheses can also be based on prior experience with similar families, problems, symptoms, and situations. A nurse's knowledge about developmental life-cycle stages and theory in general (systems, crisis, and so forth) can be connected to salient family information to generate a hypothesis. Guidelines for designing hypotheses are given in Table 3.1.

Table 3.1   Guidelines for Designing Hypotheses*

- Choose hypotheses that are useful.
- Generate the most helpful explanations of the family's behaviors at this particular time.
- Remember that there are no "right" or "true" explanations.
- Include all family components to make the hypothesis as systemic as possible.
- Link the hypothesis to the family's immediate concerns to keep the interview content relevant to their situation.
- Make the hypothesis different from the family's to help introduce new information into the system and to avoid entrapment into the family's solutions.
- Be as quick to discard unconfirmed or unhelpful hypotheses as to generate new ones.
- Do not necessarily share the hypothesis with the family.

*Adapted from Fleuridas et al., 1986.

The following example illustrates how alternate hypotheses can be generated prior to the first family meeting. A nurse working in an extended care facility noted that the family, especially the 9- and 10-year-old children, avoided visiting their 41-year-old mother with Huntington's disease, and that the patient's symptoms worsened around visiting days. The children seemed depressed and withdrawn every time they came to the nursing unit on their monthly visits. During case conferences, the staff wondered whether there might be a connection between the family's avoidance and the patient's flailing and head-banging. They generated several hypotheses to explain why the family might be avoiding the patient and why the patient's symptoms seemed to exacerbate around the time of the family visits.

One hypothesis pertained to the children's belief that head-banging and flailing were controllable. Perhaps the children felt that their mother was not trying to control herself so she could return home to care for them. This made them angry, so they avoided her. An alternative hypothesis concerned the children's conflicting loyalties toward their mother and the aunt who took care of them. Perhaps they felt that if they visited too often, their aunt might think they did not appreciate her care. Thus they spaced out their visits and acted depressed and withdrawn to demonstrate both loyalty to their aunt and affection for their mother.

Yet a third hypothesis involved the children's fears of developing Huntington's disease themselves. They avoided visiting and showed sadness because of their own expectations of contracting the disease.

Having generated several alternate hypotheses about the family and the problem in its relational context, the staff arranged a family meeting. The purpose of the interview was to seek validating information through assessment questions. Interventions would then be designed based on either confirmed hypotheses or those which seemed most salient.

Arranging a family meeting. Once a nurse decides that a particular situation would best be addressed using a family approach, she must make two important decisions: who should be present at the assessment, and where should the interview take place. These decisions are strongly influenced by the hypotheses.

The first decision is particularly critical. Although it is not necessary for every family member to be invited to the assessment, it is strongly recommended that nurses meet all members of the household at least once, preferably at the first interview. In this way the nurse can become familiar with family members' perceptions of the situation, making it less likely that the nurse will become aligned with one individual's perspective and thereby lose the *family* perspective.

Haley (1977, p. 10) states that to begin family work "by interviewing one person is to begin with a handicap." The more family members present, the more information it is possible for the nurse to gather. Sometimes the most significant accomplishment of a family assessment is bringing the whole family together simultaneously to discuss an important issue.

The nurse's second decision pertains to the interview setting. A family assessment can take place anywhere: in the family home (the kitchen, the living room, or the patient's bedroom), in the community health agency (in an interviewing room or an office), or elsewhere. There are advantages and disadvantages to conducting an initial assessment in any setting. Nurses should be flexible in choosing a setting that is appropriate for the specific purpose of the interview.

The concrete advantages to interviewing in the home have been delineated in part by Smoyak (1977). Family members of all ages are more easily able to attend. Opportunities for meeting significant but perhaps elusive family members, such as boarders or grandparents, are increased. The nurse can experience the family's social environment and observe firsthand the physical environment. Disadvantages to using the home setting for family interviews include the increased administrative and personal cost involved in traveling and the greater likelihood of interruptions. Home interviews also require increased interviewing skill from the nurse (Clark, 1978).

The greatest advantage to using the agency or hospital setting is that, often, this is the nurse's base. This is where the nurse has initial contact with at least one family member face-to-face. The nurse can therefore capitalize on this opportunity and suggest a family interview. There are generally fewer telephone calls or visitor interruptions and the nurse can structure the interview more easily. The disadvantages of the work setting usually center around issues of context. Family members can be intimidated by such professional trappings as plush furniture or complicated equipment.

Interview Guidelines

Engagement. During the engagement or first stage of the family interview, the nurse must establish and maintain a therapeutic relationship with the family. Confrontation and interpretation too early in treatment may inhibit engagement (Gurman and Kniskern, 1981). To enhance engagement, the nurse must provide structure, be active, be empathic, and involve all members of the family group. Wright and Leahey (1984) have delineated specific skills for engaging families. One of the most helpful tools in this nursing situation is the genogram; its construction is a dynamic way of involving the family in defining its own structure (Holman, 1983).

Problem definition. During this phase of the family interview, the nurse should ask the family to define its main problem or complaint. Fleuridas et al. (1986) recommend that this be done by focusing on three time frames: past, present, and future. Within each time frame the nurse can ask questions pertaining to areas of difference, areas of agreement/ disagreement, and explanations for or the meaning of the problem (Fleuridas et al., 1986). It is important to emphasize that "an effective systemic interview does not depend on the use of any one type of question or another, but on the knowledge of when, how, and to what purpose to use questions and techniques within the framework of a specific model" (Lipchik and DeShazer, 1986, p. 89).

Present. The nurse should ask each family member, including the children, to share their knowledge and understanding of the present situation. For example, the community health nurse working with a diabetic family could ask such questions as:
• What is the family's main concern *now* about John's diabetes?
• How is this concern a problem for the family *now* as compared to before?
• Who agrees with you that this is a problem?
• What is your explanation for this?

Past. In exploring the past, the nurse can again ask questions pertaining to:
• *Differences:* (How was John's behavior before his diabetes was diagnosed?)

• *Agreement/disagreement:* (Who agrees with dad that this was the main concern when the family lived in Seattle?)
• *Explanation/meaning:* (What do you think was the significance of John's decision to stop injecting his own insulin?)

Future. During the initial interview with a new family, the nurse must learn about the family's own hypotheses or beliefs about their problems (Tomm, 1984). In asking the family to explain their present situation, the nurse should consciously attempt to identify previously unrecognized connections. This might be done by asking such questions as:
• If Bill suddenly developed renal disease, how would things be different from the way they are now?
• Does Bill agree with you?
• If this were to happen, how would you explain the change in John's relationship with mom?

Children and adolescents might be reluctant to identify "problems" in the family; they may hesitate to disagree with their parents' description of the problem. Nurses may need to ask children what types of changes they would like to see in the family or how they would know if the problems went away. For example, one 7-year-old repeatedly denied that there were any difficulties surrounding his brother's diabetes and his mother's overinvolvement with the sick child. However, when the nurse asked what differences there would be in the family if his brother did not have diabetes, the 7-year-old said that he and his mother could go to hockey games after school. At the time of the family interview, the mother was reluctant to leave the house after the boys returned from school for fear that the older boy would have an insulin reaction.

In exploring the presenting problem, the nurse should obtain a clear and specific definition of the situation and identify any conflict among family members over the problem definition. If such conflict exists, then the nurse must clarify the problem further to help define the behaviors for which the family is seeking help. Rosenthal and Bergman (1986) suggest that during this stage of the initial interview the nurse should discover if the patient (whether family, couple, or individual) is committed to seeking change. In other words, is the patient a "customer" seeking the nurse's assistance to change or is the patient under duress?

Sequence of Interaction

After the problem is identified, the nurse must examine family interactions connected to it. This calls for a review of all the information obtained from the family in light of the hypotheses generated prior to the interview, and the development of additional questions. Questions focusing on interactional *behaviors* deal with three time frames: present, past, and future. Within each time frame, the nurse should once again explore differences, agreements/disagreements, and explanations/ meanings.

Present. In exploring the present situation, the nurse could ask: Who does what when? Then what happens? Who is the first to notice that something has been done?

The nurse can inquire about differences between individuals ("Who is better at getting grandmother to eat, Jose or Maria?") and between relationships ("Do your ex-husband and Sammy fight more or less than your ex-husband and Alan?"). In working with families with chronic illness, the nurse should explore differences before or after important events or milestones. For instance, the nurse could ask, "Do you worry more, less, or the same about your wife's health since her heart attack?"

In addition to exploring areas of difference, the nurse can explore areas of agreement/disagreement ("Who agrees with you that Jose is the most forgetful in attaching the SIDS monitor to the baby? Who disagrees with you?"). The nurse should also explore the family's explanation for the sequence of interaction ("How do you explain Jose's tendency to be most forgetful about the monitor? What does his behavior mean to you?").

Past. In exploring the past, the nurse uses the same types of questions to explore differences ("How was it different? How does that differ from now?"), agreement/disagreement ("Who agrees with Randy that dad is more involved in Cheryl's exercise regimen?"), and explanation/ meaning ("What does it mean to you that after all this time, things between your wife and her mother have not changed?").

Future. By focusing on the future, the nurse instills hope for more adaptive interaction regarding the presenting problem. The nurse can ask questions pertaining to:
• *Differences:* "How would it be different if your grandmother didn't side with your father against your mother in managing Katrina's Crohn's disease?"
• *Agreement/disagreement:* "Do you think your father would agree that if your grandmother stayed out of the discussions things would be better?"
• *Explanation/meaning:* "Mom, tell me why you think it would be best for your husband to stop phoning his mother for advice about Katrina's Crohn's disease."

During the interview the nurse attempts to gain a systemic view of the problem and a description of the full cycle of repeated interactions. It is not important for the nurse to "understand" the problem but rather to be able to describe the sequence of the development of the problem over time and the current contextual view of the problem interaction.

Attempted Solutions

The next task for the interviewing nurse is to explore the family's attempted solutions to their problem. The process can begin with general questions ("How has your family tried to cope with Maria's refusal to dress herself properly?"). More specific questions should then be used to identify the least and most effective strategies for achieving desired effects, and when these strategies were employed ("What was least helpful in trying to get Maria to bathe? What was most effective?"). The nurse can ask if any successful elements in the solutions are still being employed and if they are not, why not. The same types of sequence of interaction questions focusing on difference, agreement/ disagreement, and explanation/meaning can be used to explore the family's attempted solutions to the presenting problems.

In working with families with a chronically ill member, the nurse should be aware of any additional "helping agencies" involved in health care delivery. Therefore, it is important to ask appropriate questions: "What agencies have attempted to help you with this problem? What has been the most useful advice that you have received? Did you follow this advice? What has been the least helpful advice?" Leahey and Slive (1983) point out the usefulness of exploring the ideologies of the treatment systems; if there is unclear leadership or a confused hierarchy within the helping system, the family can be placed in a distressing situation, similar to that of a child whose parents continually disagree. Confusion among helping agencies can exacerbate the problem rather than alleviate it. In this way, the attempted solution (assistance by helping agencies) can become an entirely new problem.

Change Orientation

At some point during the interview, the nurse must establish what changes the family expects as an outcome of nursing intervention. Members may expect a large change, for instance, "My father will be able to walk without the aid of a cane," or a small but significant change, such as, "We will be able to leave our profoundly retarded daughter with a babysitter for one hour a week." In many cases, only a small change is necessary. "No matter how awful and how complex a situation, a small change in one person's behavior can lead to profound and far reaching differences in the behavior of all persons involved" (DeShazer et al., 1986, p. 209). Moreover, experienced nurses are aware that small changes can lead to further progress.

The nurse can clarify the family's change orientation with future/ hypothetical questions, such as, "What would your parents do differently if they did not stay at home every evening with Jennifer?" The nurse can explore future/hypothetical areas of difference ("How would your parents' relationship be different if your mom allowed your aunt to take care of Jennifer one evening a week?"), areas of agreement/disagreement ("Do you think your mom would agree that she and your dad would probably have little to talk about if they went out one evening a week?"), and explanation/meaning ("Tell me more about why you believe this would happen. What would this mean to you?").

If possible, the nurse should encourage the family to state the appearance of a specific new behavior that is incompatible with their presenting complaint ("We would like to have time for ourselves as a couple one evening a week without having to provide care for our daughter."). If the "small but significant" change is presented as *stopping* a problem behavior, then the nurse should help the family redefine the desired change "in terms of the *appearance* of a specific behavior incompatiable with the complaint" (Rosenthal and Bergman, 1986, AI. 2B).

Nurses working with families of the chronically ill often find that an expected change is too big or too vague ("We would like Tanya to feel good about herself even though she has had a colostomy."). Experienced clinical nurses know that "feeling good about onself" is very difficult to measure. The nurse could ask for a sign or for a statement defining the smallest concrete change that the patient could make on his way to the general goal. By asking for this degree of specificity about desired change early in the nurse/family relationship, it is more likely that the family and nurse can accomplish the desired change.

Planning

When a family assessment has been completed, nurses can decide whether or not to intervene. To make this decision they need to consider the family's level of functioning, their own skill level, and other resources available.

Indications for family intervention. Intervention is recommended under the following circumstances (Wright and Leahey, 1984):
• A family member presents with a chronic illness that has an obvious detrimental impact upon the other family members. For instance, a grandfather's Alzheimer's disease may result in the grandchildren being afraid of him, or a young child's acting-out behavior may be related to his mother's deterioration from multiple sclerosis.
• Family members contribute to an individual's symptoms or problems, as when lack of visitation from adult children exacerbates hypochondriasis in an elderly parent.
• One member's improvement leads to symptoms or deterioration in another family member, for example, when decreased asthma symptoms in one child correlate with increased abdominal pains in a sibling.
• A child or adolescent develops an emotional, behavioral, or physical

problem in the context of a family member's chronic illness. Perhaps a diabetic adolescent suddenly requests that his mother give him his daily insulin injections when he has been injecting himself for the past six months.
• A family member is first diagnosed with a chronic illness. If a family has no previous knowledge or experience with a particular illness, they will require information.
• A family member's condition deteriorates markedly. Whenever there is deterioration, family patterns will need restructuring and intervention as indicated.
• A chronically ill family member moves from a hospital or rehabilitation center back into the community.
• An important individual or family developmental milestone is missed or delayed, such as when an adolescent is unable to move out of the home at the anticipated time.
• The chronically ill patient dies. Even though the patient's death may be a relief, the family can be faced with a tremendous void where the caretaking role used to be.

If family intervention is to begin, and the family is not in immediate crisis, the authors recommend that sessions occur once every two weeks at most. Families, particularly those of the chronically ill, need time to incorporate interventions into entrenched patterns; too-frequent sessions may offer insufficient time for change. One cannot categorically state the optimal number of days, weeks, or months between sessions, but health care professionals should tailor visitation schedules to the needs of each client family.

Nurses' workplace context will also influence session duration and intensity. A rehabilitation nurse working with a family, for instance, might reduce session frequency the longer the patient is in the rehabilitation center. That would help avoid inadvertently fostering family dependence.

Contraindications for intervention. Family intervention is not always appropriate or required. The authors suggest the following contraindications for family intervention (Wright and Leahey, 1984):
• *All* family members request or state that they do not wish to be involved in recommended family sessions or interviews.
• The family states that all members prefer to work with another health care professional.

Generally, these contraindications are evident to the nurse following a thorough family assessment. Even when the climate for intervention seems favorable, the family might indicate a desire to terminate family treatment.

Intervention

To intervene effectively within a family system, nurses must understand some basic assumptions regarding families and chronic illness; the indicators and contraindicators for actual intervention; and some of the primary concepts of change. The authors (1984, p. 174) view change within families as a systems/cybernetic phenomenon.

> "That is, change within a family may occur within the cognitive, affective, or behavioral domains but change in any one domain will have an impact on the other domain. Interventions can be targeted at any or all of the three domains. However, we believe that the most profound and sustaining change will be that which occurs within the family's beliefs (cognition). In other words, as a family thinketh (they are so)!"

Concepts of change. Some of the major concepts of change (Wright & Leahey, 1984) are:
- Change depends upon context.
- Change depends upon the perception of the problem.
- Change depends upon realistic treatment goals.
- Understanding alone does not lead to change.
- Change does not necessarily occur equally in all family members.
- Directing change is the nurse's responsibility.
- Change can have myriad causes.

These concepts of change provide a theoretical guide for family intervention. As mentioned previously, a primary interventional goal for families with chronic illness is to change the family-created "reality" if it is problematic. Nurses can help family members interact in new ways by focusing particular techniques or interventions on the system's cognitive, affective, or behavioral domains. Such interventions can effect change by affecting family members' perceptions about the illness and about each other. Normally, nursing interventions are directed at challenging the meaning that families give to behavioral events. However, the nature of the problem for which help is sought—i.e., whether it is acute or chronic—will influence the receptivity of the family to seeing it as a problem for the family system rather than for the identified patient alone. An acute health problem, regardless of its origin (e.g., physical illness, accidental injury, etc.) by definition brings a state of disequilibrium to the family system in which it occurs. The crisis nature of the event can be useful in helping to make the family more amenable to a system intervention. On the other hand, a chronic problem in the identified patient around which the family has developed a homeostasis balance is less likely to be viewed by the family as requiring treatment exclusively for the identifieu

The nurse must remember that interventions do not begin a.
intervention stage; they are part of the total interview process, b
engagement to termination. The interventions used during the specu.
intervention stage are based upon ongoing assessment. Families who ac
not follow through with planned interventions may not be "resistant"
due to pathology but rather to a lack of an adequate engagement period.
Resistance may also indicate inadequate assessment, or the nurse
might not recognize a family as being resistant due to the so-called
suction phenomenon (Wright and Leahey, 1984).

Intervention skills. The intervention stage represents the core of the
work with a family. It provides an appropriate context in which the
family can make necessary changes. Once a thorough assessment has
been completed, family intervention is indicated; particular intervention
skills can then be utilized.

There are three basic types of intervention skills: perceptual, conceptual, and executive (see Table 3.2) (Wright and Leahey, 1984).

Types of interventions. Direct interventions focus on families' cognitive,
affective, and/or behavioral levels of functioning, and request that a
family do something different from what they have been doing.
Obviously, these interventions are most effective with compliant families
rather than noncompliant families. Most nurses assume that the family
is compliant until given reason to think otherwise, for example, when
members do not follow through with assignments or immediately state
that everything has been tried before and nothing worked. The following
interventions have been found to be most effective with compliant
families and can be implemented singly or simultaneously.

Interventions directed at the cognitive level of family functioning. Interventions directed at the cognitive level of family functioning usually give
new information or new ideas about a particular problem. If a family
cannot solve problems, it may mean that members lack sufficient information. However, when they do have the information and do not change,
the problem is different, and indirect interventions are probably indicated. Some of the more common *direct cognitive interventions* follow.
Nurses can provide:
• Information about the chronic illness: its cause (e.g., genetic concern),
progress over time, and present and potential handicaps.
• Suggestions about appropriate family responses to the illness. For example,
the nurse can discuss the need for respite, the emotional effect of chronic
illness on children, and the possible strain on a marriage. Also, the nurse can

explore with families what patient-related problems (e.g., incontinence of urine) might be most difficult for members to tolerate.

• Information about available community resources such as Meals on Wheels, rehabilitation services, and disease-specific support groups like those run by the American Diabetes Association. Information about specific equipment and/or prostheses is also very useful.

• Help with decision-making. Sometimes families need relief from the pressure of decision-making. In such circumstances the nurse should assume that responsibility, but only after the family has had the opportunity to decide for themselves. For example, it might be too painful for the family of an elderly person with a chronic illness to consider an auxiliary hospital or nursing home placement. Sometimes the nurse can recommend that the family consider such an alternative. The nurse should give a solid reason why this decision might benefit everyone concerned.

Any direct interventions which present information to families need to be presented in a context of support; this supporting atmosphere is, in some instances, even more important than the specific information provided.

Interventions directed at the affective level of family functioning. Interventions directed at the affective level are designed to modify the intense emotions that may be blocking a family's problem-solving efforts. One of the most useful interventions is validating members' emotional responses. This can alleviate feelings of isolation and loneliness by helping family members see the connection between their relative's illness and feelings of stress (Wright and Bell, 1981). For example, it is useful to show a family with a chronically ill member that it is normal for family processes to be slowed down by the illness.

Following a recent diagnosis of chronic illness, it is important to tell the family that they may feel out of control, or frightened, or sad for a period of time, but within a few months they will adjust and learn to cope. It is also important in this validation process to tell them that everybody is affected by what happens and that chronic illness is a family venture. Tucker (1984) suggests three common reactions of families to chronic illness:

• The family is overwhelmed and becomes a "disabled family."
• The family pretends that nothing has happened.
• The family balances between making an adjustment and coping well.

Many families react intensely to the initial diagnosis of chronic illness. Initially, fear, shock, and disbelief predominate; physical symptoms often appear in healthy family members. Denial is often used to cope with this initial shock; it can be a useful mechanism if it protects family members from decompensation and does not interfere with

Table 3.2   Intervention Skills

Perceptual/Conceptual	Executive
• Recognize that family systems are goal-directed and possess problem-solving abilities. For example: Believe that families are not only able to change but can also identify and implement methods for change; this helps the nurse avoid feeling overly responsible.	• Encourage family members to explore problem-solving alternatives. For example: "Mr. Sanchez, you've mentioned that your wife has become very tired lately caring for your elderly mother. Do you have any idea of what could be done to assist your wife?"
• Recognize that direct interventions will probably be most effective with compliant families, but less effective with noncompliant families.	• Intervene directly by instructing the family to do something *different*. It is expected that the family will comply.
• Recognize that direct interventions are normally focused on cognitive, affective, and/or behavioral levels of family function. It is not always necessary or even efficient to target interventions at all three levels of functioning simultaneously.	• Target direct interventions on any one or all three levels of functioning. For instance, a) cognitive—provide information to help the family perceive the chronic illness differently. b) affective—encourage different affective expression. c) behavioral—have family perform new tasks either within or outside the interview context.
• Recognize that lack of educational information can inhibit a family's attempts at problem-solving, while additional information can encourage members to devise their own solutions to problems.	• Enhance the family's knowledge and facilitate further problem-solving. For example, the nurse can provide information about the normal aging process to caretakers of an elderly parent. This type of direct intervention targets the family's cognitive level of functioning.
• Recognize that persistent and intense emotions can often hinder problem-solving. Families who predominantly experience such emotions as sadness and anger often cannot deal with problems until the emotional block is removed.	• Validate family members' emotions when appropriate, and suggest where feelings might be problematic. Example, suppressed grief over the loss of an arthritic mother's usual physical functioning may be relieved by mere confirmation of the normal grieving process. This type of direct intervention targets the family's affective level of functioning.
• Recognize that constraining repetitive behavior patterns can inhibit family creative problem-solving, and that some tasks can serve to initiate changes in the structure of the family and/or family rules.	• Assign tasks aimed at improving family functioning, e.g., instruct a mother and father with a leukemic child to have grandparents babysit for a day while they have time together. This type of direct intervention targets the family's behavioral level of functioning.
• Recognize that families are often reluctant or hesitant to discuss aspects of the future that will be affected by the chronic illness. Questions "What will happen in two years when it would have been the time for Scott to begin attending school?" might be difficult for the family to answer.	• Ask hypothetical or future-oriented questions as a way of raising sensitive core issues about chronic illness without suggesting specific family action.

treatment. If families talk about denial but behave adaptively, then the denial is not maladaptive. For example, if a young husband denies his wife's recent diagnosis of multiple sclerosis, but installs a ramp in their home for her wheelchair, then his denial is not maladaptive.

Often families with chronic illness experience intense anger, sometimes directed at the ill member because of the tremendous changes in family life that the illness has required. Overtly this anger does not last too long, if only because social norms make it unacceptable to be angry at people who are ill. At other times family members and patient may become angry at the health care system, often quite appropriately. They may feel that sufficient treatment or information is not being provided. The family's rational management of the situation and action toward making needed changes may markedly reduce the frequency of such negative responses.

Guilt is also common among families of the chronically ill. This reaction can be adaptive if it helps mobilize resources on behalf of the ill person. A useful distinction can be made between realistic and neurotic guilt.

Another emotion common in families facing chronic illness is sadness, a frequent sign of resignation and depression. This reaction may recur with every new crisis or when another developmental milestone is missed or delayed, although the pattern may become less frequent and less intense. Unfortunately, the social rituals that help families grieve after a death do not help alleviate the sense of loss associated with chronic illness, and no effective substitute is available.

Finally, there is an important point to make with regard to the affective functioning of families with chronic illness. That is, families may adapt, but they do not necessarily ever accept the chronic illness. Therefore, it is wise that nurses not demand acceptance from such families. Rather, health care professionals should simply acknowledge the fact that something sad, bad, or awful has happened, and that the family is entering a lifelong process of adapting (Tucker, 1984).

Interventions directed at the behavioral level of family functioning. Interventions targeted at the behavioral level can help family members interact more effectively and thus behave more positively in relation to one another. This goal can be accomplished by assigning specific behavioral tasks to some or all family members. Some tasks can be assigned as homework to be done between sessions, while others might be completed in the interviewing room so that the interaction can be observed.

Nurses working with families after an initial diagnosis of chronic illness must focus on the instrumental issues first, before dealing with the affective issues. This rule of thumb holds true unless a severe

blockage of affect interferes with family problem-solving. Interventions targeted at the behavioral level of family functioning require a nurse to:
• Encourage families not to make drastic adjustments in their daily life. Often families with chronic illness make major adjustments and changes immediately after diagnosis, so that they are living in a continual state of disruption (Power and Orto, 1980). Emphasize that family members continue with usual routines whenever possible and maintain their customary role responsibilities. At least one home visit is recommended when nursing a family with chronic illness in order to understand the instrumental implications within that environment. By making a home visit, the nurse can reassure the family of their own competence by stating, "Now that I have come to know your family somewhat better, I know you have the ability to cope with what is ahead of you, although it will be difficult sometimes."
• Encourage opportunities for respite. One of the caretaking family's most difficult tasks is allowing members adequate respite. Too frequently, family members feel guilty if they need or want to remove themselves from the caretaking role. Even the ill member must disengage himself from time to time from the usual caretaking and accept another person's assistance. Each family's need for respite varies. The factors affecting respite requirements include the severity of the chronic illness; availability of family members to care for the ill person; and financial resources. All of these factors must be considered and balanced before the health care professional recommends a respite schedule. Tucker (1984) reports that she advises families to buy a less expensive prosthesis and use the extra money for a family vacation. In this way, caretaking and coping are balanced. Such "time outs" or "time away" is essential for families facing excessive caretaking demands.

CHALLENGES FOR NURSES WORKING WITH FAMILIES OF THE CHRONICALLY ILL

Working with families with chronic illness poses particular nursing challenges. An awareness of possible pitfalls and problems helps nurses intervene more effectively into family systems. The first challenge pertains to nurses' understanding of reciprocal influences. She must recognize that, not only is the family a system with certain boundaries, but also that she forms a new system with the family (the nurse-family system). The nurse is, therefore, influenced by the family just as the family is influenced by the nurse. Reciprocity is an important concept to remember when working with families with chronic illness.

Because of the nature of chronic illness, nurses often have long-term relationships with patients in either rehabilitation settings or home care. Many times these relationships can be more rewarding than the brief relationships of acute care settings. However, extreme attachment and dependency can hinder the nurse, patient, and family alike. If appropriate boundaries are not maintained (e.g., if the nurse does not have a strong social network and interests outside work), then working with chronically ill patients and their families may become exhausting and intrusive.

Nurses should also recognize the triangle that forms when they work with a family with chronic illness. The triangle consists of the patient, the family, and the health care system; all of these facets interact with and influence one another. At times, the nurse may be caught between the patient and other family members; this often happens when the nurse feels that both parties want her on their side.

A second challenge relates to the depression that has been observed in health care professionals working with families with chronic illness over a long period of time. Tucker (1984) relates a study completed at the University of Illinois which attempted to help nursing students cope with this depression. It was postulated that the depression arose from the students' inability to see any progress in the families' situations. The study involved showing nursing students videotapes of client families over time in order to make the progress visible. This had a positive influence on the nursing students and made them more optimistic about nursing the chronically ill and their families. Another finding in this study was the nurses' need to work with patients at all levels of dysfunction or disability, rather than with one particular population at one particular stage of illness.

A third challenge for nurses pertains to their entry into a family system where there is a chronically ill member. Nurses should not be overempathetic, or state that they understand the patient's dilemma or suffering. Instead, a nurse should ask the family to "teach" her what to consider and what to be aware of when working with families with chronic illness. Nurses *should not* say "I know what you are going through" but rather, "Teach me about what you're experiencing."

Finally, nurses should remember that families with chronic illness normally do not present with psychiatric problems and are frequently not pathological in their functioning. Rather, they are families who are adjusting and coping with a serious health problem that disrupts their usual pattern of functioning.

CONCLUSIONS

In conclusion, family interventions are as numerous and as varied as families themselves. However, interventions should be tailored to meet each family's specific needs and problems. They should always be based on sound assessment and a recognition of certain basic assumptions relevant to all families coping with chronic illness.

REFERENCES

Blazer, D. "The Management of Chronic Physical Illness," in *Role of the Family in the Rehabilitation of the Physically Disabled.* Edited by Blazer, D., and Siegler, I.C. Baltimore: University Park Press, 1984.

Clark, C. *Mental Health Aspects of Community Health Nursing.* New York: McGraw-Hill Book Co., 1978.

DeShazer, S., et al. "Brief Therapy: Focused Solution Development," *Family Process* 25(2):207–21, 1986.

Fleuridas, C., et al. "The Evolution of Circular Questions: Training Family Therapists," *Journal of Marital and Family Therapy* 12(2):113–27, 1986.

Griffin, J.Q. "Physical Illness in the Family," in *Family-Focused Care.* Edited by Miller, J.R., and Janosik, E.H. New York: McGraw-Hill Book Co., 1980.

Gurman, A., and Kniskern, D. "Family Therapy Outcome Research: Knowns and Unknowns," in *Handbook of Family Therapy.* Edited by Gurman, A.S., and Kniskern, D.P. New York: Brunner-Mazel, 1981.

Haley, J. *Problem-Solving Therapy.* San Francisco: Jossey-Bass, 1977.

Holman, A. *Family Assessment: Tools for Understanding and Intervention.* Beverly Hills, Calif.: Sage, 1983.

Leahey, M., and Slive, A. "Treating Families with Adolescents: An Ecological Approach," *Canadian Journal of Community Mental Health* 2:21-28, 1983.

Lipchik, E., and DeShazer, S. "The Purposeful Interview," *Journal of Strategic and Systemic Therapies* 5(1 & 2):88–99, 1986.

Phipps, E., and Desplat, P. "The Intertwining of the Family System in Huntington's Disease," *Family Systems Medicine* 2(3):298–308, 1984.

Power, P.W., and Orto, A.E.D., eds. "Approaches to Family Interventions," in *Role of the Family in the Rehabilitation of the Physically Disabled.* Baltimore: University Park Press, 1980.

Rosenthal, M., and Bergman, Z. "A Flow Chart Presenting the Decision-Making Process of the MRI Brief Therapy Centre," *Journal of Strategic and Systemic Therapies* 5(1 & 2):A1.1–A1.6, 1986.

Selvini-Palazzoli, M., et al. "Hypothesizing, Circularity and Neutrality: Three Guidelines for the Conductor of the Session," *Family Process* 19:3-12, 1980.

Sluzki, C. "On Training to Think Interactionally," *Social Science and Medicine* 8:483–85, 1974.

Smoyak, S. "Homes: A Natural Environment for Family Therapy," in *Distributive Nursing Practice: A Systems Approach to Community Health.* Edited by Hall, J., and Weaver, B. Philadelphia: J.B. Lippincott Co., 1977.

Tomm, K. "One Perspective on the Milan Systemic Approach Part II. Description of Session Format, Interviewing Style and Interventions," *Journal of Marital and Family Therapy* 10(2):253–71, 1984.

Tucker, S. Personal communication. Chicago: Northwestern University, 1984.

Watzlawick, P., et al. *Change.* New York: W.W. Norton & Co., 1974.

Wright, L.M., and Bell, J. "Nurses, Families and Illness: A New Combination," in *Treating Families with Special Needs.* Edited by Freeman, D., and Trute, B. Ottawa: The Canadian Association of Social Workers, 1981.

Wright, L.M., and Leahey, M. *Nurses and Families: A Guide to Family Assessment and Intervention.* Philadelphia: F. A. Davis Co., 1984.

4 Ethnicity and families with chronic illness

Toni Tripp-Reimer, RN, PhD
Professor and Director, Office of Research
College of Nursing
University of Iowa
Iowa City, Iowa

Geoffrey M. Lauer
Project Director
Ethnic Aging Study
Colleges of Nursing and Pharmacy
University of Iowa
Iowa City, Iowa

OVERVIEW

Chronic illness, family, and ethnicity are highly dynamic and interrelated concepts. The distinctive life patterns characterizing an ethnic group may influence a family's illness behavior in a variety of ways.

This chapter considers patterned differences in American families based on national, cultural, religious, or racial identification. This identification can be examined under the more inclusive category of "ethnicity." The chapter delineates how ethnicity might mediate the experience of families with members having chronic disorders. Included will be ways in which culture affects definitions of illness and how appropriate practitioners and treatment methods are determined.

THE NURSING ISSUE: ETHNICITY

In the United States, the dominant core value promotes equality. Out of this norm developed the melting-pot myth: that all Americans are alike, the products of a blending of diverse cultures. For many years, the notion that ethnicity should be discounted or ignored influenced health and social service delivery; in some ways, this misguided notion continues to preclude sensitive understanding of clients and their families.

Definitions

People who have been raised in an ethnic group often acquire not only that group's traditional attitudes toward health and illness but also its fundamental styles of interpersonal behavior and concerns about the world (Harwood, 1981). Before addressing the relationships between ethnicity, chronic disorders, and the family, it is important to clarify the meaning of ethnicity and related terms.

Culture may be defined as values, beliefs, and customs shared by members of a social group. It may also be viewed as a set of rules of behavioral standards learned through enculturation. Thus, the term "culture" refers to learned lifestyle patterns—including both health beliefs and behaviors, and family functions and structures.

A second concept, *population* or *racial identity*, refers to biophysiological characteristics. Race has been defined as a "division of a species which differs from other divisions by the frequency with which certain hereditary traits appear among its members" (Brues, 1977, p. 1). Petersen (1981) defines race as a population group that differs from others in the frequency of one or more genes, with the significant genetic variables specified according to the context. In anthropological research, the size and determination of a race depends simply on the purpose of the particular investigator. When considering human variation, one must keep in mind that specific population characteristics may or may not be present in a given individual.

A third related concept is *minority group.* Statistically, a minority is any group (racial, religious, or other) constituting less than a numerical majority of the population. However, as Mindel and Habenstein (1976) point out, "minority" in the sociological sense relates to power or dominance, or, rather, its lack. Minority groups have unequal access to power and may be stigmatized by presumed inferior traits or characteristics. Because the term has been used in a pejorative sense, this chapter will not refer to minorities.

Parsons (1975) describes the fourth and pivotal concept, *ethnicity,* as elusive and difficult to define. Factors commonly used to determine an individual's ethnicity are: origins, concept of sociocultural distinctiveness, subcultural social relations, territoriality, kinship, and symbolic identification (Abramson, 1980), as well as geographic origin, migratory status, race, language, religion, literature, food choices, settlement patterns, and political and social interests (Thernstrom et al., 1980).

Ethnicity, in short, distinguishes collectivities on the bases of common origins and shared behavioral symbols and standards (culture); these collectivities interact within a larger social system (Harwood, 1981).

As Parsons (1975) points out, a common culture represents the core of the concept of ethnicity. Examples of symbolic cultural elements defining ethnicity include kinship patterns, physical contiguity, religious affiliation, language or dialect forms, nationality, and phenotypical features. In essence, the ethnic group is society's culture-bearing unit.

Identifying Ethnicity

Know what an ethnic group is or is not. Petersen (1981) contends that users of the term "ethnic group" often forget the distinction between a group, which by definition has coherence and solidarity, and a category, grouping, or aggregate, which denotes only patterned differentiation. Thus, "ethnic group" implies that its members interact and are aware of common interests.

While ethnicity is an important concept, remember that none of the cultural or physical characteristics used to identify an ethnic population sharply distinguish any population group. Additionally, recognize intraethnic diversity. There is as much variation within groups as between them; knowledge of this can prevent the stereotyping of members of ethnic groups.

Health practitioners in the United States often erroneously assume that Caucasians constitute a single cultural group. Recent research by Clinton (1982), while revealing that ethnic identity still determines (even through the fifth generation) much of what Americans of European descent believe and do about health, also indicated that Caucasian Americans are not homogeneous in terms of their ethnic identity and patterns of health behavior. The bias of cultural homogeneity applies no more to white Americans than to other ethnic groups.

Despite the "melting pot" myth, America has one of the most heterogeneous populations of any Western culture. This diversity of ethnic groupings calls for reexamination of "traditional" ethnic classifications and expanded consideration of nontraditional ones. For example, as Place (1981) points out, next to Native Americans, the least studied group in ethnic gerontology are the elderly of European descent. This deficit is surprising in light of their large numbers in the United States.

Many rural communities and urban neighborhoods consist of ethnic populations with demonstrated continuity. Because of the stability of these populations, health professionals should understand the relationships between ethnicity, the family, and chronic illness. A community's cultural heritage will influence values, beliefs, and behaviors. Consequently, the ways the families act and the amount of support they receive in various life circumstances will differ among ethnic groups.

Distribution of Chronic Illnesses Among Ethnic Groups

Chronic diseases are not randomly distributed within a population; most are associated with advanced age. Therefore, in Western populations, increased life expectancy has led to an increase in the rate of chronic illness.

Similarly, chronic disorders may not be randomly distributed among ethnic groups. Because many diagnostic indicators of chronic disease are not detectable without routine medical evaluation, many chronic disorders are underreported among ethnic populations with low rates of health care utilization.

The incidence of certain diseases also varies among specific populations. Nurses must be aware of these epidemiological differences, since lack of such information might lead to discriminatory screening. For example, phenylketonuria (PKU) occurs predominantly in those of European descent, but only once or so in every 12,000 births. Nevertheless, hospitals test all newborns for PKU. Screening of Black infants for sickle-cell anemia, however, is still not routine procedure in many hospitals, despite the fact that one in every 100 Black babies is affected.

Obviously, knowledge of an increased genetic susceptibility to disease among specific population groups is essential in quality health care delivery. Table 4.1 outlines these characteristic predispositions among eight major ethnic groups and subgroups.

Table 4.1   Ethnic Distribution of Disease

Population Group	Relatively High Frequency	Relatively Low Frequency
Africans		
	Sickle cell anemia	Cystic fibrosis
	Glucose-6-phosphate dehydrogenase (G-6-PD) deficiency	Hemophilia
		Phenylketonuria (PKU)
		Pseudocholinesterase deficiency
	Hypertension	Multiple sclerosis
	Thalassemia	Osteoporosis
	Tuberculosis	
	Cervical cancer	
	Esophageal cancer	
Asians		
Japanese/Koreans	Actalasia	Breast cancer
	Oguchi's Disease	Osteosclerosis
	Dyschromatosis universalis	Chronic lymphatic leukemia
	Gastric ulcer	
	Cerebrovascular accidents	

(continued)

Population Group	Relatively High Frequency	Relatively Low Frequency
Asians (continued)		
Chinese	Nasopharyngeal cancer Thalassemia G-6-PD deficiency	Chronic lymphatic leukemia
Filipinos (US)	Hyperuricemia	
Native Americans		
	Diabetes mellitus Congenital hip dislocation Gallbladder disease Tuberculosis Rheumatoid arthritis Alcoholism	Duodenal ulcer
Europeans		
Northern	Multiple sclerosis PKU Pernicious anemia Cleft palate	Sickle-cell anemia Thalassemia
Southern	G-6-PD deficiency Thalassemia Familial Mediterranean fever	Cystic fibrosis
Askenazic Jews	Tay-Sachs disease Pentosuria Niemann-Pick disease Blooms' Disease Diabetes mellitus Polycythemia vera Hyperuricemia Leukemia Ulcerative colitis	PKU Tuberculosis Alcoholism Cervical cancer

Adapted from McKusick (1967, 1973); Damon (1969).

The Importance of Ethnicity to Family Illness Management

Although particular elements vary among different ethnic groups, the concept of family is universal. The family constitutes the most important social context within which illness occurs and is resolved, and consequently serves as a primary unit in health and medical care. Indeed, most health care occurs in the family context. Kleinman (1978) and others have found that the overwhelming majority of initial health care is sought within the family, and that, in fact, the family may represent the setting in which most of the care is pursued and received.

The family is frequently involved in confirming a member's illness, selecting lay consultants or professional practitioners, ensuring compliance with prescribed therapy, and determining whether chronic illness care can be provided in the home. As Litman (1974) notes, the process of becoming a patient and using health services encompasses decisions that involve the interaction of family, friends, and professional care providers. The family's role in the process over time depends on the nature of the condition (acute, chronic, or terminal), its perceived severity, the degree of familial concern, and the member affected. The family participates in every stage of a member's illness, from diagnosis through treatment and rehabilitation or death.

A family's involvement in a member's illness is mediated by several factors, including the person's role and status within the family, and the availability of social, material, and professional support. Strong ethnic affiliation can vary these patterns dramatically.

Mindel and Habenstein (1976) note that if traditional ethnic values exist at all, they will be found in the family setting. Chrisman and Kleinman (1981) add that the labeling of sickness and its treatment among ethnic groups often involves the entire family, far more than does the similar process in a population united by factors other than heritage—for instance, middle-class American society, where individuals generally diagnose health problems and determine treatment by themselves. Ethnicity is a critical variable in a family's perceptions and treatment of its chronically ill member and of how, in turn, the family itself is viewed by the community at large. Cultural factors mediate symptom identification and interpretation, expression of pain and discomfort, the "acceptability" of a particular chronic condition, and reactions to the dependence that accompanies chronic illness. Finally, ethnicity may influence family interaction with health professionals and what practitioners must consider if their care is to be most effective.

Family structure. Family structure and organization varies widely among American ethnic groups. Remember, however, that nuclear families, isolated individuals, and extended families exist in all ethnic groups, as do male-dominated, female-dominated, and egalitarian family units. One can characterize the dominant, ideal, or modal family type within particular traditional ethnic groups, but be aware of intragroup variations.

Defining family members. Identifying the individuals who constitute a family is crucial in nursing assessment. Family composition influences what support is available, how health decisions are made, who can care for a chronically ill family member, and who is allowed to visit the ill relative.

The wide range of familial compositions in American society becomes apparent from examination of kinship systems. Among some Native American populations, first cousins are treated as siblings and children may have more than two sets of grandparents. Similarly, fictive kin, such as godparents or coparents, are often important in families of Southern Mediterranean (e.g., Greek and Italian) origin. These fictive kin may be active within the family, particularly when children are involved. A different situation, however, has been reported for Japanese Americans. Kitano and Kikumura (1976) found that, within this population's health matters, neighbors may be more important than relatives who no longer live within the household. In such cases as these, the nurse must understand that "family" may be broadly defined and that membership might not conform to conventional nuclear or legal boundaries.

Extended versus nuclear families. The "typical" American family arrangement is thought to be nuclear, consisting of parents and their young children. Yet, other patterns may be modal within specific ethnic subpopulations. For example, the Amish view the family as both a religious and a social unit. Their residential pattern consists of a large family farmhouse with an adjacent "Grossdaadi Haus," or grandparent house, to which elder parents retire after conferring farming rights to one of their children. Similarly, immigrants tend to live in extended family clusters, particularly when older members speak less fluent English than their younger relatives.

On the other hand, the prevalence of extended family households in some ethnic groups has been overestimated. For example, Jackson (1981) identifies a common notion that the extended family predominates among Blacks and that it provides for and protects its members. Jackson contends that the extended family is *not* the predominant form among either rural or urban Blacks, and that, even when present, it cannot always provide sufficient instrumental and effective aid to its members.

Male- or female-based families. The denotations of a family as patriarchal or matriarchal (male- or female-headed) is often subtler than many recognize. While the Italian-American family has been described as patriarchal, this is misleading, because it implies that the power resides in the male members of the family. In actuality, the mother generally holds the center in the Italian family and has sway over internal matters (Femminella and Quadagno, 1976). Similarly, although Mexican-American women appear subservient to the wishes of males, they often hold the primary position in household matters and are the foundation of their families' internal support systems. A different situation prevails among the Amish. While the male heads the household, notions of family and childrearing patterns are founded on shared parental responsibility. The Amish expect both parents to work together to care for the farm and children, to be almost always in the home, and to be available for mutual support (Huntington, 1976).

Contrary to popular notions about the Black family, most research indicates an egalitarian structure. In most Black families, husbands make decisions and perform household tasks. Conversely, most wives, while strong, are not dominant matriarchs, but share with their husbands the making of family decisions. Staples (1976) contends that the failure of many studies of Black family life to distinguish between the terms "dominant" and "strong" has reinforced the myth of Black matriarchy. While Black women have needed to be strong in order for their families to survive, they have not necessarily been dominant.

Matriarchy is common among many American groups, including the Navajo, Hopi, Crow, Mohawk, Seneca, Creek, and Seminole tribes. However, again, this is less clear than some believe. For example, among the Hopi, a man joins his wife's household and provides economically for her family, but he also retains ritual, leadership, and disciplinary roles in his natal household. Thus, Hopi men may make decisions for their sisters' children.

Interdependence versus autonomy. The extended family is the central, as well as the most durable and influential, social institution among Mediterranean cultures. Families visit spontaneously and maintain almost daily intergenerational contact. Children often live with their parents until marriage, and remain close afterward. During illness, Middle Easterners rely heavily on others instead of trying to cope alone.

Lock (1983) points out that the Japanese value social group harmony over individual needs and autonomy. Health professionals reared within European traditions might find this value difficult to accept. Norwegian Americans, on the other hand, value individualism and autonomy and are less interdependent in health matters, making it easier for health care providers to understand their needs.

Decision making. The factors that influence family structure and organization also affect patterns of decision making regarding health. Frequently, the decision to hospitalize is not made by the individual patient alone, but is shared with the family. For example, among many Navajo, the decision to enter a hospital is often reached only after a family conference; a woman and her husband alone may not be free to exercise discretion in this regard. Abasiekong (1981) contends that the subordination of individual decision and plans to those of the family should not be considered irrational, even by health professionals who value individual autonomy. There are important reasons for group decisions in cases dealing with medical treatment, not the least of which is that illness may become a social and economic problem for the entire family and peer network. Only when relatives and friends accept a condition as an illness can a patient be exempted from normal daily tasks. Because illness affects the entire family, it is only logical that the family participate in the decision making.

Health and Illness Behaviors

People from all cultures experience some pathological symptoms in their lifetimes. In fact, illness is a universal human experience, like birth and death (Foster and Anderson, 1978). But cultural perceptions, values, and experiences of such pathologies vary greatly. Through a process called enculturation, humans internalize cultural values, norms, and perceptions, including beliefs regarding the existence, labeling, and meaning of pathological symptoms. Family, friends, and lay practitioners, along with the symptomatic individuals, are often bound up in the process of recognizing and interpreting a specific symptom. All are involved in the negotiation that occurs between the symptomatic individual and the social group regarding expected behavioral changes.

Defining health. The first stage of the illness referral process is identifying problematic symptoms. This delineation depends, in part, on how members of the social group define a state of health.

Two parallel concepts relating to the definition and perception of self or others as diseased or ill are "health" and "normality." Perception of a "state of health" includes or excludes certain features, which can vary from culture to culture. For example, "health" for Jamaicans means a good appetite, feelings of strength and energy, performance of daily activities without problems, and sexual activity and fertility (Mitchell, 1983). Similarly, Ragucci (1981) observed that for Italian women, the ability to interact socially and perform activities of daily living (ADLs) were the most frequently mentioned indicators of health and well-being.

Obviously, many ethnic traditions can create disparity between an individual's subjective health perceptions and the scientific observations of a health care professional. Individuals may define themselves or others in their group as "healthy" even in the presence of obvious pathology (Tripp-Reimer and Dougherty, 1985). Hautman and Harrison (1982), for instance, found this true in a study of middle-income American Caucasians. Similarly, many Mexican Americans regard sweating, diarrhea, and coughing as everyday experiences easily within the range of "normal" health (Lieban, 1977).

Many health aberrations are accepted as normal because of their high frequency within a given population, but that does not mean they should be considered "good." It only means that very common symptoms may not be identified as abnormal.

Defining illness. Health care professionals, particularly physicians, have historically focused on pathological problems to the exclusion of the social dimensions of illness. New social science theories concerning the distinction between disease and illness have illuminated the social factors that influence symptom identification.

Modern Western medical taxonomy constitutes an international standard for labeling and treating "disease." As such, scientifically-trained health care professionals can agree on the nature and etiology of symptoms. In contrast, "illness" is a sociopsychological phenomenon which encompasses clients' subjective experiences as well as interactions between symptomatic individuals and their social groups.

For clients, symptom labeling and diagnosis rests not only on objective factors, but also on the degree of difference between the individual's behaviors and those the group has defined as "normal," the level of stigma attached to a particular set of symptoms, the prevalence of the pathology, and the ease of taking on the "sick role."

Often a disease pathology must have a visible impact on the individual before it is labeled an "illness." For many ethnic individuals, the point of impact is reached when the symptom interferes with customary social or personal activities, including work and household maintenance. Symptoms may be tolerated until they reach the point of individual crisis (Chrisman and Kleinman, 1981). Indeed, this is more often the rule than the exception among lower socioeconomic populations.

Among many ethnic groups, the family is often more influential in labeling persons as ill than are families from middle-class populations with European backgrounds. Factors that determine whether a family member will be perceived as moving from health to illness include age, sex, role responsibilities, and, in some cases, gender. For example, in Latin American cultures, women are often perceived as more incapacitated by disease than are men with similar symptoms (Fabrega, 1977).

Additionally, an individual's economic contribution to the family may also be a factor in illness determination. The family may be more hesitant to define as "ill" an individual upon whom everyone depends for financial support. Similarly, age may be a factor; among some urban Blacks, elderly individuals accept and cope with a terminal illness better than do young adults, who often deny a suspected terminal condition (Harwood, 1981).

After symptoms are identified and the sick role ascribed, a family lay diagnosis is made. This is the family's explanatory model of the problem and its cause; it may be based upon scientific medicine, folk theories, or a combination of the two.

Nonscientific or "folk" explanations may be divided into two categories, naturalistic and personalistic, depending upon the factors believed to cause illness (Foster and Anderson, 1978). The naturalistic model attributes illnesses to natural, nonmalevolent forces—generally, by disturbance of a natural balance. Two classic examples of naturalistic equilibrium models are the Chinese yin/yang model and the hot/cold dichotomy prevalent throughout Mexico and Central and South America.

While naturalists believe illness results from natural, explainable imbalances, believers in the personalistic model perceive illness as the result of malevolent, aggressive forces, or of supernatural entities that project harmful forces at an individual. The "evil eye" and witchcraft are two examples of personalistic forces.

Some groups pay little attention to the cause of illness. The symptom itself may be perceived as the "disease." In Jamaican culture, for example, symptoms such as diabetic skin lesions are often labeled simply as "diabetes." In such a model the disease is believed to be cured if, and when, the visible symptoms disappear. This model has important implications for scientific health care, especially in cases of chronic, intermittently active, illness. Such a model might preclude effective treatment for the source of the symptoms.

A cautionary note is required for nurses dealing with ethnic populations. Generalizations regarding ethnic beliefs about illness can obscure understanding of the individual client's personal beliefs. Thus, rather than memorizing a list of traits for each culture, a nurse should elicit an explanatory model for each patient. This individualized approach is necessary not only because no single explanatory model will apply throughout an ethnic group, but also because such a model may even change for a client during the course of his illness.

Self-care. After a symptom is identified as a problem, the first line of treatment is often self-care. All cultures have their own preferred lay or popular treatments; for example, in the United States, roughly 70% to 90% of all episodes of illness are treated first, or exclusively, through self-care (Zola, 1979). The health beliefs and practices of middle-class American clients closely approximate those of scientific health practitioners, largely because of the diffusion of the medical model through the media (television, newspapers, and magazines) and through more frequent use of scientific practitioners. Lay treatment patterns among other ethnic groups may differ dramatically, however, from scientific health practice. Health professionals are often unaware of the variety of options that may be available to ethnic clients.

Lay systems may be used for several reasons. Self-care treatments are used by all people for minor problems before they seek outside attention, especially if the symptom is perceived as minor and treatable within the home. Home therapies may also be used by ethnic clients because they cost less than treatment by an orthodox practitioner. Faced with an expensive treatment regime, it is not surprising that some people investigate alternative therapies. Nurses should note, however, that even folk remedies can be costly. For example, urban Black populations in the southeastern United States sometimes use medicinal potions that cost much more than the equivalent orthodox treatment.

Home treatments might seem attractive for their accessibility—compared to mainstream medicine care which requires traveling to a physician and then to a pharmacy. This is of particular concern in geographically isolated areas; predictably, reliance on alternative healing practices will be higher in such places than where there is ready access to professional medical care. When relatives or friends administer home remedies, it promotes health in two ways: by mobilizing the patient's social support network and by validating the trustworthiness of home therapies.

Specific illness behaviors. The activities and concerns of persons who view themselves as sick have been studied across a variety of cultures. Results indicate that cultures differ in their perception of pain, symptom evaluation, the stigma attached to various symptoms, and emotional states that precipitate or ameliorate an illness episode.

Stigma and symptom identification. There is wide cultural variation in how individuals with specific disorders are perceived and treated by others in their social network. An illness may be grounds for social ostracism or, conversely, for increased status. For example, Tripp-Reimer (1984a) traced perceptions of epileptics among different cultural groups. In Uganda, where epilepsy is considered contagious and untreatable, the epileptic is ostracized from general society. In Greece, where the epilepsy connotes family shame, members of the community may refuse to marry someone whose family has a history of the disorder. Traditional Mexican Americans, on the other hand, view the condition as the result of a physical imbalance, so it is much less stigmatic. The Hutterites view epilepsy as a trial by God; the patient who bears the burden well may gain status within the community as a faithful Christian. Consequently, among the Hutterites, the epileptic is encouraged to marry, have children, and become well-integrated into community life.

Bodily symptoms are also perceived and reported in many ways. For example, Graham (1956) found that Greek and Italian Americans reported common physical symptoms more often than did persons of Irish or British descent. Further, Greeks were more convinced that their physical complaints were evidence of disease than were the other groups studied.

Pain. Pain is a universal phenomenon. Yet its expression and interpretation vary dramatically among ethnic groups. These behaviors depend, among other things, on whether the person's culture accepts or condemns demonstrative emotional response to injury and pain. If clients do not report discomfort during painful situations, it may mean that their culture values stoicism.

Koopmen et al. (1984) investigated pain in ambulatory patients. Using American patients of Italian and Irish ancestry, they found that Italian Americans reported pain much more frequently than did their Irish-American counterparts. They concluded that the Italian Americans used pain reports to emphasize the immediacy of their somatic problems or to dramatize their attitude toward the sick role. They suggested that the Italian and Irish subgroups both coped with illness by avoidance, the Italians focusing on somatic discomfort to legitimize being cared for and the Irish denying pain.

An investigation of Black, Mexican-American, and Caucasian chronic spinal pain patients further illustrated ethnic differences in pain tolerance (Lawlis et al., 1984). Mexican-American patients reported the highest pain levels, and women of all three ethnic groups emphasized their pain more than men.

This research indicates that not only the perception of pain but also responses to it vary between cultures. Nonpatients within ethnic populations are guided by the same cultural imperatives. Among some groups, pain complaints elicit comforting attention, probably enough to reinforce the pain behavior. Additionally, ethnic differences in parental responses to children's pain have also been documented (Hartog and Hartog, 1983). American Jewish and Italian parents have been noted to be especially attentive to their children's pain ("show me where it hurts") in contrast to Protestant Americans, whose behavior more often reinforces stoicism ("you'll be all right").

Nurses should, however, note that not all research on ethnic styles of pain response has reached the same conclusions. While the studies cited above found major ethnic differences in reported pain behavior, other investigators (Flannery et al., 1981; Weisenberg et al., 1975) found few differences. These equivocal results may be explained partially by the fact that separate studies examined different ethnic groups, employed different measures of the pain experience, or were methodologically weak.

In perhaps the most complex and comprehensive study to date, Lipton and Marbach (1984) examined ethnic differences and similarities in the reported pain experience of Black-, Irish-, Italian-, Jewish-, and Puerto Rican–American pain patients. They found no significant interethnic differences for about two thirds of the variables measured. The most obvious ethnic differences were found in emotional responses to pain (stoicism vs. expressiveness) and pain-related interference in daily functioning. The pain experiences reported by the Black, Italian, and Jewish patients were found most similar; Irish and Puerto Rican patients were relatively distinct from the other groups as well as from each other.

Lipton and Marbach further attempted to identify ethnic variables that influenced the pain experience. Their results for five ethnic groups follow:
• Black patients displayed considerable dependence on lay individuals during illness. Such reliance on members of the ethnic group was strongly predictive of an expressive response to pain, as well as of disturbance in daily functioning attributable to the pain.
• For Irish patients, the reported disruption in daily functioning caused by pain and their nonexpressive response to pain seemed strongly related to membership in a long-standing Irish friendship group (an indication of a low degree of social assimilation).
• Among Italians, the duration of pain was the most useful predictor of pain response. Chronic (present for more than six months) pain was a strong predictor of both emotional response to and expression of pain as well as disruption in daily activities.
• Jewish patients' level of psychological distress seemed the most important explanation of pain response. A high level of distress was strongly predictive of an emotionally expressive pain response and of pain-related interference in daily functioning.
• Puerto Rican patients often displayed intense psychological distress and strong friendship ties and dependence on others in the ethnic group during chronic pain, all predictors of an emotionally expressive pain response and of great disruption in daily activities attributable to pain.

Interesting cultural variables also guide nursing approaches to pain. A number of investigations have compared nurses in the United States to those from abroad, indicating that nurses in other cultures display different caring behaviors based upon culturally-specific values and expectations. In the most comprehensive of such studies, conducted by Davitz and Davitz (1976, 1977, and 1978), explored cross-cultural differences in nurses' assessment of clients' physical pain and psychological stress. The first report surveyed 554 nurses in the United States, Japan, Taiwan, Thailand, Korea, and Puerto Rico. The researchers' 60-item questionnaire covered variances in such client characteristics as disease, sex, age, and illness severity. Data supported the hypotheses that nurses in different countries differed in the degree of suffering they perceived in their patients. Japanese and Korean nurses consistently inferred the greatest physical and psychological patient suffering. This finding is interesting, because many in the West consider Orientals to be stoic and less sensitive to pain. The investigations showed the need for accurate pain assessment and suggested that nurses often stereotype patient distress on the basis of what they think the patient feels. These studies indicate the importance of considering the nurse's culture as well as the client's.

In assessing pain, then, nurses should be aware of common cultural patterns of pain expression, as well as of their own cultural perspectives. Otherwise, patients might be over- or undermedicated. In addition, knowledge of the different meanings of pain can serve as the basis for effective pain control and therapy.

Nurses must also, however, avoid *over*emphasizing the role of culture in pain experiences; as Lipton and Marbach (1984) point out, the relationship is subtler than is often thought. It may be impossible to typecast any ethnic group by rigid elements of the pain experience. Rather, one could describe certain responses as only more or less characteristic of a group. Some clinicians, however, have assumed an all-or-none perspective, stereotyping particular ethnic groups' pain behavior on the basis of previous investigations or personal clinical experience.

It is important to realize that, while enormous intragroup differences exist, cultural assimilation into the mainstream, especially in the United States, is the norm. Cultural differences can certainly determine an aspect of pain response, and knowledge of this can help health care providers, but individualized, nonstereotypic assessment of each patient's responsive style is even more critical (Schechter, 1984).

Long-term care options. For at least 15 years, investigations have been conducted on ethnic groups' utilization of and access to long-term health care. This has been of special concern in gerontology; numerous investigations have found underrepresentation of Black, Hispanic, Asian, and Native American elderly relative to their presence in the overall population. This situation can be viewed from two valid perspectives: that of demand and that of access to nursing home care.

One suggested reason for lower nursing home enrollments among ethnic elderly is the presence of strong family ties. Considerable evidence indicates that familial responsibility is an important feature of many ethnic cultures. Research shows that extended family arrangements are most common among certain demographic subgroups; for example, the rural elderly, those living in inner city areas, or recently arrived immigrants of any ethnic affiliation.

Not only is long-term facility usage lower among ethnic subgroups, but different types of facilities are approached. Kart and Beckham (1976) investigated ethnic distribution in 17 categories of institutions in which aged individuals may reside. These institutions included prisons and workhouses, mental hospitals, residential treatment centers, hospitals, homes for the aged, and facilities for the mentally handicapped. They found substantial differences by institution type in the distribution of elderly Blacks and Whites. Generally, Blacks were overrepresented in state mental hospitals, while White clients predominated in nonprofit and proprietary homes for the aged. This difference is especially important because these facilities have traditionally housed the largest numbers of institutionalized elderly.

Markson (1979) suggested that institutional patterns for White ethnics are somewhat different: poverty and low socioeconomic status, coupled with foreign birth, placed these aged at a high risk for institutional care, including mental hospitalization.

Tripp-Reimer and Schrock (1982) conducted a field investigation of residential preferences for the aged among three Iowa ethnic populations of European descent: Old Order Amish, Greek, and Czech. Their report delineated the preferences of ethnic elderly themselves, as well as those of their younger relatives. Subjects in all three groups were asked where and with whom they would prefer to reside given one of these life situations: healthy and mobile, confined indoors, or confined to bed. The three groups gave significantly different answers, particularly when asked where they would prefer to reside if they were bedfast. More than three-fourths of the Amish preferred to live with relatives (the remainder would attempt to live, with assistance, at home). Half of the Greeks would live with relatives; but almost as many would prefer to live in a custodial facility. For the Czechs, 75% would prefer institutional care, with the remainder wishing to live with relatives.

These results can be explained in part by differences in the groups' value orientations. The Amish are strongly oriented toward family and the community at large. Czechs place a high value on independence; they considered the decision to move to a nursing home as a sign of self-reliance.

Preferred styles of interaction with practitioners.
Client views of the nursing role. Client-held stereotypes or ideal views of health care practitioners influence responses to the therapeutic situation. For example, Ragucci (1981) elicited the views Italian Americans

have of nurses, revealing that those views were rigid. Generally, respondents expected nurses to carry out physicians orders without making independent health care judgments. Asian immigrants have similar views, perhaps because of the structure of nursing practice in their native areas. In Asia, family members perform all support tasks—bathing, feeding, and other comfort measures—for a hospitalized person, while the nurses provide such strictly medical care as injections (Gould-Martin and Ngin, 1981).

The desired degree of intimacy. Interactions between clients and health care professionals may also depend on the client's desired degree of intimacy; it may range from very formal interactions to close personal relationships with the health professional.

For example, Southeast Asians often expect a health professional to be authoritarian or directive—socially "superior"—which might hinder communication. The emphasis on preserving social harmony may prevent the Southeast Asian client from fully expressing concerns or feelings. Such reserve may also give the health care professional a false impression that the client agrees with or understands a discussion; nodding or smiling may in fact only reflect a desire for interpersonal harmony (Tripp-Reimer, 1984b).

In contrast, Appalachian clients' traditionally close family interaction patterns often lead them to expect close personal relations with a care professional. Often their most important criterion for "quality care" is the degree to which the health practitioner interacts at a personal level. Appalachians may be uncomfortable with the impersonal, "bureaucratic" orientation of most health care institutions. In order to sustain a professional relationship with the mountaineer, the nurse may have to adopt a more personal approach (Tripp-Reimer, 1984a).

Patients of Mediterranean-area ethnic origins are generally even more insistent than Appalachians on a high degree of intimacy. They may try to draw health practitioners into the family system, involving them in personal activities and social functions. When relationships are well established, they may even feel the right to call their health care professional at any hour of the day or night (Lipson and Meleis, 1983).

Obstacles to communication. Often nurses expect all patients to behave uniformly; in the United States, that means assuming the classic Western "sick role" of undemanding compliance. However, many ethnic patients have markedly different beliefs about patient and family behavior and communication during an illness. These expectations may range from aggressive, demanding behavior to silent passivity. Hartog and Hartog (1983) point out that among American Jewish and Italian groups, complaining and making demands are often rewarded with attention. Wheat et al. (1983) found that a hospitalized Russian patient's demands and complaints were an effective coping mechanism in the Soviet system, but counterproductive in a Western health care setting.

As mentioned previously, Asian patients avoid confrontation with health care professionals, perhaps answering questions with what they believe the nurse wants to hear. Nurses working with such patients should avoid phrasing questions or statements in a manner that suggests a desired response.

Appalachian patients tend to reject interactions they perceive as "prying," due to a cultural ethic of neutrality that mandates minding one's own business and avoiding assertive or argumentative behavior.

Verbal communication. Health care professionals may overlook important information if they cannot understand a client's nonverbal behavior. Volume, speed, and directness of conversation, for instance, are all influenced by cultural values. Other important considerations include facial expression, handshaking, silence, eye contact, and proxemics.

Clark (1983) describes the impact of nursing inattention on cultural communication patterns with the case of an elderly Soviet woman who interpreted nurses' smiles as gestures of insolence and frivolity. At the other extreme, many Hispanic clients consider smiling and handshaking to be integral parts of sincere interactions and essential to establishing trust.

Ethnic interpretations of silence may vary considerably. Some individuals find silence extremely uncomfortable, and try to fill in every gap in the conversation. In contrast, many Native Americans consider silence essential to understanding, believing that a person needs to fully consider what another has said before responding. In traditional Chinese and Japanese cultures, silence does not necessarily indicate the end of a comment or conversation; it may mean that the speaker wishes the listener to consider the content of what has been said before he continues. Other cultures have still different uses for silence. The English and Arabs may use silence out of respect for another's privacy, while the Russians, French, and Spanish may interpret it as a sign of agreement. Asian cultures often use silence to demonstrate respect for elders.

Many ethnic groups, including Native Americans, Indochinese, and residents of Appalachia, consider direct eye contact impolite or aggressive, and they may avert their own eyes during an interview. This nonverbal behavior may be misunderstood by health professionals.

Speech intensity or volume may also lead to disharmony between client and nurse. Asian or Native American clients may consider health practitioners of other ethnicities to be loud and boisterous, whereas nurses treating them may interpret their more subdued tones as signs of shyness.

Many cultures value indirectness and subtlety in speech. Ethnic clients may be alienated by an American nurse's frankness. Asians may consider mainstream American behavior immature, rude, and lacking in finesse, whereas nurses might mistakenly label Asian clients as evasive and afraid to confront their problems (Sue, 1981).

Patterns of authority—information sharing. Lipson and Meleis (1983) report that clients from Mediterranean-based ethnic groups seldom question a health care professional's authority. They are not likely to ask questions or convey information that they feel could contradict or convey disrespect for the health care professional; they may avoid volunteering personal information, as they do with all strangers. Clients from these ethnic groups may even block information from family members who are patients, if they perceive the information to be negative.

Families from these groups may be unwilling to relinquish to health care professionals control over a relative/patient. For instance, they may refuse to allow caregivers to make decisions that imply that a patient's condition is bleak, out of the belief that such decisions imply a loss of faith in God's power to intervene.

Cultural Assessment

Cultural assessment is vital in caring for families with chronic disease. Within the health care literature, numerous guidelines for the content and process of cultural assessment can be found. While it is beyond the scope of this chapter to further explicate these processes, the reader is referred to a number of helpful readings (Aamodt, 1978; Affonso, 1979; Brownlee, 1978; Kay, 1978; Leininger, 1978; Orque, 1983; Tripp-Reimer, 1984a; Tripp-Reimer et al., 1984).

While these guidelines are helpful, it is essential to place the individual client and family into the appropriate context. Understanding the complete cultural context—the values, beliefs, customs, and family patterns—in which families are enmeshed can provide important background data for assessments and intervention planning.

However, nurses must recognize the limitations of assumptions based on such background data. The reactions of a particular client or family to chronic illness or its treatment cannot be predicted with certainty simply on the basis of ethnicity. It is critical not to stereotype individuals on the basis of their ethnic affiliation.

Assessment by nurses must consciously maintain a culturally relativist stance from which they can try to understand and accept ethnic clients' behavior without making value judgments. The culturally relativistic nurse tries to view clients in their own cultural context.

There are problems with relativism that merit attention, however. First, the client's traditional customs may not promote health. Indeed, some culturally-based behaviors can be harmful. Folk remedies, for example, might be either effective or toxic. Similarly, advice given by lay providers or folk practitioners may be inappropriate. Consequently, a nurse must assess the effect of specific customs and behaviors on the client's health, reinforcing those that are benign or effective and discouraging those that are harmful.

Secondly, and perhaps more importantly, blind relativism may preclude effective nursing care. Unquestioning acceptance of a client's cultural system easily becomes patronization. The client might not want traditional beliefs and customs incorporated into his care if alternative approaches are acceptable. Ethnic clients may not wish to remain unassimilated; indeed, it may simply perpetuate another form of stereotype to assuming that all members of an ethnic group subscribe to the culture's most conservative position.

This traditionalist fallacy may even deny such clients' equal access to care. Morrison (1982) for example, coined the phrase "cultural aversion hypothesis" to describe health providers' assumptions that ethnic families wish to care for the elderly at home, and find the prospect of long-term care unsuitable. This view, she points out, may result in health providers failing to provide needed services to families who cannot or would not like to care for an elderly person at home.

Similarly, as pointed out previously, each ethnic group has acculturated members, and acculturation rates within any single group differ in a variety of ways. The degree to which any individual or family adheres to his traditional culture often depends on age, sex, education, and generation of immigration.

The point of relativism is to sensitize nurses not only to the fact that their clients have cultures that guide their attitudes and responses, but also to their own predefined values, beliefs, customs, and perceptions.

CONCLUSIONS

Zola (1979) contends that everyone has a cultural heritage which largely influences "the family" and individual health practices. He insists, however, that the most practical nursing approach is not to master the infinite varieties of culture, but to recognize these varieties and how they affect health practices. Nurses should be sensitive to the patient's heritage, their own heritage, and to what happens when different heritages meet.

REFERENCES

Aamodt, A. "Culture," in *Culture, Childbearing, Health Professionals.* Edited by Clark, A. Philadelphia: F.A. Davis Co., 1978.

Abasiekong, E. "Familism and Hospital Admission in Rural Nigeria—A Case Study," *Social Science and Medicine* 15B:45-50, 1981.

Abramson, H.J. "Assimilation and Pluralism," in *Harvard Encyclopedia of American Ethnic Groups.* Edited by Thernstrom, S. Cambridge, Mass.: Harvard University Press, 1980.

Affonso, D. "Framework for Cultural Assessment," in *Childbearing: A Nursing Perspective,* 2nd ed. Edited by Clark, A. Philadelphia: F.A. Davis Co., 1979.

Brownlee, A. *Community, Culture and Care: A Cross-Cultural Guide for Health Workers.* St. Louis: C.V. Mosby Co., 1978.

Brues, A.M. *People and Races.* New York: Macmillan Publishing Co., 1977.

Chrisman, N.C., and Kleinman, A. "Health Beliefs and Practices," in *Harvard Encyclopedia of Ethnic Groups.* Edited by Thernstrom, S. Cambridge, Mass.: Harvard University Press, 1981.

Clark, M. "Cultural Context of Medical Practice," *Western Journal of Medicine* 139:806–10, 1983.

Clinton, J. "Ethnicity: The Development of an Empirical Construct for Cross–Cultural Health Research," *Western Journal of Nursing Research* 4:281–300, 1982.

Damon, A. "Race, Ethnic Group, and Disease," *Social Biology* 16(2):69–80, 1969.

Davitz, L.L., and Davitz, J.R. "Black and White Nurses' Inferences of Suffering," *Nursing Times* 74:708–10, 1978.

Davitz, L.L., and Davitz, J.R. "Cross-Cultural Inferences of Physical Pain and Psychological Distress," *Nursing Times* 73:521-23, 556–58, 1977.

Davitz, L.L., and Davitz, J.R. "Suffering as Viewed in Six Different Cultures," *American Journal of Nursing* 76(8):1296–97, 1976.

Fabrega, H. "Group Differences in the Structure of Illness," *Culture, Medicine, and Psychiatry* 1:379–94, 1977.

Femminella, F., and Quadagno, J. "The Italian American Family," in *Ethnic Families in America: Patterns and Variations.* Edited by Mindel, C., and Habenstein, R. New York: Elsevier, 1976.

Flannery, R., et al. "Ethnicity as a Factor in the Expression of Pain," *Psychosomatics* 22(1):39–50, 1981.

Foster, G., and Anderson, B. *Medical Anthropology.* New York: John Wiley & Sons, 1978.

Goldberg, G., et al. "Issues in the Development of Neighborhood Health Centers," *Inquiry* 6:37–47, 1969.

Gould–Martin, K., and Ngin, C. "Chinese Americans," in *Ethnicity and Medical Care.* Edited by Harwood, A. Cambridge, Mass.: Harvard University Press, 1981.

Graham, S. "Ethnic Background and Illness in a Pennsylvania County," *Social Problems* 4:76–81, 1956.

Hartog, J., and Hartog, E. "Cultural Aspects of Health and Illness Behavior in Hospitals," *Western Journal of Medicine* 139:910–16, 1983.

Harwood, A. "Introduction," in *Ethnicity and Medical Care*. Edited by Harwood, A. Cambridge, Mass.: Harvard University Press, 1981.

Hautman, M.A., and Harrison, J. "Health Beliefs and Practices in a Middle Income Anglo–American Neighborhood," *Advances in Nursing Science* 4(3):49–64, 1982.

Huntington, G.E. "The Amish Family," in *Ethnic Families in America: Patterns and Variations*. Edited by Mindel, C., and Habenstein, R. New York: Elsevier, 1976.

Jackson, J.J. "Urban Black Americans," in *Ethnicity and Medical Care*. Edited by Harwood, A. Cambridge, Mass.: Harvard University Press, 1981.

Karno, M., and Edgerton, R. "Perception of Illness in a Mexican-American Community," *Archives of General Psychiatry* 20:233-38, 1969.

Kart, C., and Beckham, B. "Black-White Differentials in the Institutionalization of the Elderly: A Temporal Analysis," *Social Forces* 54:901–10, 1976.

Kay, M. "Clinical Anthropology," in *The Anthropology of Health*. Edited by Bauwens, E. St. Louis: C.V. Mosby Co., 1978.

Kitano, H., and Kikumura, A. "The Japanese American Family," in *Ethnic Families in America: Patterns and Variations*. Edited by Mindel, C., and Habenstein, R. New York: Elsevier, 1976.

Kleinman, A. "International Health Care Planning from an Ethnomedical Perspective: Critique and Recommendations for Change," *Medical Anthropology* 2:71-94, 1978.

Kleinman, A. "Sickness as Cultural Semantics: Issues for an Anthropological Medicine and Psychiatry," in *Toward a New Definition of Health*. Edited by Ahmed, P.I., and Coelho, G.V. New York: Plenum Press, 1979.

Koopman, C., et al. "Ethnicity in the Reported Pain, Emotional Distress and Requests of Medical Outpatients," *Social Science and Medicine* 18:487–90, 1984.

Lawlis, G., et al. "Ethnic and Sex Differences in Response to Clinical and Induced Pain in Chronic Spinal Pain Patients," *Spine* 9(7):751–54, 1984.

Leininger, M. "Culturological Assessment Domains for Nursing Practices," in *Transcultural Nursing: Concepts, Theories and Practices*. Edited by Leininger, M. New York: John Wiley & Sons, 1978.

Lieban, D.W. "The Field of Medical Anthropology," in *Culture, Disease and Healing*. Edited by Landy, D. New York: Macmillan Publishing Co., 1977.

Lipson, J., and Meleis, A. "Issues in Health Care of Middle Eastern Patients," *Western Journal of Medicine* 139:854–61, 1983.

Lipton, J., and Marbach, J. "Ethnicity and the Pain Response," *Social Science and Medicine* 19:1279–98, 1984.

Litman, T. "The Family as a Basic Unit in Health and Medical Care: A Social–Behavioral Overview," *Social Science and Medicine* 8:495–519, 1974.

Lock, M. "Japanese Responses to Social Change—Making the Strange Familiar," *Western Journal of Medicine* 139:829–34, 1983.

Markson, E. "Ethnicity as a Factor in the Institutionalization of the Ethnic Elderly," in *Ethnicity and Aging: Theory, Research and Policy*. Edited by Gelfand, D., and Kutzik, Z. New York: Springer Publishing Co., 1979.

McKusick, V.A. "Ethnic Distribution of Disease in Non-Jews," *Israel Journal of Medical Science* 9:1375–82, 1973.

McKusick, V.A. "The Ethnic Distribution of Disease in the United States," *Journal of Chronic Diseases* 20:115–18, 1967.

Mindel, C.H., and Habenstein, R. "Introduction," in *Ethnic Families in America: Patterns and Variations*. Edited by Mindel, C.H., and Habenstein, R. New York: Elsevier, 1976.

Mitchell, M. "Popular Medical Concepts in Jamaica and Their Impact on Drug Use," *Western Journal of Medicine* 139:841–47, 1983.

Morrison, B. "Sociocultural Dimensions: Nursing Homes and the Minority Aged," *Journal of Gerontological Social Work* 5:127–45, 1982.

Orque, M. "Orque's Ethnic/Cultural System: A Framework for Ethnic Nursing Care," in *Ethnic Nursing Care: A Multicultural Approach*. Edited by Orque, M., et al. St. Louis: C.V. Mosby Co., 1983.

Parsons, T. "Some Theoretical Considerations on the Nature and Trends of Change of Ethnicity," in *Ethnicity: Theory and Experience*. Edited by Glazer, N., and Moynihan, D. Cambridge, Mass.: Harvard University Press, 1975.

Petersen, W. "Concepts of Ethnicity," in *Harvard Encyclopedia of Ethnic Groups*. Edited by Thernstrom, S., et al. Cambridge, Mass.: Harvard University Press, 1981.

Place, L.F. "The Ethnic Factor," in *The Dynamics of Aging*. Edited by Berghorn, F., and Schafer, D. Boulder, Colo.: Westview Press, 1981.

Ragucci, A.T. "Italian Americans," in *Ethnicity and Medical Care*. Edited by Harwood, A. Cambridge, Mass.: Harvard University Press, 1981.

Schechter, N. "Recurrent Pains in Children: An Overview and an Approach," *Pediatric Clinics of North America* 31(5):949–68, 1984.

Staples, R. "The Black American Family," in *Ethnic Families in America: Patterns and Variations*. Edited by Mindel, C., and Habenstein, R. New York: Elsevier, 1976.

Sue, D. *Counseling the Culturally Different: Theory and Practice*. New York: John Wiley & Sons, 1981.

Thernstrom, S., et al. "Introduction," in *Harvard Encyclopedia of American Ethnic Groups*. Edited by Thernstrom, S., et al. Cambridge, Mass.: Harvard University Press, 1980.

Tripp-Reimer, T. "Cultural Assessment," in *Nursing Assessment: A Multidimensional Approach*. Edited by Bellack, J., and Bamford, P. Monterey, Calif.: Wadsworth Health Sciences, 1984a.

Tripp-Reimer, T. "Cultural Diversity in Therapy," in *Mental Health–Psychiatric Nursing*. Edited by Beck, C., et al. St. Louis: C.V. Mosby Co., 1984b.

Tripp-Reimer, T., and Dougherty, M.C. "Cross-Cultural Nursing Research," *Annual Review of Nursing Research* 3:77–104, 1985.

Tripp-Reimer, T., and Schrock, M. "Residential Patterns and Preferences of Ethnic Aged: Implications for Transcultural Nursing," in *Proceedings of the 7th Annual Transcultural Nursing Society*. Edited by Uhl, C.N., and Uhl, J. Salt Lake City: Transcultural Nursing Society, 1982.

Tripp-Reimer, T., et al. "Cultural Assessment: Content and Process," *Nursing Outlook* 32:78–82, 1984.

Weisenberg, M., et al. "Pain: Anxiety and Attitudes in Black, White, and Puerto Rican Patients," *Psychosomatic Medicine* 37:123–35, 1975.

Wheat, M., et al. "Aspects of Medical Care of Soviet Jewish Emigres," *Western Journal of Medicine* 139:900–04, 1983.

Zborowski, M. "Cultural Components in Response to Pain," *Journal of Social Issues* 8(4):16–30, 1952.

Zborowski, M. *People in Pain.* San Francisco: Jossey–Bass, 1969.

Zola, I.K. "Culture and Symptoms—An Analysis of Patients' Presenting Complaints," *American Sociological Review* 31:615–30, 1966.

Zola, I.K. "Oh Where, Oh Where has Ethnicity Gone?" in *Ethnicity and Aging: Theory, Research and Policy.* Edited by Gelfand, D., and Kutzik, A. New York: Springer Publishing Co., 1979.

SECTION II

Assessing Families with Chronic Illness

5 Assessing families of infants with congenital defects

June Leifson, RN, MS, PhD
Professor and Dean,
College of Nursing
Brigham Young University
Provo, Utah

OVERVIEW

This chapter describes the parents' reactions to the birth of an infant with a handicap; it discusses major family crisis theories and presents specific family assessment models. A case example demonstrates assessment of such families' immediate needs, structure, developmental stage, strengths, and functioning during crisis, specifically when an infant is born with a handicapped condition.

When a family crisis occurs in a clinical setting, what is the appropriate nursing role? Is there a clear conceptual model nurses can adopt to assess and intervene with families presenting such problems as the birth of a handicapped child? This chapter presents models to help nurses complete a family assessment, applies a case study to a family assessment model, and describes briefly the planning process.

THE NURSING PROCESS

Assessment

The health problem: Children with handicaps. Health professionals have expressed increasing concern about the rising number of children born with congenital anomalies caused by environmental pollutants, prenatal drug use, and infectious agents. However, accurate statistics are difficult to obtain. First, many congenital conditions go unrecognized at birth and do not present until the child is older. These and other birth defects often go unreported on birth certificates, having been intentionally or unintentionally omitted by the physician(s).

Given the limited accuracy of data, the United States National Center for Health Statistics reported for 1978 a rate of 855.8 anomalies per 100,000 live births, an increase from the 1974 rate of 821 anomalies for every 100,000 births. (U.S. Department of Health, Education, and Welfare [HEW], 1985). Statistics, however, do not convey the impact and trauma of birth anomalies on individual families nor do they address the social circumstances or far-reaching implications of the child's problem.

Parental reactions. Parental adjustment to their infant's congenital defect progresses through stages: grief, anger, anxiety, and family/lifestyle adaptation (Cohen, 1962). Through a study encompassing a variety of infant malformations, Drotar et al. (1975) identified five stages of parental reaction—shock, denial, sadness and anger, adaptation, and reorganization—and concluded that early crisis counseling is crucial in parental attachment and adjustment. Leifson's (1979) work with 47 families identified no constant single pattern of reactions; a "blurring" of emotional responses was more common. However, even these could be categorized by primary reaction: shock, depression, anxiety, grief, guilt, denial, anger, fear, acceptance, and the need to resolve problems.

Researchers disagree on parental reactions to the specific crisis of bearing a handicapped child. Westphal (1982) cites numerous authors who believe coping stages are predictable in length and emotional intensity and that the normal process is of limited duration and coexists with a family goal of eventual acceptance. On the basis of a literature review, Fortier and Wanlass (1984) proposed a five-stage model of family crisis: impact, denial, grief, focus outward, and closure.

Olshansky (1962), on the other hand, described a parental reaction of "chronic sorrow," a recurring unpredictable emotion experienced throughout the child's life. Wikler et al. (1981) and Russell (1974) report particular family stress during the time a healthy child might walk, talk, begin school, enter puberty, and reach the age of majority. Horan (1982) hypothesizes that the more the parents feel they could have prevented the defect, the more guilt they feel.

Major crisis concepts, theories, and models. During the past three or four decades, the volume of family crisis research has increased. More recently, that research has focused on families giving birth to a child with a handicap.

Family crisis research. Angell (1936) was among the first to document family crisis and the recovery process, identifying integration and adaptability as important determinants of a family's recovery. Family integration has been defined as bonds of coherence and unity. Family adaptability is viewed as "variation in the ability of a family to change its structure or way of operating with little psychic or organizational discomfort" (Burr, 1973, p. 264). Cavan and Ranck (1938) and Hill (1949) and Koss (1948) all observed that a family's past experience with the previous methods of managing a crisis preconditioned them to future upheavals. Therefore, if the family endured a previous crisis successfully, the next crisis would probably have a positive outcome.

One major formulation described in the family crisis literature is Hill's (1949) ABCX Model. A is the *event* interacting with B, the family crisis-meeting *resources,* which in turn interact with C, the *definition the family made of the event.* The interactions between A, B, and C produce X, the *crisis.* Hill (1949) also devised the classic definition of crisis: "any sharp or decisive change for which old patterns are inadequate" (p. 51).

Placing the situation of bearing a handicapped infant into the context of Hill's model, A would be the *birth of the child;* B would be the family's *resources,* such as medical insurance, availability of specialized care, and nurses educated in holistic family nursing; C would be the family's *definition of the happening*—does the family perceive the child's handicap as a crisis, or as a small inconvenience; and X is the *combination of these factors,* the family *crisis.*

Another major focus in family crisis research has been family processes or patterns in stress situations. Hansen and Hill (1964) illustrated stages of family activity under stress with the analogy of a truncated roller coaster. The relationship between the four components of their Family Adjustment Model, the crisis event, periods of disorganization, recovery, and reorganization is illustrated in Figure 5.1. As families confront crisis and define and assimilate its implications, their functioning is temporarily disorganized; members are in shock, numbed by the impact of the event(s). Recovery time varies with each family, and the level of reorganization depends upon their ability and resources. In his synthesis of family crisis propositions, Burr (1973) identified factors influencing regenerative power and vulnerability to stress. Regenerative power, he states, denotes variation in families' abilities to recover from crisis. Among the propositions identified were:
- amount of crisis in the family system
- family definition of the seriousness of the change
- externalization of blame
- anticipated time changes
- anticipated socialization
- presence of extended family
- marital adjustment
- wife's social activity
- amount of consultation.

Burr's model is fairly abstract. Its propositions need testing to see if additional contingent variables influence the effect and to identify additional variables if necessary.

Figure 5.1 Common Patterns of Family Adjustment to Crisis

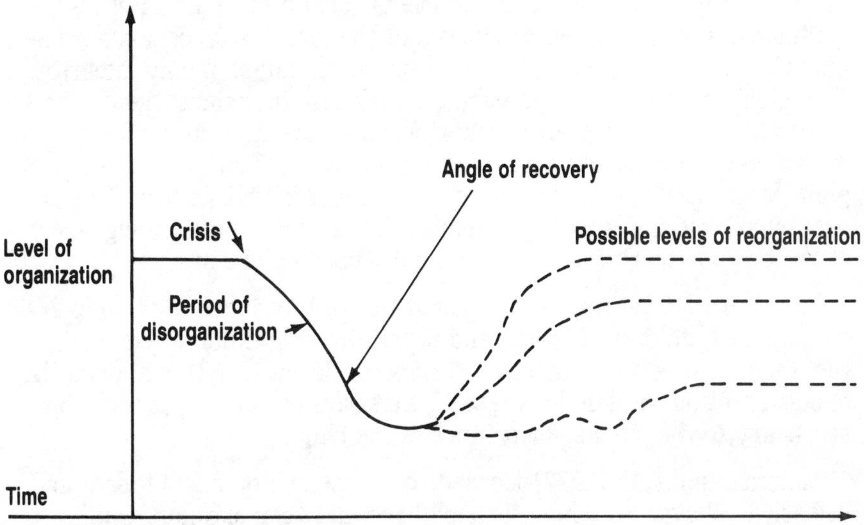

Source: Hansen and Hill, 1964. Reprinted with permission from *Handbook of Marriage and the Family.* Edited by Christensen, H.T. Chicago: Rand McNally, 1964.

Numerous unanswered questions about family crisis remain. In rethinking family stress, Hansen and Johnson (1979) contributed to a new synthesis of family crisis concepts by asking, "Why is it that some families that are 'vulnerable' lack 'regenerative power,' while other 'vulnerable' families quickly recover? Why do some that are disrupted by severe stresses recover quickly, while others show little 'regenerative power' once they have fallen into disarray? Hansen and Johnson's provocative ideas included the time linkage concept, disruption maintenance in family interaction, negotiation of new family patterns, definitional aspects of family interaction under stress, family communication patterns and behavior, and family personal and positional resources. Each of these concepts opens additional research possibilities. For instance, in time linkage, Hansen and Johnson question why some people endure debilitating stress while others seem to revel in the swiftness of change. They discuss the rate of change in the family, and the effects of the rate when the change is perceived to be desirable or under control.

Family crisis research—Handicapped children. Farber (1960) was the first to focus on family crisis related to handicap. He studied the psychological and social impact of caring for a mentally retarded child on mothers, concluding that mothers suffered a greater emotional trauma than fathers at the time of diagnosis, especially when the mothers were not in good health.

Berggreen's (1971) study of the mental health of relatives of 20 multihandicapped children revealed that the initial diagnosis is a stunning blow that strains family resources and threatens family integrity. This problem proved to be dynamic, continuing throughout the child's lifetime and influencing all family members. Parents were found to receive much unsolicited advice, which contributed to the tension and guilt. Marriages and family life were threatened; siblings were frequently subjected to gross, but seldom deliberate, neglect, owing solely to the overpowering nature of the handicapped child's needs.

Langford's (1961) research explored the guilt common in families of handicapped children. Parents and physically sick children felt that the illness was a punishment for their sins. Cohen (1962) examined the child's effect on the family, stressing that parents see the handicap as secondary to the overall importance of the child.

Mattson and Agle (1972) focused their research on adaptational and defensive behavior in young hemophiliacs and their parents. Guilt, sadness, and fear were common attitudes in this situation; these attitudes caused families to withdraw, affecting the child's personality development. Haggerty and Alpert (1963) also found that parents consistently assume blame for the child's illness.

Kew (1975), in another study of handicapped children and their parents, found guilt and anxiety to be common emotions. He also noted that despite growing interest in this area, many of the problems posed by handicapping conditions have not yet been identified, much less corrected.

McCubbin et al. (1983) described the coping patterns of parents with a handicapped child. Given the predictable demands of caring for such children at home and parents' natural tendency to invest much of their personal self and energy in their children, the researchers say that such parents should balance childcare with personal investment in themselves and in the family as a whole; they should also understand the medical situation completely. This research also stressed the importance of the father's role and the value of his coping efforts. These findings emphasize the need to view coping as an integral part of family stress theory.

Brantley and Clifford (1980), comparing a group of mothers of children with cleft lips and palates with a control group of physically normal children, found that mothers of the children with deformities reported fewer positive feelings toward and greater anxiety about their children. Socioeconomically privileged mothers displayed more negative affect than mothers from lower classes. In studies with direct implications for nursing practices, Park (1977) mentions the need to assess the strengths of the parents and to be aware of available family and social supports; Fortier and Wanlass (1984) stress the need for health workers to prepare families for the crisis of having a defective child. Parents do not want to believe this can happen to them—it happens, they think, only to other parents.

In a recent review of the family crisis literature, Longo and Bond (1984) focused on four major areas: parents' psychological well-being, marital stability, sibling welfare, and overall family functioning. They detected no universal summation of the handicapped child's impact on parents' psychological well-being. The data they reviewed, however, indicated that fathers may be more at risk than mothers. Their most amazing finding, however, was that so many investigators found that marriages remained stable regardless of the child's disability. Despite the added strain and challenge, couples could maintain their relationships, a finding that contradicts public opinion.

The influence of a handicapped child's birth on siblings is inconclusive. Longo and Bond (1984) found several studies suggesting that the handicapped child's presence hinders sibling welfare and adjustment; more optimistic findings suggested that such siblings are no more at risk than children in families without a handicapped child. Overall, family functioning is characterized as adequate by the majority of investigators reviewed.

While most of the family research literature focuses on the family crisis, Longo and Bond (p. 57) conclude, "Few clinicians, however, are prepared to assess families who demonstrate high degrees of adaptability and who function extremely well after the diagnosis has been presented and the initial grief reaction has passed." In the clinical setting, do nurses adequately assess families in crisis? The next section presents various models that can help the nurse make a valid assessment of families who present in crisis.

Family assessment models. A family assessment model can be overwhelming, and therefore nonfunctional, if it has too many components. The nurse must select one model, or component parts of several models, to make a functional tool (see Table 5.1). The following models indicate workable examples. Many of these models are complex and still in development, and are explained cursorily. Sample questions for the nurse are presented in Table 5.2.

Table 5.1 Summary of Family Assessment Models: Components for Assessment

Calgary Family Assessment	McMaster	Circumplex	CHIP	FSF
Structural Internal	Problem solving	Cohesion	Family integration	Love
External	Communication	Adaptability	Cooperation	Religion
Developmental stages	Roles	Communication	Optimism (definition of situation)	Respect
Tasks	Affective			Communication
Attachments	responsiveness		Social support	
				Individually
Functional	Affective		Self-esteem	
Instrumental	involvement			
Expressive			Psychological	
	Behavior control		stability	
			Understanding of medical situation	

The Calgary Family Assessment Model (CFAM). CFAM consists of three categories:
• *Structural,* which allows the nurse to examine family composition, members of the household, rank, order, and position of family members, and the unit's subsystems and boundaries.
• *Developmental,* which is based on life-cycle stages and then specific tasks.
• *Family functioning,* which focuses on instrumental and expressive aspects (Wright & Leahey, 1984).

McMaster model. The McMaster family assessment model has evolved over 25 years of research and clinical application. The developers do not claim that it encompasses all aspects of family life, but that it covers the areas essential to understanding family functioning (Epstein et al., 1978; Epstein et al., 1984). Designed as a screening instrument, this tool draws information on various systemic structural and organizational dimensions directly from family members. The model conceptualizes six major functional dimensions—problem solving, communication, roles, affective responsiveness (individual), affective involvement (with other family members), and behavior control (in physically dangerous and interpersonal situations)—within a systems theory approach. The nurse applying the McMaster model to the family of a child with a congenital handicap could ask questions developed around these six major dimensions (Table 5.2).

Circumplex model. The circumplex model, which is still being clarified, refined, and modified (Olsen et al., 1984), is based on three dimensions of family behavior and seven hypotheses. The three major dimensions emerged from a conceptual clustering of over 50 concepts that describe marital and family dynamics. They are:
• Family cohesion
Emotional bonding between family members. Concepts include emotional bonding, boundaries, coalitions, time, space, friends, interest, decision making. Four levels—disengaged, separate, connected, enmeshed.

• Family adaptability
Family's ability to change power structure, role relationships, and relationship rules in response to situational and developmental stress. Concepts include negotiation styles, relationship roles, and rules. Four levels—rigid, structured, flexible, chaotic.

• Family communication
Facilitating dimension that allows the families to function within the other two dimensions. Concepts include positive and negative communication skills (empathy, reflective listening, double messages, double binds).

The seven hypotheses follow:
• Couples/families with balanced (two central levels) cohesion and adaptability generally function more adequately across the family life cycle than those at the extremes of these dimensions.
• Balanced family types have a larger behavioral repertoire and are therefore more able to change than extreme family types.
• If a couple or family's normative expectations support extreme behaviors in one or both circumplex dimensions, the unit will function well. (All members must accept these expectations.)
• Couples and families function most adequately if there is a high level of congruence between all members' perceived and ideal descriptions of their situation.
• Balanced couples/families tend to have more positive communication skills than do extreme families.
• Positive communication skills enable balanced couples/families to change their levels of cohesion and adaptability more easily than those at the extremes.
• Balanced families change their cohesion and adaptability to deal with situational stress and developmental change across the family life cycle whereas extreme families resist change over time.

Table 5.2 Sample Questions: Family Assessment Models

Model	Concept	Ask Self	Ask Family
CFAM	Family structural assessment	Is the newborn accepted in the family system by the mother, by the father?	Could you tell me the members of your immediate family?
	Family developmental assessment	How will the family encourage the handicapped child's development?	What activities have you planned to stimulate your child's development?
	Family functioning	Have daily routines changed due to the birth of the handicapped child?	How has having this child changed your family's daily activities?
McMaster	Problem solving	Can the family problem-solve during this crisis?	Do you need help finding medical resources?
		Does the family accept the child's problem and can they investigate conflicting ideas?	Are you able to think of solutions at this time, or do you need time to collect your ideas and thoughts?
	Communication	How does the family exchange information? Are they expressing their concerns, their feelings?	Are you able to obtain the information you desire concerning your child's problem?
		Do they hesitate to handle the problem?	What are your feelings now? Are you angry, hurt, disappointed?
	Roles	What role changes/supplementations are taking place in the family?	Are you assuming new responsibilities since the child's birth?
		How does the family allocate responsibilities and handle accountabilities?	Are there any changes in your household activities since this baby's birth?
			Who is caring for your children while you are at the hospital?
	Affective responsiveness	What feelings are the parents displaying?	What reactions are you feeling to the birth of this child?
	Affective involvement	What support are the family members providing for one another?	How are your social activities and that of members of your family now, compared to before this crisis?

(continued)

Model	Concept	Ask Self	Ask Family
McMaster *(continued)*	Behavior/control	What behavior patterns are the family demonstrating during this crisis?	How are you interacting with one another at this time?
		Have the established patterns of socialization and daily activity changed?	How are your family members interacting with neighbors and friends since the birth of this child?
Circumplex	Cohesion	What is the degree of unity and coalition in the family?	Has the birth of this child made a difference in the family's closeness?
	Communication	How does the family communicate during crisis?	How well do you communicate? Has it changed since the child was born?
	Adaptability	Does this family adapt readily and accept challenges?	How are you adjusting to the changes imposed on you by the birth of this child?
		Do they like the excitement of unknown pathways?	
CHIP	Family integration/ cooperation/ optimism	Do family members display a cooperative, optimistic attitude?	How will this child's problem influence your family in the future?
		What coping strategies are demonstrated by this family?	What do you see as your child's future opportunities?
	Social support/ self-esteem/ psychological stability	What are the family's external resources? Are they maintaining their self-esteem?	Who are you able to call on to assist you: are there friends, neighbors, relatives? Has having this child with a handicap influenced how you feel about yourself?
	Understanding medical situation	Does the family understand the child's medical condition?	Do you understand the child's medical condition?
		Do these parents seek information from other parents and health personnel?	Have you talked to other parents who have children with a similar problem as your child? Do you fully understand what the physician is saying when he explains your child's medical conditions?

(continued)

Table 5.2 Sample Questions: Family Assessment Models
(continued)

Model	Concept	Ask Self	Ask Family
FSF	Strengths	What are the family's strengths?	What do you see as your major family strengths?
		Is this family aware of the range of its strengths and resources?	
	Potentials	What are the family's latent potentials?	What do you see as the family's potential strengths?
		How can the family be helped to develop and use its strengths, including latent strengths and potentialities?	

The Circumplex model is dynamic, allowing for family changes over time; that is, it accepts that families move in different directions in different situations and in the various stages of the family life cycle. This model's assessment tools are designed to evaluate the family cohesion and adaptability dimension. For families in crisis with the birth of a handicapped child, the nurse would focus on the three dimensions of family behavior: cohesion, adaptability, and communication.

Coping Health Inventory for Parents (CHIP). The CHIP is not presented as a model; however, in the context of assessing families with handicapped children, it helps describe the coping patterns that emerge as parents try to manage family life and health in the face of a child's chronic illness (McCubbin et al., 1983). The research was based on work with parents of children with cystic fibrosis. The nurses could evaluate families in terms of three parental coping patterns:
• Maintaining family integration, cooperation, and an optimistic definition of the situation.
• Maintaining social support, self-esteem, and psychological stability.
• Understanding the medical situation through communication with other parents and consultation with medical staff.

Also, the assessing nurses could establish criteria for validating the family's adaptive life pattern: cohesiveness, expressiveness, conflict reduction, organization, and control. CHIP research notes that some families may be considered at high risk: single parent families, families with older children who have cystic fibrosis, and low income families.

The developers of this instrument claim that their findings constitute empirical support for its use in family assessment; they state that it provides a reliable depiction of parental efforts to manage stressful situations. See Table 5.2 for sample assessment questions.

Family Strength Framework. Although the Family Strength Framework (FSF) is not developed as a model, some of its concepts can help assess families with handicapped children. During a crisis, such families often forget their own strengths; the nurse's assessment can help them recognize those strengths and abilities (Otto [1973] defines family strengths as factors or forces that contribute to [family] unity and solidarity). FSF guidelines can also help health professionals make more consistent and concentrated use of family strengths. Strength-oriented assessment is a major focus; the nurse is encouraged to evaluate the following:

- physical, emotional, and spiritual needs
- child-rearing practices and discipline
- communication
- support, security, and encouragement
- internal and external growth-producing relationships and experiences
- responsible community relationships
- growing with and through children
- self-help and acceptance of help
- flexibility of family functions and roles
- mutual respect for members' individuality
- use of crisis for growth
- family unity, loyalty, and internal cooperation
- flexibility of family strengths.

The nurse must assess these criteria with care because the family strength factor can sometimes be an impediment rather than an asset. For example, families who try to rely on self-help alone may deprive themselves of community resources. It is also important to note that family strengths are not isolated variables; they are dynamic, fluid, and interrelated, varying at different stages in the family life cycle. See Table 5.2 for sample FSF questions.

Empirical work on family strengths is still developing. Stinnett et al. (1981) isolated five strength categories: love, religion, respect, communication, and individuality. Davis (1980) defines family pride as a family variable contributing to strengths. The important point, however, is that all families do have strengths. Promoting the use of these positive factors during crisis could buffer the effects of the crisis, thus facilitating family adjustment and adaptation.

CASE STUDY

As Steve Smith watched his young wife, Ann, bring their first child into the world, he hoped, as every parent hopes, that his baby would be well and whole. But his wishes were shattered when he looked at the child—the baby girl had a cleft lip and palate. A thousand thoughts at once rushed through his mind. Would his wife accept the baby? Could *he* love and accept the baby? Would the child be able to play and dance and sing and date and...? He looked at the doctor, but the doctor seemed to look everywhere but at Steve. The nurses were busily taking care of the technical aspects of the postdelivery process. Tears rolled down the cheeks of one nurse. Even though these professionals were obviously aware of the problem, they seemed to be caught up in the mechanics of the situation, neither assessing the parents' needs nor offering necessary support.

At the birth of their handicapped child, both parents were subjected to extensive stress. Even though the nurse did not have extensive family information, nor would she be able to obtain all the information she would like to, family assessment was initiated in the hospital delivery room. The nurse began by assessing Steve's and Ann's immediate needs; she realized the importance of communicating with them immediately. Working from the CFAM model, she:
- explored the parents' feelings about and responses to the crisis
- asked what questions they had
- demonstrated emotional support
- inquired whether or not their parents were sitting in the waiting room to give them support
- answered their questions about the medical help available for their child
- informed them of the availability of social and financial resources.

During the acute phase of care, family assessment gives the nurse insight into the family—their knowledge, capabilities, strengths, and potentials.

CFAM—Structural Assessment

Internal Structure. The Smith family consists of the wife, husband, and their newborn child. The *rank order* of the child is known—firstborn and female; if the nurse had known the parents' rank order during the crisis situation, it could determine the priority of the information exchanged.

The family *boundary* in this setting is not clear. Who accepted the newborn into the family system? The father, the mother? The nurse observed each parent's interactions with the handicapped child to determine how the family defined its boundary.

External Structure. A crisis situation can hinder a complete assessment of external family structure. Often, parents are not in a responsive frame of mind; they are focusing on "here and now" concerns. Therefore, the nurse pursues whatever areas can be assessed.

Steve mentioned during his wife's labor that he was a college graduate in a new job. Ann spoke about her joy in teaching elementary school students in the third grade and said that she planned to return to work within a month of the baby's birth. The couple did not share the fact that both were second-generation Icelanders, with the strong work orientation, sensitivity, and family attachment characteristic of that nationality. Nor did the nurse know they were active in their church and came from upper-middle-class families. (Steve and Ann both had average-paying jobs with adequate hospital insurance. They probably did not investigate the insurance coverage for the birth of a handicapped child.)

Further, the nurse did not know that the couple had just moved into an unfinished home in the same city as Steve's parents. Ann's parents lived in another state, some distance from them. Parents of the couple supported the marriage and pregnancy. Also unknown was that Steve's father had been born with cleft lip and palate.

This background information would have given the nurse valuable insights for use in future family planning. For example, if she had known of Ann's plans to return to work within a month, the nurse could have helped the new mother teach the baby's caregiver to use the special feeding technique the infant would require. Such an action would help Ann return to her third-grade teaching position as desired.

Developmental Assessment

Because this is the Smith family's first child, the nurse places them in developmental Stage II: Early Childbearing (Duvall, 1977). Most parents in this stage are excited, anxiously awaiting the birth of a healthy, normal child. In this situation, even though they may have considered the possibility of an abnormal birth, the Smith family was not sufficiently prepared when the abnormal birth happened.

One of the major developmental tasks of families at the Smiths' life-cycle stage is having, adjusting to, and encouraging infant development. When the child is born with a handicap, it adds to this existing family stress.

Another major task in Stage II is accommodating new parenting roles; these roles are made more complex by the presence of a handicapped child. Parents may begin to question their attitudes toward parenthood, their lack of experience, and the many unknowns they face. The 24-hour responsibility of caring for their child may seem overwhelming.

Maintaining the marital bond is an additional Stage II developmental task. Steve is concerned for Ann, who is in turn concerned about him. Will Steve feel guilty knowing that his father had this same handicap? They are young, inexperienced parents; what impact does this factor have upon their crisis?

Even before leaving the delivery room, Steve wondered how he and his wife would accept the baby. The eventual answers to these questions will determine whether the couple develops adaptive or maladaptive attachments to the infant or to one another. Will they overprotect the child at the expense of their marital relationship?

CFAM—Family Functioning

While it is too early in the Smith family's crisis to measure the impact of the child's handicap on family functioning, the following questions will assist in evaluation:
- Have there been changes in task allocation, role assignments, and daily routines due to the handicapped child?
- How well does the family communicate? Is interaction productive, nonverbal, problem-solving?
- Is the family's behavior appropriate to the crisis situation?
- What are the family's strengths and needs during this crisis situation?

Planning

Overall performance improves when the nurse has a formal, systematic planning approach for family crisis associated with the birth of a handicapped child. In such a situation, plans must address both the parents' and the child's immediate needs, as well as their secondary needs. Critical thinking about the child's present and future condition will aid in plan development, implementation, and evaluation.

Nursing care plans should be based on assessment of and communication with child and family. As previously stated, parents may focus only on the immediate crisis. The nurse must open communication, and make the family comfortable and trustful enough for them to share information and feelings. Sensitivity to parents' needs is fundamental to the planning process.

The nurse should also help parents obtain immediate specialty care for their infant, arrange home care for healthy siblings if present, and obtain the minister's and extended family's support, if desired. Care plans must be flexible and enable adaptation to changing crisis situations. Although some handicaps are not life threatening, many are, and the child's and parents' immediate needs may change rapidly.

Once immediate needs have been met, secondary goals can be established. Such advance planning is vital in family recovery from crisis. Pertinent questions are: What new knowledge will the family need to care for the child? What equipment and supplies? What arrangements must be made to prepare for home health care? What community resources can assist? Should the nurse help the family set up home equipment before the child's arrival? Will the nurse need to supervise the child at home? If so, how often should the nurse visit during the first week, the second week, the first year? What community resources can help the family meet psychological, social, and financial needs?

Planning gives specific direction to intervention. The family assessment provides the information and insight needed for strategic planning in the case of a family crisis at the birth of a handicapped child.

CONCLUSIONS

When assessing a family during crisis, the nurse should gather as much information as possible during the acute stage. The nurse must listen to and interact with the family, and allow each member to react to the crisis in his own way. Such families require assurance that they are not alone, that they have support and direction. Clearly, however, these basics do not cover all of the wide-ranging implications of family assessment. The family assessment is an ongoing process in an acute situation. It helps the nurse gain insight into family structure, family development, communication processes, family function, relationships, strengths, and needs.

REFERENCES

Angell, R.C. *The Family Encounters the Depression.* New York: Charles Scribner and Sons, 1936.

Berggreen, S.M. "A Study of the Mental Health of the Near Relatives of Twenty Multihandicapped Children," *Acta Paediatria Scandinavia* (Supple. 215):5–16, 1971.

Brantley, H., and Clifford, E. "When Any Child Was Born: Maternal Reactions to the Birth of a Child," *Journal of Personality Assessment* 44:620–23, 1980.

Burr, W.R. *Theory Construction and the Sociology of the Family.* New York: Wiley-Interscience, 1973.

Cavan, R.A., and Ranck, K.H. *The Family and the Depression.* Chicago: University of Chicago Press, 1938.

Cohen, P. "The Impact of a Handicapped Child on the Family," *Social Casework* 43:137–42, 1962.

Davis, E.S. "The Assessment of Family Pride," Unpublished doctoral dissertation. Madison, Wis.: University of Wisconsin–Madison, 1980.

Drotar, D., et al. "The Adaptation of Parents to the Birth of an Infant with a Congenital Malformation: A Hypothetical Model," *Pediatrics* 56(5):710–17, 1975.

Duvall, E. *Marriage and Family Development,* 5th ed. Philadelphia: J.B. Lippincott Co., 1977.

Epstein, N.B., et al. "The McMaster Model of Family Functioning," *Journal of Marriage and Family Counseling* 40:19–31, 1978.

Epstein, N.B., et al. "McMaster Model of Family Functioning," in *Family Studies Review Yearbook,* vol. 2. Edited by Olsen, D.H., and Miller, B.C. Beverly Hills, Calif.: Sage, 1984.

Farber, B. "Family Organization and Crisis: Maintenance of Integration in Families with a Severely Mentally Retarded Child," *Monographs of the Society for Research in Child Development* 75(1):25, 1960.

Fortier, L.M., and Wanlass, R.L. "Family Crisis Following the Diagnosis of a Handicapped Child," *Family Relations* 33:13–24, 1984.

Fox, D.H., and Fox, R.T. "Strategic Planning for Nursing," *The Journal of Nursing Administration* 13(5):11–16, 1983.

Haggerty, R.J., and Alpert, J.J. "The Child, His Family and Illness," *Postgraduate Medicine* 34:228–33, 1963.

Hansen, D.A., and Hill, R. "Families under Stress," in *Handbook of Marriage and the Family.* Edited by Christensen, H.T. Chicago: Rand McNally, 1964.

Hansen, D.A., and Johnson, V.A. "Rethinking Family Stress Theory: Definitional Aspects," in *Contemporary Theories about the Family.* Edited by Burr, W.R., et al. New York: Free Press, 1979.

Heuser, R.L. Personal communication, 1985.

Hill, R. *Families under Stress.* New York: Harper & Row Publishers, 1949.

Horan, M.L. "Parental Adjustment to the Birth of an Infant with a Defect: An Attributional Approach," *Advances in Nursing Science* 5:57–68, 1982.

Kew, S. *Handicap and Family Crisis.* London: Pitman Publishing, 1975.

Koss, E.L. "Middle-Class Family Crisis," *Marriage and Family Living* 25–40, 1948.

Langford, W.S. "The Child in the Pediatric Hospital: Adaptation to Illness and Hospitalization," *American Journal of Orthopsychiatry* 31:667–85, 1961.

Leifson, J. "Family Crisis: The Handicapped Child," Unpublished doctoral dissertation. Provo, Utah: Brigham Young University, 1979.

Longo, D.C., and Bond, L. "Families of the Handicapped Child: Research and Practice," *Family Relations* 33:57–65, 1984.

Mattson, A., and Agle, D.P. "Therapeutic Processes and Observations of Parental Adaptation to Chronic Illness in Children," *American Academy of Child Psychiatry* 11:558–71, 1972.

McCubbin, H.I., et al. "CHIP—Coping Health Inventory for Parents: An Assessment of Parental Coping Patterns in the Care of the Chronically Ill Child," *Journal of Marriage and the Family* 45:359–70, 1983.

Olsen, D.H., et al. "Circumplex Model of Marital and Family Systems," in *Family Studies Review Yearbook*, vol. 2. Edited by Olsen, D.H., and Miller, B.S. Beverly Hills, Calif.: Sage, 1984.

Olshansky, S. "Chronic Sorrow: A Response to Having a Mentally Defective Child," *Social Casework* 43:190–94, 1962.

Otto, H.A. "A Framework for Assessing Family Strength," in *Family Centered Community Nursing*. Edited by Reinhart, A.M. St. Louis: C.V. Mosby Co., 1973.

Park, R. "Parental Reactions to the Birth of a Handicapped Child," *Health and Social Work* 2:51–66, 1977.

Russell, C.S. "Transition to Parenthood: Problems and Gratifications," *Journal of Marriage and Family* 36:294–302, 1974.

Stinnett, N., et al., eds. *Family Strengths 3: Roots of Well-Being.* Lincoln, Neb.: University of Nebraska Press, 1981.

U.S. Department of Health, Education, and Welfare. *Congenital Anomalies and Birth Injuries among Live Births: United States, 1973–1974.* Hyattsville, Md.: U.S. Government Printing Office, 1985.

Westphal, J. "Reactions of the Family at the Birth of a Newborn with a Congenital Defect," Salt Lake City: Mental Retardation and Medical Genetics Symposium, March 24–25, 1982.

Wikler, L., et al. "Chronic Sorrow Revisited: Parent vs. Professional Depiction of the Adjustment of Parents of Mentally Retarded Children," *American Journal of Orthopsychiatry* 51:63–70, 1981.

Wright, L.M., and Leahey, M. *Nurses and Families: A Guide to Family Assessment and Intervention.* Philadelphia: F.A. Davis Co., 1984.

6 Assessing families of children with developmental disabilities

Margaret Register Bean, RN, MN, MS
District Clinical Coordinator of Nursing
Georgia Department of Public Health
District 1, Unit 1
Rome, Georgia

OVERVIEW

The presence of a child with developmental disabilities causes major alterations in family structure, roles, and functions. Therefore a complete family assessment is the first step in the nursing process. This chapter discusses several theories and models to facilitate this process. A model is proposed using assessment tools in relation to established standards. The nurse's role in planning is reviewed, especially in light of changes in health care delivery which affect this process. A case study depicts assessment and planning with the family of a developmentally disabled child with Down syndrome.

NURSING PROCESS

Assessment

The health problem: Developmental disability. Family assessment is mandatory in nursing families of children with developmental disabilities. The term "developmental disability" covers a wide variety of conditions; Thompson and O'Quinn (1979) present a detailed description of developmental disability as defined by public law 94–103. Their definition includes such conditions as "mental retardation, cerebral palsy, epilepsy, or autism" which present before age 18. It also includes conditions similar to mental retardation which result in "impairment of general intellectual functioning or adaptive behavior" (Thompson & O'Quinn, 1979, p. 13). This definition is used throughout this chapter. In addition, the term "developmental disabilities" is used to describe a specialty area of nursing.

The prevalence of developmental disability in children varies widely. Thompson and O'Quinn (1979, p. 4) report that, in 1962, the President's Panel on Mental Retardation estimated that 5.4 million children were mentally retarded. According to Jones (1983, p. 41), the current incidence of cerebral palsy ranges "from 0.6 to 5.9 per thousand live births." Discussing epilepsy, Nealis (1983, p. 75) notes that "the disorder is extraordinarily common—varying between 2 and 18.6 seizure sufferers per 1,000...and generally affects children." Lyle (1983, p. 100) states that muscular dystrophy "affects approximately 200,000 people in the United States." According to Bricker (1983, p. 222), "approximately 1 percent of children have congenital heart disease." These are just the most common conditions with potential developmental implications.

Need for family assessment. The nurse encounters families of developmentally disabled children in a variety of settings; assessment may therefore begin as part of a multidisciplinary team evaluation or as an individualized measure in a health department, nursery, or preschool setting. The comprehensiveness of the assessment depends on organizational goals and available intervention strategies.

Nursing assessments for families with developmentally disabled children are necessitated by disability-related changes in family structure, roles, and functions. K.P. and L. Meadow (1971, p. 21) note that "socialization to the role of parent of a handicapped child is usually a traumatic and conflict-producing experience." It is "influenced by the socioeconomic status, age, religion, and physical characteristics of the parents and by the sex and birth order of the child." Barnard and Kelly (1980, p. 37) quote Farber, pointing out "that the presence of a child with a severe handicap can affect age and sex roles in the family, community relationships, and the social mobility of parents and siblings."

Schild (1982, p. 204) identifies four problems common to parents of retarded children: "parental expectations and feelings of competency and self–worth; value conflicts that arise because of the parent's maturation, particularly those involved in the decision for institutional care; life transitions such as changes in family structure of the emerging independence of the child; and environmental transactions that leave parents socially isolated." Zuzich's (1980, p. 120) discussion of role change resulting from society's conflicting attitudes toward the handicapped child points out that "the parent faces the dilemma of either accepting the role of devalued member of society along with the handicapped child, rejecting the devalued child, or assuming the role of advocate for all handicapped, devalued persons."

Along with structure and roles, a wide range of family functions are altered dramatically by the birth of a developmentally disabled child. The affected functions include:
- reproductive
- affect

- socialization
- status confirmation
- role confirmation
- health care/promotion
- family coping
- economic stability (Young and Mack, 1962).

For example, the reproductive function includes parental expectations for the unborn child; when these expectations are not fulfilled due to the infant's handicap, "parents need to mourn the loss of their perfect child before they can begin their attachment to their imperfect child" (Lepler, 1978, p. 32). In developing these attachments, the affective functions of "holding, caressing and bonding...are as essential to the parents of a malformed child as they are to the parents of a normal child" (Clark, 1982, p. 336).

The infant's functional limitations can also reverberate throughout the family unit. A child who cannot respond to a parent, elicit maternal caretaking behavior, or engage in socializing activities may impair the parents' adaptive abilities. Socialization for both parties can also be inhibited by parental overprotection and refusal to allow the child to interact with others. As such children grow older, their community status is influenced by the parents' acceptance of their child's limitations and by their own abilities to maintain prior contacts with outside groups.

Parents of a developmentally disabled child must set realistic expectations for him, while simultaneously helping him develop the security, self-esteem, and trust necessary to maximize potential. K.P. and L. Meadow (1971) discuss how socioeconomically well-off parents often find it difficult to accept the limitations of a handicapped child. Others describe how health care and promotion functions can overwhelm families of the developmentally impaired. For example, according to Wyatt, "Alfred Wood suggests that families have difficulty assimilating information relating to phenylketonuria and that the dietary restrictions are a source of intrafamilial stress" (Wyatt, 1978, p. 297). Coyner (1983) further relates the stress caused by the handicapped child's health problems to child abuse.

In short, family stress associated with health and other problems may impair parental coping skills and threaten the solidarity of the family unit (Burton, 1975, p. 4). Yet another burden on family coping behavior is the economic hardship that arises from the handicapped child's extra medical and educational bills (Lepler, 1978).

Family assessment models and theories. Various theories and models can be applied to family assessment in developmental disability. Reinhardt and Quinn (1973, p. 117) present Hill and Hansen's summary

of five conceptual frameworks for studying family interaction:
- interactional
- structural–functional
- situational
- institutional
- developmental.

The first framework examines interaction between family members alone and excludes the outside community. The structural–functional approach focuses on structure and "analyzes the functions which the family performs for society as a whole." In discussing this approach, Friedman (1981, p. 83) notes that it "provides a meaningful way of studying family linkages to other institutions." In the situational approach, the important feature is "the situation itself, or the individual's behavior in the situation" (Reinhardt and Quinn, 1973, p. 117). When looking at the institutional approach, "individual and cultural values are the prime concern." The developmental approach focuses on family life stages in relation to "changing developmental tasks and role expectations of parents and children" and "developmental tasks of the family."

Friedman (1981, p. 44) discusses another framework, the systems approach. Under this model, "the family is viewed as an open social system with boundaries, self–regulatory mechanisms, interacting and superordinate systems, and subcomponents."

Wright and Leahey's (1985) Calgary Family Assessment Model (CFAM) integrates some of these frameworks. "It is a multidimensional framework consisting of three major categories (structural, developmental, and functional)" (p. 182). The structural category includes both internal and external components; the developmental section refers to life stages through which the family progresses, including such tasks as socialization and attachment between family members. The functional category refers to instrumental activities of daily living. Expressive functions include "emotional communication, verbal communication, nonverbal communication, circular communication, problem solving, roles, control, beliefs, and alliances/coalitions" (p. 193).

Meister (1977, p. 43) utilized Tapia's five family levels which are drawn from child growth and development terms—Level 1, Infancy; Level II, Childhood; Level III, Adolescence; Level IV, Adulthood; and Level V, Maturity; to develop an assessment tool for family functioning. This tool presents "measurable behavioral indices or characteristics for each family level" in a graph with nursing activities (pp. 46–48). This model allows more efficient nursing "identification and documentation for both long- and short-term intervention with families" (p. 48).

Barnard (1978a) developed yet another model, this one including more specific techniques for measuring parent/child interaction. Referred to as the Child Health Assessment Interaction Model (CHAIM), it represents three basic components—environment, mother, and child—as circles. The three components are both independent and overlap through interaction. The environment includes inanimate, animate, and supporting features. The child's circle includes temperament and adaptation, while the mother's incorporates adaptation style (Barnard, 1978a, p. 19). The model is accompanied by four scales, enabling the nurse to gather specific and quantifiable data on parent/child interaction.

These scales are:
- "Nursing Child Assessment Sleep/Activity (NCASA) record"
- "Nursing Child Assessment Feeding Scale (NCAFS)"
- "Nursing Child Assessment Teaching Scale (NCATS)"
- Bettye Caldwell's "Home Observation for Measurement of the Environment (HOME)."

Interactional, structural–functional, and developmental models, including the CFAM and Child Health Assessment Interaction Model, have proven helpful in cases of childhood developmental disability. Through the interactional model, the nurse gains information about the family's "internal dynamics" (Friedman, 1981, p. 45). Other data relevant to "role playing, status relations, communication patterns, decision making, coping patterns, and socialization" are also gained. Issues the nurse might address are found in Table 6.1.

The structural/functional approach supplements interactional evaluations by focusing on the client family's relationships with outside groups. This data is very important since parents of developmentally disabled children call on several agencies to help meet their child's needs, and relationships with community groups affect family adjustment.

The developmental approach helps identify both the family's life-cycle stage and the alterations imposed by the child's disabilities. For instance, parents may become fixed at one developmental point because they are afraid that their child might not become self–sufficient. The nurse should encourage long–term parental planning so the child's physical needs will be met when parents cannot do so themselves.

The CFAM (Wright and Leahey, 1985) incorporates information on interaction, structure, and functions into a systematic, comprehensive framework for care planning. This model includes assessment tools helpful in the area of developmental disabilities. CFAM's structural assessment tool, the genogram, can be expanded to elicit genetic data which may shed light on the origins of the child's disorder. Another tool, the ecomap, helps the nurse visualize the nature of extra-family relationships which may either facilitate or inhibit adjustment to the child's disability. The Calgary model also includes schemas (developed

Table 6.1   Family Assessment Questions

Do the parents interact with the child through touch, eye contact, and vocal behaviors?

• Do they cuddle the infant during feeding or maintain distance by positioning the baby on a bed or in an infant seat?

• Do the parents touch or stroke an older child who is fed in a high chair other than during actual feeding activities?

• During feeding, dressing, and play, do the parents periodically make direct eye contact with the child?

• Do the parents talk to the child and respond positively to vocalizations?

Do the parents include the child in regular family activities?

• Do they take the child to the grocery store, on outings, or to visit relatives?

• Do they involve the child and other siblings as a family unit in home activities?

How do the parents perceive the child's limitations and developmental potential?

• Do the parents discuss the fact that the child's activities will be limited?

• Are the parents setting realistic goals for their child?

• Do the parents include the child in activities with their friends?

Are parents able to communicate their feelings about the child's problems to each other?

• Do they discuss their own feelings of guilt about the child's problems, or do they tend to blame each other or someone or something else?

• Can the parents discuss their fears about the child's problems and future?

Are the parents able to meet the disabled child's siblings' needs?

• Do the parents give some of their time to healthy siblings on a one-to-one basis?

• Are siblings' health care needs being met? Is the family able to make appropriate decisions?

• Do the parents make realistic decisions for managing the handicapped child's problems, or do they overextend their time and the family budget to meet the child's perceived needs?

• Do the parents direct energy toward preventive health care for the entire family?

by Tomm) for diagramming communication interactions. These help the nurse identify communication problems common in families of children with developmental disabilities.

Barnard's (1978a) CHAIM allows assessment of parental, child/ patient, and environmental strengths and weaknesses, and provides additional scales to assist in planning and intervention. A unique feature of Barnard's model is that the scales provide baseline data and can therefore be readministered at the end of nursing intervention to see what changes have occurred.

Tools for assessing families with a developmentally disabled child. The
most helpful assessment for developmental disability would permit
scoring of *all* pertinent family data in relation to acceptable standards.
Necessary categories to be addressed are interactional, structural/
functional, and individual/environmental. Necessary quantifiable assessment tools include: a crisis assessment framework related to the parental adjustment process; a descriptive profile including interactional
and structural/functional information; and specific individual and environmental data. All of these indices should be measurable relative to
established standards. For example, a crisis theory–adjustment scale
would include data in all areas affected by family crisis, including
integration of the disabled child into the family, constructive management of parental feelings, appropriate relationships with siblings/healthy
children and outsiders, and parental managerial competence (Barnard
and Kelly, 1980, pp. 40, 45). These areas were developed and expanded
upon by the Nationally Organized Collaborative Project as goals for
"families of atypical infants" (Barnard and Kelly, 1980, pp. 40, 45).
After family intervention, this data could be reevaluated to detect any
improvement. Descriptive tools should provide significant interactional
and structural/functional components in relation to recommended standards; this information would help the nurse assess whether each
component was contributing to or inhibiting adjustment. Bernard also
describes feeding, teaching, and HOME scales, all of which measure
specific situations and gather data on individual characteristics and
interaction. These scales should be readministered after intervention to
measure outcomes.

Planning

Once the assessment is completed and a nursing diagnosis and/or
problem list developed, the nurse must begin to plan intervention strategies. In the case of developmental disability, the nursing diagnosis
should be a statement about the parents' response to the child's handicap and their potential for seeking treatment (Winslow, 1985). The
problem list represents the index for any planning framework (Kline,
1985), since strategies must be developed for resolving each specific
problem. These may include such things as inappropriate parent/child
interactions, inadequate linkage to other agencies, difficulties in role
performance, inability to meet the child's physical needs, or parental
overprotectiveness. As the problems are resolved, they are dated and
marked through. Other health care providers can use the problem list
as an up-to-date profile of the child's progress.

Also to be considered in care planning for families with developmentally disabled children are the family's strengths; the problems resolva-
ble by nursing and those to be referred to other resources; priorities

in problem solving; long- and short-term family goals; and evaluation of family outcomes.

Nurses may become overwhelmed by the problem list sometimes, and may forget about the parents' resources. On the contrary, it is amazing how many parents can care for a child's multiple problems while maintaining normal family routines (Burton, 1975). Therefore a nurse should consider how the parents perceive the child's problems—and how those perceptions might differ from her own. Strategic planning should mobilize family resources and promote parental independence (Tudor, 1978).

To determine whether a problem requires direct nursing intervention or referral to another health provider, the nurse must clearly understand her functions, as described by Bean (1985), in caring for the developmentally disabled. According to that author, the nurse intervenes through "teaching, supporting, coordinating, counseling, and advocating" (p. 379). East (1983, p. 70) refers to several roles played by the nurse, which include "teaching new skills; behavioral work; response to crisis; preventive work; and drug monitoring." East further notes that "the modern concept of mental handicap nursing is rapidly changing from custodian to therapist and enabler" (p. 71).

Parents often need referral to several providers and/or agencies. K.P. and L. Meadow (1971) discuss the therapeutic value of interacting with other parents whose children have developmental disabilities. In setting treatment goals, the nurse should remember the one that Lawson (1977, p. 54) cites from Yancey's list: "...prevent the illness, treatment regime, and people involved from disrupting the family." Indeed, Power (1985) cites a study which shows that when the nurse can help the family cope she can also demonstrate an improvement in the child's outcome.

The nurse's priorities should derive from the family's long- and short-term goals. Aggleton and Chalmers (1984, p. 61) note that, in planning, "the nurse negotiates with the patient immediate, intermediate, and long-term goals. These may also be ranked on order of importance." Tudor (1978, p. 25) emphasizes the need to "help the family to set realistic objectives and long-term goals for their infant, while at the same time working in the present—constantly checking to see if the quality of the infant's and family's lives has been compromised for a future, intangible goal."

In planning, as in assessment, a nurse must always make plans to determine eventual family outcomes. The nurse must be able to demonstrate a positive change in the family's situation as a result of nursing interventions (Bean, 1985). One key to success is early planning, since delay decreases the chance of changing outcome (Zuzich, 1980). Continued assessment is essential since the original plan may become inappropriate and new approaches become needed (Young, 1977).

Changes in health care delivery which affect planning. Several changes in health care delivery affect planning for families with a developmentally disabled child. According to Koop (1983, p. 105), "over the past four decades, revolutionary transformations in medical technology... have altered the prognosis for innumerable children with grave medical problems." Koop goes on to say, "but while modern American society has geared itself to almost unlimited support of medical technology, there has been a significant lag in the development of essential support services for children with handicaps and particularly for their families." In family care planning, the nurse must keep in mind the need for this type of service. In discussing "the technologic explosion in health care," Leavitt (1984, p. 84) refers to the "increased demand for more humanistic care" and to the family as a "more rational resource to rehumanize health care." These concepts should be applied in all planning for families of the developmentally disabled.

The current trend toward shorter hospital stays, which has resulted in the discharge of handicapped children still in need of highly skilled nursing care, places new pressures on parents and nurses alike. Nurses usually need special training and sometimes even certification to intervene in such situations, and parents need intensive guidance to provide even part of this skilled assistance.

CASE STUDY

The Mancini family's first child, Joe, was born with Down syndrome, a "genetic imbalance (which) causes the alterations of growth and development seen in the child...and is the most important factor in determining what his potential will be.... Down syndrome is the most common serious problem in development seen in a newborn" (Smith and Wilson, 1973, p. 1).

The parents were 23 and 24 years of age, respectively, at their child's birth, and both school teachers. They came from similar (upper-class) socioeconomic religious backgrounds. The pregnancy was well planned and the prenatal course was normal.

The Mancinis had eagerly anticipated the birth of their first child; immediately after delivery, however, the pediatrician diagnosed the infant's condition as Down syndrome. He met with the Mancinis immediately and referred them to a multidisciplinary evaluation clinic for further studies, counseling, and educational planning.

Assessment

Theories/models. Components of the interactional and structional/functional approaches (Reinhardt and Quinn, 1973), as well as Barnard's CHAIM were used to assess this family. Initially, both parents experienced denial and difficulty interacting with each other. Both felt guilt even after the pediatrician explained the cause of Joe's disorder, and refused to consider the fact that their son would always have limited intellectual functioning.

The couple's first interactions with Joe were cautious, but through increased eye contact and touching they soon felt comfortable relating to the infant. His alertness helped the parents to respond. Although Joe did have some difficulty sucking, due to poor muscle tone, his parents talked to him in response as he attended to them with his eyes.

Both parents had extended family members who lived nearby and were very supportive. They also had many contacts with outside groups but maintained much solidarity in the nuclear unit. At the time of the evaluation, the parents found it difficult to maintain relationships with outside social groups, because they feared that others would perceive them as incompetent parents. They did manage to avoid one common concern of families in their situation. Since they were well established financially, they were not overwhelmed by the numerous medical bills.

Assessment tools. Barnard's (1978b, p. 14) Nursing Child Assessment Teaching Scale (NCAST) was administered in the home setting. The tool measured the mother's "*sensitivity* to the infant's cues, ability to *alleviate the infant's distress,* and the ability to mediate the environment for the infant in ways that *foster(ed) cognitive and social/emotional development*," and Joe's "ability to *produce clear cues* for the caregiver and the ability to *respond to the caregiver.*" The family's overall score on this test was 69 out of a possible 73, which demonstrated, in this particular situation, good mother/infant interaction. Another useful assessment tool used was the genogram, which indicated no cases of Down syndrome through the past three generations of either parent's family.

Planning

Planning was based on the family strengths and problems identified in the assessment, relative to available services, priority needs, family goals, and outcome criteria. The major identified problems included denial of Joe's limitations, parental guilt, poor understanding of Joe's feeding problems, and fear of rejection by friends. Nursing expectations were that the parents would learn to cope with Joe's disability and recognize and use available resources to help their infant achieve his maximum potential.

The assessing nurse had identified numerous family strengths, including extended family support, financial stability, nuclear family solidarity, early diagnosis/counseling/referral, and a desired pregnancy. Initial nursing interventions consisted of counseling the Mancinis in managing Joe's feeding problems, and referring them to a nursery program for Down's syndrome children. There they could receive support from other parents and health care professionals. They were also taught methods of providing developmental stimulation for Joe. Through these activities, the Mancinis were able to work toward their goal of making educational opportunities available to their son.

As Joe developed new skills, his parents became more accepting of him as an individual, a perception which helped them feel better about themselves as parents, and became more willing to reenter old social groups and develop new ones. Continued counseling with the pediatrician was recommended to help relieve ongoing guilt about the etiology of Joe's problem and to provide guidance for meeting Joe's medical needs.

The Mancinis were able to work through the denial process and adjust to Joe's disability. Financial security and other family strengths enabled the parents to keep Joe in special programs until school age when he entered a class for the educable mentally retarded.

CONCLUSIONS

Family assessments are vital to nursing families whose children have developmental disabilities, due to the pronounced family-wide changes in structure, roles, and functions necessary to deal with the handicap.

In planning, the nurse needs to use the problem list as an index in outlining intervention approaches. The value of incorporating other factors (e.g., problems to be referred to other resources) with a comprehensive family assessment was illustrated in the case example of the family of a child with Down syndrome.

REFERENCES

Aggleton, P.J., and Chalmers, H. "The Riehl Interaction Model," *Nursing Times* 80(45):58–61, 1984.

Barnard, R. *Instructor's Learning Resource Manual.* Seattle: University of Washington, 1978a.

Barnard, R. *Nursing Child Assessment Teaching Scale.* Seattle: University of Washington, 1978b.

Barnard, R., and Kelly, J.F. "Infant Intervention: Parental Considerations," in *Guidelines for Early Intervention Programs.* Edited by Meservy, D. Salt Lake City: University of Utah, 1980.

Bean, M. "Nursing Role in Developmental Disabilities," in *Community Health Nursing: Keeping the Public Health,* 2nd ed. Edited by Jarvis, L.L. Philadelphia: F.A. Davis Co., 1985.

Bricker, J.T. "Heart Disorders," in *Physical Disabilities and Health Impairments: An Introduction.* Edited by Umbreit, J. Columbus, Ohio: Charles E. Merrill Publishing Co., 1983.

Burton, L. *The Family Life of Sick Children.* London: Routledge & Kegan Paul, 1975.

Clark, L.W. "The Importance of Touch with an Anacephalic Baby," *Maternal Child Nursing* 7(5):336–37, 1982.

Coyner, A.B. "Meeting Health Needs of Handicapped Infants," in *Developmentally Disabled Infants and Toddlers: Assessment and Intervention.* Edited by Zelle, R.S., et al. Philadelphia: F.A. Davis Co., 1983.

East, P. "Supporting the Family," *Nursing Times* 79(39):70–71, 1983.

Friedman, M.M. *Family Nursing: Theory and Assessment.* East Norwalk, Conn.: Appleton-Century-Crofts, 1981.

Jones, M.H. "Cerebral Palsy," in *Physical Disabilities and Health Impairments: An Introduction.* Edited by Umbreit, J. Columbus, Ohio: Charles E. Merrill Publishing Co., 1983.

Kline, M. Personal communication, July 31, 1985.

Koop, C.E. "Meeting the Health Care Needs of Children with Disabilities," *Public Health Reports* 98(2):105–07, 1983.

Lawson, B.A. "Chronic Illness and the School-Aged Child: Effects on the Total Family," *Maternal Child Nursing* 2(1):49–56, 1977.

Leavitt, M.B. "Nursing and Family-Focused Care," in *Nursing Clinics of North America.* Edited by Sheila, S.A., and Leavitt, M.B. Philadelphia: W.B. Saunders Co., 1984.

Lepler, M. "Having a Handicapped Child," *Maternal Child Nursing* 3(1):32–33, 1978.

Lyle, R.R. "Muscular Dystrophy," in *Physical Disabilities and Health Impairments: An Introduction.* Edited by Umbreit, J. Columbus, Ohio: Charles E. Merrill Publishing Co., 1983.

Meadow, K.P., and Meadow, L. "Changing Role Perceptions for Parents of Handicapped Children," *Exceptional Children* 38(1):21–27, 1971.

Meister, S.B. "Charting a Family's Developmental Status—For Intervention and for the Record," *Maternal Child Nursing* 2(1):43–48, 1977.

Nealis, J.G.T. "Epilepsy," in *Physical Disabilities and Health Impairments: An Introduction.* Edited by Umbreit, J. Columbus, Ohio: Charles E. Merrill Publishing Co., 1983.

Power, P.W. "Family Coping Behaviors in Chronic Illness: A Rehabilitation Perspective," *Rehabilitation Literature* 46(3–4):78–82, 1985.

Reinhardt, A.M., and Quinn, M.D., eds. *Current Practice in Family Centered Community Nursing.* St. Louis: C.V. Mosby Co., 1973.

Schild, S. "Beyond Diagnosis: Issues in Recurrent Counseling of Parents of the Mentally Retarded," *Social Work in Health Care* 8:81–93, 1982. (From *Psychological Abstracts,* 1983.)

Smith, D.W., and Wilson, A.A. *The Child with Down's Syndrome (Mongolism).* Philadelphia: W.B. Saunders Co., 1973.

Thompson, R.J., and O'Quinn, A.N. "Evolution of the Concept of Developmental Disabilities," in *Developmental Disabilities.* Edited by Thompson, R.J., and O'Quinn, A.N. New York: Oxford University Press, 1979.

Tudor, M. "Nursing Intervention with Developmentally Disabled Children," *Maternal Child Nursing* 3(1):25–31, 1978.

Winslow, B. Personal communication, March 26, 1985.

Wright, L.M., and Leahey, M. "Family Assessment," in *Community Health Nursing: Keeping the Public Healthy,* 2nd ed. Edited by Jarvis, L.C. Philadelphia: F.A. Davis Co., 1985.

Wyatt, D.S. "Phenylketonuria: The Problems Vary During Different Developmental Stages," *Maternal Child Nursing* 3(5):296–302, 1978.

Young, R., and Mack, R.W. "The Family," in *Systematic Sociology.* Edited by Young, R., and Mack, R.W. New York: American Book Co., 1962.

Young, R.K. "Chronic Sorrow: Parents' Response to the Birth of a Child with a Defect," *Maternal Child Nursing* 2(1):38–42, 1977.

Zuzich, A.M. "Grief in Parents in a Child with a Birth Handicap," in *Grief Response to Long-Term Illness and Disability.* Reston, Va: Reston Publishing Co., 1980.

7 Assessing families of children with cystic fibrosis

Debra P. Hymovich, RN, PhD, FAAN
Lecturer/Consultant in Chronic Illness
and Pediatric Nursing
Gulph Mills, Pennsylvania

OVERVIEW

This chapter reviews recent advances in theory and tool development for families of children with cystic fibrosis. It describes the Hymovich model for assessing and intervening with families of chronically ill children, and provides an example of its use with a family whose child has cystic fibrosis. The model has seven major components—the precipitating event, system, mediating variables, capabilities, needs, time, and intervention—and is intended to help nurses develop well-organized care plans based on specific family needs.

CASE STUDY

The Turners are a family of six: four children (Joey, 13 years; David, 10 years; Kara, 6 years; Kyle, 4 years) and Karen and Lloyd, who have been married 15 years. They relocated four months ago because Lloyd, an architect, was "offered an excellent position" in a new city. They are renting a house while looking for a suitable home to purchase. The family is being assessed at a cystic fibrosis center because Kyle, whose condition was diagnosed three years ago, has had a fever of 102° F. and has experienced difficulty raising sputum for the past two days. He has received health care since the family move. Family information was obtained through an initial interview and administration of the CICI:PQ questionnaire (Hymovich and Baker, 1985).

NURSING PROCESS

Assessment

Health problem: Cystic fibrosis. Cystic fibrosis (CF) is a genetically transmitted, chronic progressive disorder of the exocrine glands. It occurs in approximately one in 2000 live Caucasian births (Matthews and Drotar, 1984), and can present with a wide variety of symptoms and growth patterns. Thick mucus in the lungs, secreted in larger than normal amounts, leads to air trapping, mucal stasis, and lung infections, which in turn cause airway obstruction. Affected children often display chronic cough with purulent sputum, barrel chests, clubbing fingernails and toenails, dyspnea with increased activity, and cyanosis. Most suffer pancreatic insufficiency because thick mucus in the duodenum prevents pancreatic enzyme excretion. Absorption of proteins, fats, and fat-soluble vitamins is impaired. CF children may also have diarrhea, steatorrhea, protuberant abdomens, and large appetites with poor weight gain. Bowel obstruction (meconium ileus) may occur at birth or during childhood; elevated chloride and sodium levels in the sweat creates the potential for excess salt loss during febrile periods or hot weather. A small number of CF victims develop clinically significant diabetes mellitus, portal hypertension, or rectal prolapse. In 1981, the projected average life expectancy for recently diagnosed CF children was 21 years (Cystic Fibrosis Foundation, 1981).

Since CF has no cure, treatment is essentially supportive and individualized according to the degree of involvement and disease severity (Cystic Fibrosis Foundation, 1981). Therapeutic goals are to prevent and treat complications. Treatments may include physical therapy (postural drainage, breathing exercises), physical activity to help raise sputum, aerosol therapy, intermittent positive pressure breathing (IPPB), expectorants, bronchodilators, antihistamines, pancreatic replacements, and salt supplementation. Surgery may be necessary for meconium ileus and certain other CF complications.

Need for family involvement. The diagnosis of cystic fibrosis produces significant psychosocial stress in all members of the child's family. The need for family involvement in the affected child's care is cited frequently in the literature (Hymovich, 1981; Matthews and Drotar, 1984; Patterson, 1985). Since CF is a chronic condition with which the family must cope for many years, an ongoing relationship of trust with the health care system should be established as early as possible. Providing comprehensive care based on family perceptions and needs is essential, but it has been made difficult in the past by the lack of a relevant theoretical framework of assessment tools. Recent progress in nursing has allowed more effective assessment, planning, interventions, and evaluation in the care of all families of chronically ill children, including those with CF.

Models for family assessment in chronic illness. Numerous models and guidelines have been proposed for family assessment and for adaptation to chronic illness (Craig and Edwards, 1983; Hymovich, 1979; Lawrence and Lawrence, 1979; McCubbin and Patterson, 1983; MacVicar and Archibald, 1976), but their clinical usefulness has rarely been documented. Each of the three overlapping stages of Lawrence and Lawrence's (1979) chronic illness adaptation model has a beginning but no end. Stage I is characterized by shock, disbelief, denial, and independent behavior; Stage II involves developing awareness, anger, and dependent behavior; Stage III encompasses loss resolution, identity and role transition, and both dependent and independent behaviors. Adaptation requires the interaction of all three stages and is characterized by self-reliance, hope, and bargaining.

Another model, developed by Craig and Edwards (1983), describes chronic illness adaptation from the perspectives of humanity, caring, and health. MacVicar and Archibald (1976) proposed a framework based on Hill's crisis model, within which the nurse examines the characteristics of the illness/crisis, the family's perception of threat, and the family's resources and past experience with similar situations. McCubbin and Patterson (1983) expanded Hill's model into the double ABCX model which considers the event's postcrisis variables. This model focuses on family stressors and strains, coping, and resources, and has been used recently in research with CF families (Patterson, 1985). Lefton and Lefton's (1979) model emphasizes the concepts of teamwork and team relationships in care delivery for chronic illnesses. This model stresses the need for more than just medical treatment of chronically ill patients and their families.

In 1979, Hymovich suggested a three-part framework for assessing families with chronically ill children, encompassing individual and family developmental tasks, impact variables (perceptions, resources, coping abilities), and necessary interventions. Subsequent revisions have used Glaser and Strauss's (1967) approach for developing grounded theory. The latest version (1984) is this chapter's model for nursing assessment of CF families.

Hymovich model for family assessment in chronic childhood illness. Successive versions of Hymovich's original model have been used by nurses working with children having a variety of chronic illnesses; modifications of it continue to be made with ongoing clinical use and testing. In CF cases, the model directs the nurse to assess family members individually and as a unit. The assessment approach should be systematic and thorough, and requires extended interaction with the family. The accuracy of collected data should be checked with the family members; such tools as the CICI:PQ (Hymovich and Baker, 1985) can be used to illuminate the needs, concerns, and coping strategies of CF parents.

The Hymovich model is intended to help nurses plan and organize effective intervention programs. A nursing care plan that responds to specific family needs can be shared readily with all health team members, thus enhancing comprehensive care.

The model has seven major components: the system, precipitating event, mediating variables, capabilities, needs, time, and intervention (see Figure 7.1).

Figure 7.1

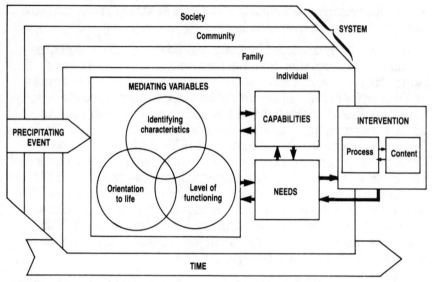

Source: Debra P. Hymovich © 1985

System. The model's first component relates to the system with which the nurse is working: individual family members; the family unit; the community in which the family lives (including friends, neighbors, and agencies); and society at large (including state and federal agencies and their policies). Since care for CF children may involve resources beyond the family, it is important to include all relevent systems in the assessment.

The system of primary concern for the Turner family are the individual members, the family unit, and the new community in which they reside.

Precipitating event. The model's second component is the precipitating event—any stressor or potential stressor creating a need for outside (nursing) assistance.

Two events prompted the Turner family's entry into the health care system: the relocation to a new city and need to obtain ongoing care for Kyle; and Kyle's fever and difficulty raising sputum.

Mediating variables. Mediating variables are factors that influence the effect that the precipitating events may have on the system; they fall between the precipitating event and the system's capabilities and needs. Three mediating variables are common to every system: (1) identifying characteristics, (2) orientation to life, and (3) functional level.

A complex array of characteristics help identify and define each system. Among those most relevant in nursing care planning and intervention are system structure, developmental level, race, roles, economic resources, relationships, and experiences, as well as characteristics of individual members such as age, sex, temperament, cognitive abilities, and educational level.

In the Turner case, the nurse defined a constellation of relevant characteristics. The family can be described as White, Episcopalian, and of middle income, with children at the preschool, school age, and early adolescent developmental levels. Mr. Turner, who has a master's degree in architecture, is the only employed family member; the three older children attend school while Kyle remains at home with his mother. Mrs. Turner describes the family as "close, a very happy family, we're very children-oriented. Almost everything we do, the whole family does." She feels close to all of her children but closest to Joey and Kyle. Both parents describe Joey as "very withdrawn"; David as "athletic and spontaneous"; Kara as "smart as can be and a little jealous of Kyle"; and Kyle as "contained and quiet." Mrs. Turner describes herself as shy and withdrawn while Mr. Turner sees himself as "more outgoing and tending to lose my temper easily."

The second mediating variable refers to the system's world view, and includes family values, attitudes, and beliefs regarding life, death, health, illness, and health care. Sometimes a precipitating event challenges these values and forces members to change their beliefs in order to make sense of their experiences. Burton (1975) noted that parents' abilities to maintain a positive outlook on their situation seemed to increase their ill child's longevity.

Lloyd and Karen report "having a lot of fun as a family." They believe in giving each of their children individual time and ensuring that the children "have a happy life without a whole lot of worries." They believe Kyle "was given to us for a very special reason, because he is a very special child. We live more and enjoy each thing we do a little bit more because we realize it might be the last time for any of us." The Turners value their health and have always sought professional health care when they needed it; most of their experiences with the health care system have been "Okay, especially with the CF center."

The third mediating variable, the functional level, describes how the system deals with its developmental and situational tasks, its stressors, and its coping strategies. It should be examined from the standpoints of individuals and their family units.

Developmental tasks. Developmental tasks arise at critical times in individual and family life and must be accomplished in order to progress

to subsequent life-cycle stages (Duvall, 1977). For instance, all parents must (Hymovich and Chamberlin, 1980, pp. 23-29):
• Meet their family's basic physical needs (i.e., for food, health care, shelter, money).
• Help all family members fulfill individual developmental tasks.
• Meet all family members' emotional needs.
• Maintain and adapt family organization and management to meet group needs.
• Function within the community.

Children also have developmental tasks to accomplish (Hymovich & Chamberlin, 1980, p.15):
• Develop and maintain healthy growth and nutrition patterns.
• Learn to manage the body satisfactorily.
• Learn to understand and relate to the physical world.
• Develop self-awareness and a satisfying sense of self.
• Learn to relate to others.

Gauging the extent to which all children in the CF child's family have accomplished their developmental tasks is an important consideration in the family nursing assessment. As Matthews and Drotar (1984, p. 146) point out, "key developmental transitions often become focal points for the expression of psychological distrubances." These points cluster around school age and around both early and late adolescence.

Situational tasks. Families of chronically ill children face tasks related to their child's illness and superimposed on normal developmental tasks. The most important of these situational tasks are listed in Table 7.1.

Table 7.1 Situational Tasks of Families with Chronically Ill Children

Parents	• Learn to understand and manage the child's illness. • Help the children understand and cope with the chronic illness. • Understand the impact of the chronic illness on all family members. • Develop a feeling of control over the situation. • Develop a life-orientation that allows coping with illness-related stressors.
Ill Child(ren)	• Understand the illness and necessary care procedures. • Cope with illness-related stressors. • Accomplish developmental tasks within the limits imposed by the disorder.
Siblings	• Understand the illness and its impact on the family. • Cope with illness-related stressors. • Accomplish developmental tasks.

The Turners try to meet all family members' appropriate developmental tasks. Lloyd and Karen also try to help Kyle understand his illness and his need for treatments; he is beginning to question them. At the moment, they do not feel that they have adequate control over their situation because they are new to the community and the CF center and do not yet know their care personnel. Before the move, both parents were involved in local activities, but they are not yet familiar with the organizations in their new city. Mr. and Mrs. Turner say that, of the siblings, only Joey has extensive knowledge of Kyle's illness. The major task for the older children is adjusting to a new school and friends.

Stressors. Any environmental or internal events that are strange enough to strain or surpass adaptive resources can significantly impair both family function and nursing care in chronic illness. For assessment purposes, any areas identified by family members as problematic, for themselves or others, can be labeled stressors.

Common stressors among parents of CF children include concern about their child's future comfort or happiness; the responsibilities of child care; the effect of the weather on their child's activities; the need for adequate insurance; and uncertainty about proper care for their child (Hymovich and Baker, 1985). Other stressors include excessive demands on parents' time and energy, marital strain, periodic hospitalization of the ill child, physicians' visits, the child's physical deterioration (Travis, 1976), and guilt about their child's condition (Geyman, 1983). They may also be concerned about their child's longevity, the family's ability to manage the situation, and what their child's approaching death will mean to the family (Clifford, 1979).

Research has shown that even very young children comprehend the seriousness of their illness without being told directly (Bluebond-Langer, 1977; Kübler-Ross, 1969; Waechter, 1971) and, moreover, that parental inability to discuss the situation openly makes the child feel lonely and isolated (Buckingham, 1983; Geyman, 1983). Still further stress arises when ill children feel they must pretend to be unaware of their condition's seriousness and protect their parents by not discussing it. Other stressors include disease- and treatment-related physical changes, altered family and peer relationships, feelings of helplessness, pain, anticipatory anxiety (Ross and Ross, 1984), and parental refusal to set limits (McEvoy et al., 1985).

Stressors for siblings include the fear of becoming ill (Kruger et al., 1980) and of being "protected" from unpleasant facts (Siemon, 1985), chores, family financial strain, altered family relationships (Harder and Bowditch, 1982), and changes in family activities.

Stressors initially identified by the Turners included a lack of friends in their new neighborhood, poor interfamily communication ("We get along fine but I wish we had more communication"), and uncertainty about Kyle's future development. Mrs. Turner reported additional stress from her 13-year-old son's questions about sex, saying she did "not know how to treat boys."

Coping strategies. Knowledge of the ways in which family members minimize or relieve the distress caused by perceived stressors can help nurses make useful recommendations or advise family members about child care. Such knowledge may also alert the nurse to the need for further family education in alternative coping strategies.

Parents often cope with a child's chronic illness by participating in care and seeking information. This relieves stress and enhances their ability to master the tasks they face. The most common coping strategy cited by CF parents (Hymovich and Baker, 1985) was asking direct questions of physicians, nurses, and other parents. When asked how stresses such as marital tension affected their coping routine, the same parents reported using prayer, talking with someone/asking for help, and distracting themselves with other activities. Less common strategies included "getting away," exercising, and ignoring the problem.

Young children communicate both verbally and symbolically through play, drawings, or stories (Kübler-Ross, 1969). They usually learn about illnesses by questioning other children and eavesdropping on adult conversation (Bluebond-Langer, 1977). Coping strategies during school-age differ from child to child, or even from situation to situation (Ross & Ross, 1984). While many children want to discuss their illness with someone, some prefer to deny its seriousness (Geyman, 1983). Others regress, which is a means of coping that can occur at any age. During adolescence, an intellectual coping style appears dominant. Overall, most children cope relatively well with CF or other chronic illness (Drotar et al., 1981).

Mr. and Mrs. Turner's established coping strategies are community involvement, anger with one another, overeating, and requesting help from the CF center personnel when indicated. Mrs. Turner also cries and goes to church more often.

Capabilities. The Hymovich model's fourth major component is capabilities, or the net balance of a system's strengths and limitations. Families caring for chronically ill children must identify and maximize their strengths in order to carry out the tasks associated with normal development and their child's special situation. In addition, health professionals can build on strengths while helping the family minimize its limitations. Traditionally, nursing assessment has centered on limitations and problems, with little focus on families' abilities to develop coping strategies adequate to their needs.

The nurse assessing the Turner family identified many strengths, including the ability to seek help when needed; an understanding of Kyle's condition and developmental needs; and finances adequate to cover the cost of his illness. Limitations identified initially were inadequate knowledge of the new community and the CF center; poor communication between the parents; and Karen's inability to respond adequately to Joey's questions about sex.

Needs. Needs, as defined here, are developmental or situational deficits requiring assistance or relief; they are related to precipitating event(s), mediating variables, and capabilities. The more specific and well-defined the system's needs, the easier it is to determine appropriate nursing intervention.

CF parents must develop trust in their own ability to manage difficult situations and in the availability and adequacy of the health care system if they are to accomplish their developmental and situational tasks. They also need information, guidance, and support through all phases of their child's illness (Hymovich, 1976). All family members need to feel that support and comfort will be available when needed (Siemon, 1985).

Chronically ill children have many of the same needs as adults (Buckingham, 1983). In addition to symptom relief and physical care (Gates, 1982), children often need freedom to choose when and what to eat and what activities they want to do, thus exercising some control over their situation. They need to communicate openly and honestly with their families, to ask questions and receive direct, helpful answers. Children need an open relationship with the health care team and confidence that those professionals will inform them about their condition and treatment and answer their questions. They also need established limits in order to establish a sense of control (McEvoy et al., 1985). Ill children need careful explanations of the causes of their illness and the need for treatment procedures (Pattison, 1978); they need to accomplish appropriate developmental tasks and do things that give them satisfaction, including involvement in activities and with friends.

Healthy siblings share the ill child's need for open communication and knowledge of the condition, as well as for understanding of the changes taking place in their family. They need to feel wanted and to have the opportunities and guidance necessary to help them accomplish their developmental and situational tasks.

Needs identified by the Turner parents are to:
- obtain knowledge of their new community and the CF center
- purchase a house
- obtain medical care for Kyle
- learn how to answer Joey's questions about sex.

In addition, they would like further information about Kyle's expected physical, emotional, and intellectual development, and guidance in explaining Kyle's condition to his siblings.

Time. Although they interact with family systems in the present, nurses should be acquainted with each client group's past and anticipate its future. Since CF care often continues for many years, intervention must be based on knowledge of the family's background and future goals.

At initial assesssment, little was known of the Turners' history prior to their recent move. Mr. Turner's job opportunity arose suddenly, and the parents felt that an immediate decision was important; within two months they had moved. It was known that Mr. Turner's mother died one year before assessment, and that his father, who had lived with the family after her death, refused to relocate with them. Their immediate goals are to obtain adequate care for Kyle, to find an affordable house in a good school district, and to obtain a part-time job for Mrs. Turner. Over the longer term, they hope to improve the family's financial status and send the children to college. They express uncertainty regarding Kyle's future and hesitate to make long-range plans for him.

Family assessment and intervention questions for nurses. Comprehensive family nursing care requires attention to a number of important questions (see Table 7.2).

Table 7.2   Questions to Consider in Family Assessment and Intervention

- Who are the recipients?
- What are the goals?
- When is the appropriate time?
- Where should assessment and intervention take place?
- What nursing strategies are needed?
- How will the outcome be measured?

It is, for instance, important to determine whether the intervention is for the child with CF, the child's siblings, the parents, or the entire family unit. It may also be necessary to intervene with members of the community, such as school personnel. Assessment and intervention must be carefully directed toward helping the family acquire the skills and knowledge needed to cope with CF-related stressors and accomplish developmental and situational tasks. Objectives should be devised in light of the family's perceived needs.

Assessment timing is also important, and should be based on evaluation of each family member's unique needs and readiness. Some interventions may be needed immediately; others might be used more appropriately at a later date. Assessment/intervention location(s), for instance, in the home, outpatient unit, hospital, or school, must also be selected with an eye to family requirements.

Assessment strategies in CF nursing might include observation, structured and unstructured interviews, developmental testing, and family-completed written or oral assessment instruments. Useful intervention strategies include physical caretaking, teaching, counseling, supporting, or making referrals. As always, specific evaluation criteria must be established in order to monitor the success of nursing efforts.

Family assessment tools. Written or oral questionnaires are one suggested family assessment tool. Unfortunately, such tools, especially those related to chronic childhood disorders, are still scarce.

Holt and Robinson's (1979) Family Assessment Tool was designed for nurses working in school systems, and includes both assessment guidelines and suggestions for developing a care plan. Guidelines suggested by Edison (1979) provide for open-ended yet comprehensive assessment and are useful in a variety of clinical settings.

The Feetham Family Functioning Survey (FFFS) (Roberts & Feetham, 1982) was more specifically conceived for parents of chronically ill children, with 21 items related to relationships within the family and with the environment. Designed for two-parent families, it can serve as the basis for an interview or be self-administered, although people with less than a high school education may have difficulty with the format. It was constructed using the Porter Format, and measures current family functioning (How much is there now?), the desired status (How much should there be?), and the importance of the item (How important is this to me?). For example, using a 7-point scale from "Little" to "Much," parents respond to such statements as "Amount of time you spend with your other children." The discrepancy between the current situation and what is desired is thus easily determined.

The Wellness of the Family System Assessment Tool (WFSAT) described by Kandzari and Howard (1981) is an 81-item, nurse-completed instrument that assesses how family members relate to one another, function as a unit, and relate to the community. McCubbin and colleagues (1983) developed the CHIP—Coping Health Inventory for Parents—to assess parental coping strategies. This 45-item checklist reveals how parents perceive their management of family life with a chronically ill child.

Hymovich (1981, 1984) developed the Chronicity Impact and Coping Instrument: Parent Questionnaire (CICI:PQ) to measure the perceived overall impact of chronic childhood illness on a family; how parents cope with the impact; and their perceived needs. The CICI:PQ is self-administered and takes 20 to 25 minutes to complete.

The instrument used most often with children is the Piers-Harris Self-Concept Scale (PHSCS) (Piers, 1969). This tool's 80 items probe children's feelings about themselves, yielding a total self-concept score and subscales rating intellectual and school status, physical appearance/attributes, popularity and happiness, behavior, anxiety, and satisfaction.

Planning

Following assessment, a written family-centered care plan should be completed and interventional goals established mutually by nurse and family. The plan itself should incorporate each family members' goals and needs, and should be shared with the entire CF team.

Mutually-established short-term goals for the Turners were to treat Kyle's current illness, regularly assess his physical condition and developmental level, and provide information and guidance to the parents about Kyle's expected development, as well as helping the children understand Kyle's illness and handling Joey's questions about sex. The family agreed to meet with the social worker at the CF center to obtain information about the community. The nursing strategies employed included teaching, counseling, referral, and family support. Long-term goals included reinforcing the family's strengths and helping them improve communication skills.

CONCLUSIONS

This chapter describes the Hymovich model of nursing practice and illustrates its application to families of children with cystic fibrosis. The model was developed to help nurses design comprehensive, well-organized nursing care plans that respond to family members' specific needs. These plans can be transmitted to all team members, thus contributing to effective and efficient care. Family assessment should include each member's perceptions of the precipitating event, mediating variables, stressors, capabilities, and needs. Interventional goals should be agreed upon by nurse and family, and aimed at helping the family members minimize stress and enhance their coping abilities by completing necessary developmental and situational tasks.

REFERENCES

Bluebond-Langer, M. "Meanings of Death to Children," in *New Meanings of Death*. Edited by Feifel, H. New York: McGraw–Hill Book Co., 1977.

Buckingham, R.W. *The Complete Hospice Guide*. New York: Harper & Row Publishers, 1983.

Burton, L. *The Family Life of Sick Children. A Study of Families Coping with Chronic Childhood Disease*. Boston: Rutledge & Kegan Paul, 1975.

Clifford, I.M. "Comprehensive Planning for Home Care and the Home Health Agency," in *Home Care Living and Dying*. Edited by Prichard, E.R., et al. New York: Columbia University Press, 1979.

Craig, H.M., and Edwards, J.E. "Adaptation to Chronic Illness: An Eclectic Model for Nurses," *Journal of Advanced Nursing* 8(5):397–404, 1983.

Cystic Fibrosis: A Summary of Symptoms, Diagnosis, and Treatment. Rockville, Md.: Cystic Fibrosis Foundation, 1981.

Drotar, D., et al. "Psychosocial Functioning of Children with Cystic Fibrosis," *Pediatrics* 67(3):338–42, 1981.

Duvall, E.M. *Marriage and Family Development*. Philadelphia: J.B. Lippincott Co., 1977.

Edison, C.E. "Family Assessment Guidelines," in *Family Health Care*, vol. 1, 2nd ed. Edited by Hymovich, D.P., and Barnard, M.U. New York: McGraw–Hill Book Co., 1979.

Gates, G.R. "Terminal Care in Country Practice," *Australian Family Physician* 11:338–42, 1982.

Geyman, J.P. "Dying and Death of a Family Member," *Journal of Family Practice* 17(1):125–34, 1983.

Glaser, B.G., and Strauss, A.L. *The Discovery of Grounded Theory: Strategies for Qualitative Research*. Chicago: Aldine, 1967.

Harder, L., and Bowditch, B. "Siblings of Children with Cystic Fibrosis: Perceptions of the Impact of the Disease," *Children's Health Care* 10(4):116–20, 1982.

Holt, S.J., and Robinson, T.M. "The School Nurse's 'Family Assessment Tool,'" *American Journal of Nursing* 79(5):950–53, 1979.

Hymovich, D.P. "Assessment of the Chronically Ill Child and Family," in *Family Health Care*, vol. 1, 2nd ed. Edited by Hymovich, D.P., and Barnard, M.U. New York: McGraw–Hill Book Co., 1979.

Hymovich, D.P. "Assessing the Impact of Chronic Childhood Illness on the Family and Parent Coping," *Image* 13:71–74, 1981.

Hymovich, D.P. "Development of the Chronicity Impact and Coping Instrument: Parent Questionnaire," *Nursing Research* 33:218–22, 1984.

Hymovich, D.P. "Parents of Sick Children: Their Needs and Tasks," *Pediatric Nursing* 2:9–13, 1976.

Hymovich, D.P., and Baker, C. "The Needs, Concerns and Coping of Parents of Children with Cystic Fibrosis," *Family Relations* 34:91–97, 1985.

Hymovich, D.P., and Chamberlin, R.W. *Child and Family Development: Implications for Primary Health Care*. New York: McGraw–Hill Book Co., 1980.

Kandzari, J.K., and Howard, J.R. *The Well Family: A Developmental Approach to Assessment*. Boston: Little, Brown & Co., 1981.

Kruger, S., et al. "Reactions of Families to the Child with Cystic Fibrosis," *Image* 12(3):67–80, 1980.

Kübler–Ross, E. *On Death and Dying.* New York: Macmillan Publishing Co., 1969.

Lawrence, S.A., and Lawrence, R.M. "A Model of Adaptation to the Stress of Chronic Illness," *Nursing Forum* 18(1):33–43, 1979.

Lefton, E., and Lefton, M. "Health Care and Treatment of the Chronically Ill: Toward a Conceptual Framework," *Journal of Chronic Disease* 32:339–43, 1979.

MacVicar, M.G., and Archibald, P. "A Framework for Family Assessment in Chronic Illness," *Nursing Forum* 15(2):180–94, 1976.

Matthews, L.W., and Drotar, D. "Cystic Fibrosis: A Challenging Chronic Disease," *Pediatric Clinics of North America* 31(1):132–52, 1984.

McCubbin, H., and Patterson, J. "The Family Stress Process: The Double ABCX Model of Family Adjustment and Adaptation," in *Advances and Developments in Family Stress Theory and Research.* Edited by McCubbin, H., et al. New York: Haworth, 1983.

McCubbin, H., et al. "CHIP—Coping Health Inventory for Parents: An Assessment of Parental Coping Patterns in the Care of the Chronically Ill Child," *Journal of Marriage and the Family* 45:359–70, 1983.

McEvoy, M., et al. "Therapeutic Play Group for Patients and Siblings in a Pediatric Oncology Ambulatory Care Unit," *Topics in Clinical Nursing* 7(1):10–18, 1985.

Patterson, J.M. "Critical Factors Affecting Family Compliance for Children with Cystic Fibrosis," *Family Relations* 34:79–89, 1985.

Pattison, E.M. "The Living-Dying Process," in *Psychosocial Care of the Dying Patient.* Edited by Garfield, C.A. New York: McGraw-Hill Book Co., 1978.

Piers, E.V. *Manual for the Piers-Harris Children's Self-Concept Scales.* Nashville, Tenn.: Counselor Recordings and Tests, 1969.

Roberts, C.S., and Feetham, S.L. "Assessing Family Functioning Across Three Areas of Relationships," *Nursing Research* 31(4):231–35, 1982.

Ross, D.M., and Ross, S.A. "Stress Reduction Procedures for the School-Age Hospitalized Leukemic Child," *Pediatric Nursing* 10(6):393–95, 1984.

Siemon, M. "Thinking of Siblings," in *Meeting Psychosocial Needs of Children and Families in Health Care.* Edited by Fore, C., and Poster, E.C. Washington, D.C.: Association for the Care of Children's Health, 1985.

Travis, G. *Chronic Illness in Children.* Stanford, Calif.: Stanford University Press, 1976.

Waechter, E.H. "Children's Awareness of Fatal Illness," *American Journal of Nursing* 71:1168–72, 1971.

8 Assessing single-parent families with physically disabled children

Sharon Ogden Burke, RN, PhD
Associate Professor and
National Health Research Scholar
Health and Welfare Canada

School of Nursing
Queen's University
Kingston, Ontario, Canada

OVERVIEW

This chapter documents the special risks and stresses experienced by single-parent families who have a physically disabled child. The special needs of the mother, the handicapped child, and the normal siblings are highlighted, and the ways in which the extended family can be a source of either support or stress is examined. Because the single-parent situation is often limited in duration, families in various stages of transition are described along with case-specific nursing concerns. A family assessment model details additional risks to health and development, stresses, supports, and protective factors. By assessing the type of single-parent family with a handicapped child and using the family assessment model, the nurse can tailor nursing practice to individuals and families, thus reducing risk factors, eliminating sources of stress, and maximizing protective and supportive factors.

NURSING PROCESS

Assessment

The health problem: Physical disability in children with single parents.
The term "single-parent family" (SPF) applies to a wide range of situations, and some generalizations are possible. But the nurse must also be able to identify each family's unique characteristics.

This chapter defines SPF broadly—as a parent and at least one child living in the same household. A physically disabled child is identified as one whose genetic or physical condition limits normal activity. The word "handicap" refers to the disability's impact on the child's general development, health, and daily functioning. Childhood handicaps can be physical, mental, or both; all will be included here. The term "single-parent family with a handicapped child" (SPFHC) encompasses all of the above; a two-parent family with a handicapped child (TPFHC) refers to the same type of child living with two parents.

Single-parent family statistics. North American census statistics estimate conservatively that 18% to 20% of all families with children at home are single-parent families (see Table 8.1). These rates vary considerably with community ethnicity; for example, figures are much higher among blacks. An estimated 40% to 50% of all children will live in an SPF before reaching adulthood (Guidubaldi and Perry, 1984).

Most custodial single parents are females (U.S. Bureau of the Census, 1983; Census of Canada, 1983); not surprisingly, almost all research on single parenthood has focused on female-headed families. The proportion of male-headed SPFs is growing as a result of the women's movement and changes in custody legislation and its interpretation (Tankson, 1979), but it is not likely to approach that of female-headed SPFs. Most single fathers differ from single mothers in the stresses they experience, their use of social support, and their financial resources (Todres, 1975; Hughes and Scoloveno, 1984). However, as long as the nurse considers these factors individually in family assessment and interventions, this chapter's guidelines should apply to both single-father and single-mother situations.

There is considerable uncertainty about the incidence of handicaps among children; the National Center for Health Statistics (NCHS), the principal source of data, reports that 3.8% of all children who are under age 17 and living at home have some degree of activity limitation (Newacheck et al., 1984).

Table 8.1   Percentages of Single-Parent Families

Percent of Total Families with Children Living at Home

	Total	Female-headed	Male-headed
U.S.A.[1]	17.9	14.3	3.6
Canada[2]	19.8	16.4	3.5
Clinic Populations[3]	up to 40 or more		

[1]1980 U.S. Bureau of the Census, 1983.
[2]1981 Census of Canada, 1983.
[3]Kalnins, 1983.

SPFs and health care services. Professionals working with handicapped children report much higher ratios of SPFs in their caseloads than the NCHS figures imply; some report ratios as high as 40% (Kalnins, 1983). There are three viable explanations for this phenomenon:
- higher divorce rates among families with handicapped children
- higher service use rates among single-parent families
- larger numbers of single-parent families than reported in census data.

Although the idea seems plausible, there is little data to confirm the presence of higher divorce rates among families with disabled children. Kalnins (1983) reviewed 20 studies of divorce and separation among families of handicapped, chronically ill, or life-threatened children and observed that the best of them implicated no variation in divorce rate from that of the general population. Also, parents who separated rarely attributed their problems to the child's condition. Conversely, 20% to 50% of couples surveyed said their child's health problem strengthened their marriage.

The second hypothesis, that SPFHCs use services more frequently, is a better reason why nurses see more of these families than population statistics suggest they should. The author's work (Ogden, 1975) and that of others (Goldberg et al., 1984) supports this notion; the remaining question is why do SPFHCs use health and social services more? There are at least three interrelated explanations for this. First, there may be more stressors and fewer sources of support for these families, resulting in more problems requiring care. Ample empirical evidence supports this (Ogden, 1975; Burke, 1978; McLanahan, 1983). Second, the SPFHC often lacks the familial "staff" to manage problems a two-parent family would handle itself, thus forcing the SPF into the health care system (Weltner, 1982). Lastly, mothers report confidentially that there are serendipitous advantages to professional services, for example, better lunches in a special school or the provision of a respite for a single mother when a child's hospitalization is extended for a day (Ogden, 1975).

SPFHCs utilize hospitals more frequently than the general handicapped family population, especially when the children are aged 9 months to 5 years; their total in-hospital time and average length of stay are greater. Single mothers view their children's health problems as more serious and longer lasting than those of two-parent children. Although the type of medical care given to these two groups does not seem different, two-parent children see their doctors more often on an outpatient basis.

Finally, underreporting and narrow professional definitions of SPF help account for the large ratio of such families on health service rolls. There remains a cultural bias in North America toward the (now mythical) "typical" two-parent, two-child, father-works, mother-stays-at-home family. Census data could be biased by a hesitancy to report against the norm, especially when marital status is not certain. Studies in which children are asked directly, "How many parents live with you?" indicate much higher SPF rates than comparable census data (Wright and Dhanota, 1981).

In summary, every diverse clinic, community, or ward population probably has at least one single-parent family in every five family units; of these, about 4% of the children could have a handicap. The nurse whose clients are primarily handicapped children can expect nearly half to be living in an SPF at some time before adulthood, and there is considerable evidence that the number of SPFHCs is increasing. Two of the factors behind this increase are rising divorce rates and falling mortality rates for some handicapping conditions (e.g., spina bifida), which increases the number of survivors (Kalnins, 1983). This prevalence of SPFHCs can change both the nature and number of nursing problems.

Types of single-parent families. Because the SPF is not necessarily stable, a continuum has been developed (Burke, 1983) to reflect the wide range of SPF types as well as the tendency for families to cycle from one type to another over time. Although this continuum does not necessarily mean that a family *will* experience all stages, some families will, often more than once. (See Figure 8.1 for the continuum and its relationship to two-parent families.)

Figure 8.1   The Single-Parent Family Continuum and Its Relationship to Two-Parent Families

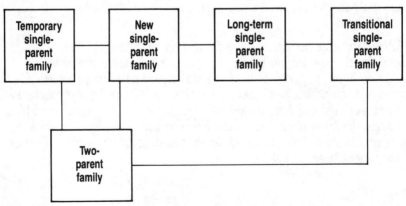

Source: Burke, 1983.

Temporary SPFHCs. SPFHCs in which a parent is temporarily absent from the home are often overlooked. Parents may be apart because of a trial separation, weekly commuting to another city, extended work assignments away from home (for instance, the military), or other such time-limited separations, including imprisonment. How well these families manage is extremely variable.

Assessment of these families must include:
• the amount and nature of continuing contact with the absent parent
• previous family experience with separation
• perceptions of past coping effectiveness
• the existence of special supports (i.e., companies that might provide return passage for a husband located in another country or formal/ informal support groups, such as those for military and prisoners' wives)
• the extent of the absent parent's usual involvement in the care of the handicapped child and other family roles.

The nature, and thus the impact, of nursing interventions can vary widely in temporarily single SPFHCs. Many families interpret the intervention as a memorable growth experience in which the family successfully copes with a major crisis.

Newly single SPFHCs. Most nurses see newly single parents and their children disproportionally more often than other SPFHCs, simply because their separation has suddenly thrown them into stress or crisis. However, some newly single individuals and families experience tremendous relief and a desire to get on with their lives if, for example, a now-dead parent had suffered a lingering illness, or if the absent parent has been a negative force in the family. These families fall roughly into four parental categories: widowed, separated or divorced, unmarried, and adoptive.

Widowed and divorced parents. A newly widowed parent and divorced parents accustomed to coping with their child's handicap respond well to standard nursing approaches. Wallerstein and Kelly (1980) and Wallerstein (1983) have done excellent longitudinal, research-based work on children's reactions, and on therapist and parent interventions of divorced parents. Kessler (1975) outlined phases of divorce: disillusionment, erosion, detachment, physical separation, mourning, second adolescence and exploration, and hard work. Yet since accumulating evidence suggests that people often do not fit neatly into identified stages of crisis behavior (Rutter, 1983), it might be wise to view these categorizations with skepticism.

Adoptive parents. Single persons wishing to adopt are often given the option of adopting either an older or a handicapped child, thus forming another group of SPFHCs. Fairly extensive preadoption counseling, as well as advance contact with other parents who have adopted such children, may facilitate adjustment. A typical pattern is that of the working woman in her late thirties or early forties, who wishes to have children but sees no prospects for marriage. These inexperienced mothers have to manage massive changes in both their family roles and their day-to-day lives; even with the best preparation and support there will be many stresses and crises in the new family, especially after the so-called honeymoon period wears off for the family and social constellations. A period of high stress often follows as new patterns develop and new roles are learned.

Unmarried parents. Many unwed mothers are adolescents, whose needs and concerns are complex. Such parents require expert emotional and physical care even if the baby is normal; an infant's handicap only adds to the problem. Rarely can the young mother alone manage the combined concerns of adolescence and mothering, not to mention the social stigma of their child's disability. In the author's experience, the only such parents who can keep their child successfully at home are those for whom someone else (usually their mother) assumes substantial responsibility in parenting. In fact, the maternal grandmother is often the primary parental figure in such families. Nurses interacting with unmarried single-parent families must assess the nature of all parenting roles and the relationships between those who hold them. Interacting primarily with the adolescent mother, for example, might not only be ineffective, but could also build resentment in the dominant figure, the maternal grandmother.

Of course, the older single woman who decides to have a child without marrying is a marked exception to the guidelines just described. These mothers probably resemble conventional adoptive mothers more than they do the younger mothers just discussed.

Long-term single parenting. In most cases, single parenting becomes a way of life; when the nurse sees them, such families are maintaining status quo; they are no longer in the initial crisis phase nor considering becoming a two-parent family. This group's typical problems are:
• role strain and altering generational boundaries
• social stigma and isolation
• reduced financial status
• child rearing
• emotional, school, and health problems in both handicapped and normal children.

Role strain and altering generational boundaries. Role strain is often most evident in the mother, but studies of siblings of handicapped children indicate that the older children, particularly females, can also be affected (Vadasy et al., 1984). Besides missing the strong religious and cultural traditions that sanction two-parent families, SPFs must cope with the reality that most family functions require more than one person to execute them effectively (Weltner, 1982). Many newly single mothers work permanent overtime, and soon complain of "burn-out" and exhaustion. This coping strategy often proves ineffective over time, leaving parents frustrated, confused, and guilty, as well as exhausted. Of course, a few women can maintain this routine for extended periods; for them the term "supermom" is apt. By telling single mothers that it is normal for them not to be able to do everything they would like, the nurse can reduce their feelings of failure, paving the way for more effective approaches.

Most single parents first attempt to compensate for their family's executive understaffing within their nuclear family boundaries. This usually means that established roles and generational boundaries relax as older children assume parenting and homemaking duties. The disadvantages of this approach are that the parent often neglects such traditional parenting functions as limit-setting, nurturance, and advice-giving, making it harder for the children to complete developmental tasks. In some families, however, this situation can lead to maturity and a closeness between parent and child that each treasures and respects. Nursing assessment of any SPFHC should include a developmental assessment of all the children. Studying the social development of the older siblings can provide the data needed to discuss the situation with the entire family, assess its impact, and indicate needed changes.

If individual role accommodation alone cannot restore family equilibrium, extended family members may help out; it is not unusual to find a grandparent involved and often living with such families. Therefore nursing practice must focus on the extended family unit. The social and financial support the grandparent can bring to the family must be assessed in relation to the additional responsibilities and stresses on the extended family. The situation must be viewed from the family's cultural norm. The nurse assessing a SPFHC should determine the extent and helpfulness of the family's social support network. The family stress level is another important consideration. Realistically, it may be impossible to affect the network's extent, but it is possible to increase its helpfulness and its ability to reduce family stress.

The SPFHC will also use health care and social services more often in attempting to fulfill executive role functions. It is unreasonable to expect such families to fulfill their obligations as clients the way TPFHCs do. For example, the rate of visits to pediatricians for emotional and behavioral problems is higher for SPFs, as is the referral rate (Goldberg et al., 1984).

Social stigma and isolation. Single parents often complain of social isolation and loneliness. Social interaction requires time and energy, and these are rare commodities for single parents. Consciously or unconsciously, many of them decide to give priority to their children's needs, and limit opportunities to meet their own social needs. Such parents should realize that meeting their own needs for social inter- course and support will enhance their parenting abilities. The nurse can awaken the parent to these unconscious decisions and provide informa- tion on self-help groups, recreational, and support groups; she can also encourage brainstorming that might enhance the meaning and value of existing social interactions. SPFHCs are more likely to develop new friends than to rely on old friends as their families dramatically change (Ogden, 1975).

The nurse can also help reduce the social stigma that may accompany SPFHC status. As a professional and authority figure, the nurse's interactions with other people and services on behalf of the family will set the tone. Labels like "broken home" are clearly inappropriate. One discusses these families with others in relation to the issues at hand; prefacing such discussions by saying, "This is a single-parent family" or "This is a handicapped child family" is clearly inappropriate. The best strategy is to focus on the individual(s) and family first, and then on the relevant factors, which may or may not include the number of parents in the home or the health status of one of the children.

Reduced financial status. Female-headed single-parent families are likely to have incomes insufficient to meet family needs. The financial drain associated with housing, transporting, and supplying medical services to a handicapped child further strains meager resources. The nurse can direct such families to specialized resources and services for the child, and maximize their usefulness. Governmental and private income sup- plementation programs may be needed, and assistance with obtaining job training or paying for day-care might enable a mother to improve her financial situation. Counseling on family budgeting could also ease the impact of the problem.

The importance of careful attention to financial matters is illustrated in Figure 8.2. Low income is associated with additional problems no matter how many parents are in the home; since most SPFHCs have lower incomes they will most likely have more problems. The intervening variable is probably family stress.

Child rearing. The author knows of no evidence that SPFHCs' child- rearing attitudes or behaviors differ from those of any other family. Her (Ogden, 1975) study found no differences in parenting attitudes be- tween mothers in SPFHCs and TPFHCs; however, mothers not having a second parent with whom to share their burdens, especially those with a handicapped child, are more concerned about their sole responsibility for child rearing. This heightened role awareness can lead to greater parental understanding. A nurse can aid by offering books, counseling, or courses on child rearing and managing children with problems.

Single mothers with a disabled child do not differ from married mothers in their perceptions of the amount of time required for child care or in the nature or handling of problems between the disabled child and siblings. However, the single women do have lower educational expectations for their disabled child. Furthermore, their disabled children (matched for severity of handicap) are more likely to be in special schools and classrooms. The single mothers favor these schools and classes because they provide better services beyond education, such as free door-to-door transportation and school lunches, which enable the mother to spend more time with the other children or to work.

Figure 8.2   Relationships Between Income and Number of Problem Areas Reported by Single- and Two-Parent Families with Handicapped Children

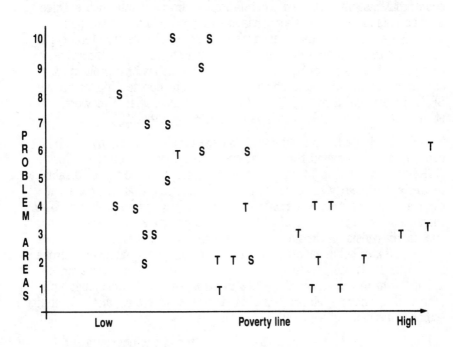

S = Single-parent family

T = Two-parent family

n = 15

Source: Ogden, 1975.

There is a small but growing body of research (Vadasy et al., 1984) on the siblings of handicapped children. The handicapped child's needs and the mother's concerns can easily overshadow those of the siblings. The normal developmental needs of the older female sibling are of particular concern. Some evidence suggests, however, that sibling involvement in day-to-day care and planning for the handicapped child benefits the entire family.

A wide range of family dynamics relating to the normal sibling may be in place, so the nurse must collect data carefully from the sibling(s) as well as parents and, if indicated, from others such as teachers. Boyle's (1985) recent work contains an excellent interview guide and analysis for siblings.

Emotional, school, and health problems in both handicapped and normal children. Most children in SPFHCs function within acceptable limits. Still, a slightly higher percentage of them will display health, developmental, school, or behavior problems than will children of TPFs. These two types of families are *not* comparable, however, in many of the other sociodemographic factors—such as income—that are linked to such problems, so statistical correlations emerging from such studies may be biased, if these other variables are not taken into account. If one is cautious and uses research findings not to justify stereotyping, but rather to heighten awareness of risk, it is helpful to summarize these variables. Accidents, particularly burns, behavioral problems, school problems, and child abuse have all been reported higher among SPFs (Libber and Stayton, 1984; Goldberg et al., 1984; Wadsworth et al., 1983, 1984, 1985; Guidubaldi and Perry, 1984).

There is also a body of literature on the problems faced by handicapped children beyond those that stem from their disabilities. Pless's (1983) review of this literature revealed that the severity of disability relates curvilinearly to psychosocial consequences; that is, those with the least *and* most severe disabilities tend to have more severe problems than those with moderate disabilities. This phenomenon, rather than specific diagnosis, is the more important psychosocial factor. The increased risk of behavior problems among handicapped siblings is probably 1.5 to 2.5 times greater than that of normal siblings. However, it is important to remember that 70% to 80% of these handicapped children will *not* have such problems. Moderate to severe cosmetic disability seems to be more of a problem for girls than for boys.

Finally, family stress appears to be a factor in the developmental progress of children in all families—single- and two–parent, with and without a handicapped child (see Figure 8.3). Stress does seem to be more of a factor with normal than with handicapped children, for whom the disability itself has an effect (Burke, 1978).

Figure 8.3 Differences in Children's Developmental Quotients by Family Type

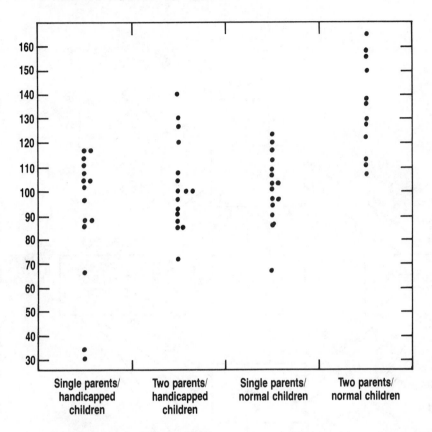

Family assessment model. The author has developed an assessment model that might improve nursing practice with SPFHCs. It has been applied to SPFs (Burke and Mensah, 1985) and to handicapped children (Burke, in press a and b); it is presented here as applied to SPFHCs (see Figure 8.4). The model's theoretical underpinnings are detailed in earlier publications.

No order of events is implied. The solid lines represent major directions of relationships. Since the model is an open system, the constructs are most often interactional, i.e., affecting each other; thus the total effect within the system is a unique combination of individual cell and interactive effects. The weaker relationships are represented by dotted rather than solid lines (Burke and Mensah, 1985).

Risk factors. The risk factors illustrated in the model are (a) the single parent, (b) childhood disability, and (c) SPFHC status. Of course, these are not the only risks; any long-term family or individual situation

Figure 8.4   A Family Assessment Model: Single-Parent Families with Handicapped Children

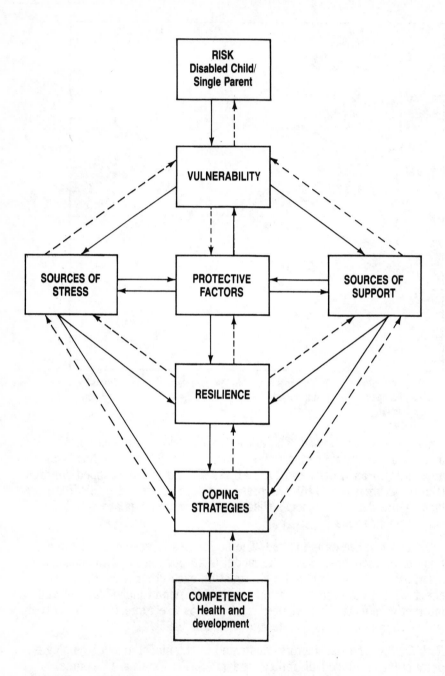

Sources: Burke, 1985; Burke and Mensah, 1985.

could increase relative vulnerability. For example, both chronic poverty (Garmezy, 1976) and chronic mental illness (Anthony, 1974) have demonstrated this effect.

Risk factors can be assessed through use of stressful life events questionnaires or open-ended interview questions such as, "Most families have ongoing problems; what would you say yours are?"

Vulnerability, resilience, and competence. The model does not view the closely interrelated concepts of vulnerability, resilience, and competence as absolute states or traits. Rather, relative vulnerability is the most stable and competence the most variable.

Vulnerability can be identified only indirectly, through observation of health or developmental outcomes or competences. It can be defined conceptually as conscious or unconscious perceptions of hazard and of relative capacity for dealing with challenging events, situations, or environments (adapted from Burke, 1980; Burke and Wiskin, 1983; Clarke and Driever, 1983; Burke and Mensah, 1985; Burke, 1985). Since vulnerability is an emerging concept, agreement in the nursing literature remains elusive.

Among SPFHCs, high vulnerability is characterized by difficulty coping with predictable stresses and everyday situations, as well as with major crises. Highly vulnerable families and individuals feel that their coping mechanisms are inadequate (adapted from Clarke and Driever, 1983; Burke and Mensah, 1985).

Most SPFHC families and their members display vulnerability. Few nurses will encounter clients with lowered vulnerability, whom Garmezy (1976) has termed "invulnerable." The proportion of invulnerable SPFHCs is not known, but in view of other risk populations 10% to 15% seems a reasonable estimate. These families thrive on the challenges of stressful life events. See Burke and Wiskin (1983) for a review of studies of invulnerability. They consider their coping mechanisms to be superior and expect to react competently (adapted from Clarke and Driever, 1983; Burke and Mensah, 1985).

Relative resilience is defined conceptually as consistent response to stress and support. Assessment of families' relative vulnerability and resilience is based on open-ended interview questions based on the definition in the previous paragraphs.

Competence is defined conceptually as the behavioral manifestation of the interplay between stress, support, and protective factors. It reflects the ability to bounce back from stressful events and to use support sources effectively in a wide range of domains. Werner and Smith (1982) describe competent people as those who work well, play well, love well, and expect well. Although competence fluctuates and has predictable, especially developmental, shifts, it shows considerable consistency over time. Competence is multidimensional—both domain–specific and global—and includes health and development. It guides nursing actions.

Two competence assessment tests currently in use are Achenbach and Edelbrock's (1983) Child Behavior Checklist and Harter's (1985) Self-Perception Profile for Children.

Sources of stress. Stress can be defined as disequilibrating events requiring change or adaptation. It is not simply a checklist of individual events. The impact of the stresses and crises affecting SPFHCs—death, separation, divorce, adoption, unmarried motherhood, diagnosis, relapse, social stigma—are considered part of the construct of stress. These individuals and families often (but not always) experience increased, often unfamiliar, stresses. Although such cumulative stresses are commonly associated with illness (Cassell, 1975; Sarason et al., 1979), most recent thinking discounts the notion of cumulative events exclusively leading to higher levels of general stress, and points to more specific and idiosyncratic individual effects (Rutter, 1983). Burns (1984) provides a good overview of the stress of hospitalization for the single-parent family.

Major stressful events or crises may have predictable phases, although supporting research evidence of this remains controversial. Studies have been performed on grief over the death of a spouse (Williams, 1979), the childhood developmental implications of parental divorce (Wallerstein, 1983), and living with a handicapped child (Blacher, 1984). Knowledge of these phases allows the nurse to give both parents and children anticipatory guidance.

Evidence that indicates a curvilinear relationship between the number of stresses and favorable treatment outcomes might apply to SPFHC nursing. Studies of relative stress levels associated with family problems have concluded that subjects reporting only a few stresses seemed to display overall resilience in facing problems (Werner and Smith, 1982; Pless, 1983).

The same schedule of stressful life events used to assess risk factors can help the nurse evaluate overall stress levels. A procedural modification of these schedules called the Visual Life Events Schedule (VLES) provides a method of retrospective examination of clusters of stressful events and their impact and meaning to the family over a period of as long as 10 years (Burke, in press, a; tool available on request from Burke).

Protective factors. Protective factors are individual or family characteristics which buffer stress effects; their mechanisms are not always clear. Numerous protective factors (problem-solving skills, high self-esteem, and willingness to take calculated risks) noted in the literature on handicapped children have been validated (Burke and Wiskin, 1983). The author (1978) has also found hopefulness, and planning for the future to be instrumental in reducing family stress. The fact that developmental status also affects stress management abilities reemphasizes the importance of doing developmental assessments on all children in SPFHCs.

Sources of support. Sources of support are usually social, but can also be financial or environmental. All can buffer many stress effects (Lindblad-Goldberg and Duke, 1985; Dimond and Jones, 1983). Sources of support, like sources of stress, are highly situational and individual; in other words, what helps one SPFHC may not help another. Nevertheless, some generalizations have emerged. For example, their own mothers are an important resource for child care and other aspects of family functioning. Single-parent groups of "Big Brothers"–type groups are also important in some SPFHC situations. People who had previously been "joiners" continued to use this avenue of support; those with no history of group membership were unlikely to use this coping approach (Burke, 1978).

For the child, the parent is a key source of support. Werner and Smith (1982) note that early and stable involvement of grandparents also affects the development of resilience in children. Siblings are another potential supportive factor. Nurses can aid in the development and maintenance of all these relationships.

Children whose fathers are actively involved in their SPF upbringing, and those whose mothers are "in transition" on the single-parent family continuum (that is, who are involving a new partner in child rearing), tend to make slightly better developmental progress. Conversely, an inaccessible, rejecting, or hostile custodial parent can do more harm developmentally than one who is absent altogether. The key elements in normal childhood development appear to be family function, parental support, and the long-term stability of the home (Burke, 1978); the term "islands of stability" was coined to denote these stabilizing elements amid apparent stress (Burke and Wiskin, 1983).

The Family Systems Strain Schedule (Burke, 1980) and the Family APGAR (Smilkstein et al., 1982) are among the many tools for assessing family function. The sources and effectiveness of social support can be measured using such instruments as the Norbeck Social Support Scale (Norbeck et al., 1981). Caldwell and Bradley's (1980) HOME is also valuable for assessing support.

Coping. Coping is defined conceptually as conscious and unconscious action-oriented or intrapsychic efforts to manage environmental and internal demands and conflicts, including those exceeding personal or familial resources. Coping approaches vary over time, situation, and context (Lazarus and Launier, 1978; Ritchie et al., 1983; Burke and Mensah, 1985). The conceptual structure of coping is generating much interest and some assessment tools are emerging (Jalowiec and Powers, 1981; McCubbin et al., 1983; Ritchie et al., 1983).

Planning

The nurse's goals in working with SPFHCs evolve directly from the model just described. They are (Burke and Mensah, 1985):
* Reduce or minimize risk factors
* Reduce sources of stress
* Maximize protective factors
* Facilitate development/use of effective support sources.

A COMPOSITE "CASE STUDY"

This composite picture of an SPFHC is based on two of the author's studies, in which a total of 30 SPFHC mothers, 30 mothers raising similarly handicapped children in two-parent families, and 30 mothers of all normal children (15 SPF and 25 TPF) were interviewed. The families resided in Toronto, Canada, and were selected by random and by matching. Two- to four-hour interviews were conducted utilizing both open-ended and structured questions, as well as questionnaires. Community health nurses who knew the children and families provided additional information.

Most of the single mothers were separated or divorced, but a few were unmarried or widowed. The children had medical diagnoses of cerebral palsy and related diseases (50%), spina bifida and/or hydrocephalus (about 25%), muscular dystrophy and other neuromuscular diseases (about 12.5%), and other physical handicaps (the final 12.5%). All had been diagnosed at least one year before the interviews. In general, the children's medical diagnoses seemed less important in presenting developmental status than did family management of the situation.

In general, the single mothers reported more areas of concern and rated these concerns as more severe than did the married mothers. Parenting attitudes did not differ between the groups of mothers. The financial situation among the single-parent families was much worse than for the two-parent families and seemed closely related to the number of reported problems (see Figure 8.1); SPFHC housing was generally inferior as was the group's day-care access and use. Single mothers relied more on grandmothers and neighbors for alternate childcare because it is less expensive; interestingly, however, when matched for age and severity of their child's handicap, SPFHC mothers were more likely to feel that they could leave their child unattended and for longer periods of time.

SPFHC mothers did not differ noticeably from TPFHC mothers in reported personal health, frequency of going out, closeness to friends, use of parent support groups or associations, or perceived closeness to their own parents. There were differences at more specific levels, however. Both groups cited "nerves" as their most common health problem, but only single mothers (20% of the sample) reported using tranquilizers to cope with it. SPFHC mothers also reported being closest to relatively new friends, whereas TPFHC mothers tended to be closer to friends of longer standing.

Looking back to when they first learned of their child's handicap, single women were more likely to think that the father had misgivings about his ability to handle the situation; many of the divorced mothers recalled their former husbands either blaming them for "getting the measles on purpose," behaving as if the child's condition was a "living death," or withdrawing and staying away most of the time. The married women also reported intense shock, disappointment, and guilt among their husbands at the child's diagnosis, but they also offered such explanations as "it's harder for a man to accept." Interestingly, the groups of mothers were divided equally on whether or not having a handicapped child interfered with their relationships with men.

As the women reflected on the relative merits of marriage, those in SPFHCs answered in terms of relieving parental responsibility and having help with discipline and child care. Several of these now single women said, "It's better for me to do it alone," or words to that effect. In contrast, the married women usually spoke of marriage in terms of emotional support and companionship; several volunteered that they could not raise a family on their own.

When asked what made them especially happy at this time in their lives, the single women primarily alluded to their motherhood roles, while the married women's answers related primarily to the role of wife, and only secondly to that of mother.

The presence of a handicapped child in a family proved associated with high levels of familial strain and lowered developmental outcomes in normal siblings.

Single parenthood seems associated with slightly lowered developmental outcomes in two ways: direct influence on the child and high familial strain. The number of parents in the home is probably more accurately described as a continuous rather than a dichotomous variable. Children in transitional single-parent families, that is, those progressing toward two-parent status, exhibit fewer negative developmental effects than children whose SPFs have no such hopes or plans (see Figure 8.3).

CONCLUSIONS

To summarize, nursing for SPFHC individuals and families should reflect assessment of the type of SPFHC, of any additional risks to health and development, and of stresses, supports, and protective factors. Provisional care for these families is usually so varied that only very large centers can support special SPFHC programs (Feldman et al., 1983). Thus, modifying nursing practice for these individuals and families will be based on the special risks and stresses highlighted in this chapter.

REFERENCES

Achenbach, T., and Edelbrock, C. *Manual for the Child Behavior Checklist and Revised Child Behavior Profile.* Burlington, Vt.: Department of Psychiatry, University of Vermont, 1983.

Anderson, J., and Ogden, S.L. "Twenty Fatherless Families," *Canadian Welfare* 51:14-15, 1975.

Anthony, E.J. "The Syndrome of the Psychologically Invulnerable Child," in *The Child in His Family: Children at Psychiatric Risk III.* Edited by Anthony, E.J., and Kaupernich, C. New York: John Wiley & Sons, 1974.

Baird, S.F. "Crisis Intervention Strategies," in *High Risk Parenting: Nursing Assessment and Strategies for Families at Risk.* Edited by Johnson, S.H. Philadelphia: J.B.Lippincott Co., 1979.

Blacher, J. *Severely Handicapped Young Children and Their Families: Research in Review.* Orlando, Fla.: Academic Press, 1984.

Boyle, I. "Siblings of Disabled Children: Perceptions of Interfamilial Relationships," Unpublished masters thesis. Halifax, Nova Scotia: Dalhousie University, 1985.

Burke, S.O. "Developmental Risk and Competence in Children," *Canadian Journal of Public Health* (in press, a).

Burke, S.O. "Familial Strain and the Development of Normal and Handicapped Children in Single- and Two-Parent Families," Unpublished doctoral dissertation. Toronto: University of Toronto, 1978.

Burke, S.O. "Helping One-Parent Families Cope," *Canadian Nurse* 79(10): 33-37, 1983.

Burke, S.O. "The Invulnerable Child," *Nursing Papers,* 12:42-43, 48-54, 1980.

Burke, S.O. "Resilience, Vulnerability, and Risk in Children: A Conceptual Model." *Proceedings of the National Nursing Research Conference.* Toronto: University of Toronto Press (in press, b).

Burke, S.O., and Mensah, L.M. "Single Parents and Their Children: Individual, Family, and Aggregate Level Care," *Community Health Nursing in Canada.* Edited by Stewart, M. Toronto: Gage Publishing, 1985.

Burke, S.O., and Wiskin, N. "Invulnerable Handicapped Children: Clinician Validation of Characteristics and Amenability to Change," *Nursing Papers* (Special Supplement) October 12-14, 1983.

Burns, C.E. "The Hospitalization Experience and Single-Parent Families," *Nursing Clinics of North America* 19:285-93, 1984.

Caldwell, B.N., and Bradley, R.H. *Home Observation for Measurement of the Environment.* Little Rock: University of Arkansas, 1980.

Cassell, J. "Social Science in Epidemiology: Psychosocial Processes and the 'Stress' Theoretical Formulation," in *Handbook of Evaluation Research,* vol. 1. Edited by Strevening, E.L., and Guttentag, M. Beverly Hills, Calif.: Sage Publications, 1975.

Census of Canada (1981). *Census of Families in Private Households: Selected Characteristics.* Ottawa: Statistics Canada, 1983.

Chinn, P.L., and Jacobs, M.R. *Theory and Nursing: A Systematic Approach.* St. Louis, C.V. Mosby Co., 1983.

Clarke, H.F., and Driever, M.J. "Vulnerability: The Development of a Construct for Nursing," in *Advances in Nursing Theory Development*. Edited by Chinn, P.L. Rockville, Md.: Aspen Systems Corp., 1983.

Critchley, D.L. "The Child as Patient: Assessing the Effects of Family Stress and Disruption on the Mental Health of the Child," *Perspectives in Psychiatric Care* 19:144-55, 1981.

Dimond, M., and Jones, S.L. "Social Support: A Review and Theoretical Integration," in *Advances in Nursing Theory Development*. Edited by Chinn, P.L. Rockville, Md.: Aspen Systems Corp., 1983.

Feldman, W.S., et al. "A Behavioral Parent Training Program for Single Mothers of Physically Handicapped Children," *Child: Care, Health and Development* 9: 157-68, 1983.

Garmezy, N. "Stressors of Childhood," in *Stress, Coping and Development in Children*. Edited by Garmezy, N., and Rutter, M. New York: McGraw-Hill Book Co.,1983.

Garmezy, N. "Vulnerable and Invulnerable Children: Theory, Research and Intervention," *Catalog of Selected Documents in Psychology* 6:96, 1976.

Goldberg, I.D., et al."Mental Health Problems Among Children Seen in Pediatric Practice: Relevance and Management," *Pediatrics* 73:278-92, 1984.

Guidubaldi, J., and Perry, J.D. "Divorce, Socioeconomic Status, and Children's Cognitive-Social Competence at School Entry," *American Journal of Orthopsychiatry* 54:459-68, 1984.

Harter, S. *Manual for the Self-Perception Profile for Children (Revision of The Perceived Competence Scale for Children)*. Denver: University of Denver Press, 1985.

Hughes, C.B., and Scoloveno, M.A. "The Single Father," *Topics in Clinical Nursing* 6:1-9, 1984.

Jalowiec, J., and Powers, M.J. "Stress and Coping in Hypertensive and Emergency Room Patients," *Nursing Research* 30(1):10-16, 1981.

Johnson, S.H. *High-Risk Parenting: Nursing Assessment and Strategies for Families at Risk*. Philadelphia: J.B. Lippincott Co., 1979.

Kalnins, I.V. "Cross-Illness Comparison of Separation and Divorce Among Parents Having a Child with a Life-Threatening Illness," *Children's Health Care* 12: 72-77, 1983.

Kazak, A.E., and Linney, J.A. "Stress, Coping, and Life Change in the Single-Parent Family," *American Journal of Community Psychology* 11:207-20, 1983.

Kelly, J.B., and Wallerstein, J.S. "Brief Interventions with Children in Divorcing Families," *American Journal of Orthopsychiatry* 47:23-39, 1977.

Kessler, S. *The American Way of Divorce*. New York: Nelson-Hall, 1975.

Lazarus, R.S., and Launier, R. "Stress-Related Transactions Between Persons and Environment," in *Perspectives in Interactional Psychology*. Edited by Pervin, L.A., and Lavis, M. New York: Plenum Press, 1978.

Lazarus, R.S. "The Stress and Coping Paradigm," in *Competence and Coping During Adulthood*. Edited by Bond, L.A., and Rosen, J.C. Hanover, N.H.: University Press of New England, 1980.

Libber, S.M., and Stayton, D.J. "Childhood Burns Reconsidered: The Child, Family, and the Burn Injury," *Journal of Trauma* 24:245-52, 1984.

Lindblad-Goldberg, M., and Duke, J.L. "Social Support in Black, Low-Income, Single-Parent Families: Normative and Dysfunctional Patterns," *American Journal of Orthopsychiatry* 55:(1):42-58, 1985.

McCubbin, H.I., et al. CHIP—Coping Health Inventory For Parents: An Assessment of Parental Coping Patterns in the Care of the Chronically Ill Child," *Journal of Marriage and the Family* 45:359-70, 1983.

McLanahan, S.S. "Family Structure and Stress: A Longitudinal Comparison of Two-Parent and Female-Headed Families," *Journal of Marriage and the Family* 2:347-57, 1983.

Newacheck, P.W., et al. "Trends in Childhood Disability," *American Journal of Public Health* 74: 230-36,1984.

Norbeck, J.S., et al. "The Development of an Instrument to Measure Social Support," *Nursing Research* 30:264-69, 1981.

Ogden, S.L. "Single and Dual Parents with Handicapped Children: Expressed Concerns, Coping Behaviors, and Attitudes Toward Child Rearing," Unpublished master's thesis. Toronto: University of Toronto, 1975.

Pless, I. "Adjustment of the Young Chronically Ill," *Research in Community and Mental Health* 1:61-85, 1979.

Pless, I.B. "Effects of Chronic Illness on Adjustment: Clinical Implications," in *Advances in Behavioral Medicine for Children and Adolescents*. Edited by Firestone, P., et al. Hillsdale, N.J.: Lawrence Erlbaun Assoc., 1983.

Ritchie, J.A., et al. "Coping in Preschool Hospitalized Children: Toward the Development of an Observation Instrument," *Nursing Papers* (Special supplement) October 12-14, 1983.

Rutter, M. "Stress, Coping and Development: Some Issues and Some Questions," in *Stress, Coping, and Development in Children*. Edited by Garmezy, N., and Rutter, M. New York: McGraw-Hill Book Co., 1983.

Sarason, I.G., et al. "Assessing the Impact of Life Changes," in *Stress and Anxiety*. Edited by Sarason, I.G., and Spellbury, C.S. New York: John Wiley & Sons, 1979.

Smilkstein, G., et al."Validity and Reliability of the Family: APGAR as a Test of Family Function," *Journal of Family Practice* 15(2):303-11, 1982.

Tankson, E.A. "The Single Parent," in *High-Risk Parenting: Nursing Assessment and Strategies for Families at Risk*. Edited by Johnson, S.H. Philadelphia: J.B. Lippincott Co., 1979.

Todres, R. "Motherless Families," *Canadian Welfare* 51:11-13, 1975.

U.S. Bureau of the Census. *General Population Characteristics (1980): United States Summary*. Washington, D.C.: U.S. Department of Commerce, 1983.

Vadasy, P.F., et al."Siblings of Handicapped Children: A Developmental Perspective on Family Interactions," *Marriage* 33:155-67, 1984.

Wadsworth, J., et al."Family Type and Accidents in Preschool Children," *Journal of Epidemiology and Community Health* 37:100-04, 1983.

Wallerstein, J., and Kelly, J. *Surviving the Break-Up*. New York: Basic Books, 1980.

Weltner, J.S. "A Structural Approach to the Single-Parent Family," *Family Process* 203-10, 1982.

Werner, E.E., and Smith, R.S. *Vulnerable, But Invincible*. New York: McGraw-Hill Book Co., 1982.

Williams, J.C. "The Terminally Ill Parent," in *High-Risk Parenting: Nursing Assessment and Strategies for Families at Risk*. Edited by Johnson, S.H. Philadelphia: J.B. Lippincott Co., 1979.

Wright, E.N., and Dhanota, A.S. *The Grade Nine Student Survey: Fall 1980*. Toronto: Board of Education, 1981.

9 Assessing families of adolescents with Crohn's disease

Fabie Duhamel, RN, PhD
Private Practice
Calgary, Alberta, Canada

OVERVIEW

This chapter focuses on the family nursing assessment of an adolescent diagnosed as having Crohn's disease. The biophysical component of this health problem is discussed, as are the developmental tasks normally associated with adolescence. The reciprocal nature of the relationship between an adolescent's illness and the family is explained and assessed through a family nursing assessment model; the need for family involvement in the case of a chronically ill adolescent is further substantiated by a literature review. The case of a family whose adolescent has Crohn's disease illustrates two fundamental aspects of the nursing process: assessment and planning. A list of relationship questions is included to help the family nurse assess the impact of chronic illness on adolescents and their families as well as the impact of family dynamics on the course of the illness.

Throughout, the chapter emphasizes the unique challenges of nursing chronically ill adolescents, and is intended to help nurses understand the major issues that can influence the care they provide. Some of the salient questions addressed are: What impact does a chronic health problem have on the lives of adolescents and their families? How does chronic illness affect the relationship between adolescents and their families? And how does the family affect the course of an adolescent's illness?

NURSING PROCESS

Assessment

The health problem: Crohn's disease
Symptoms and effects. Crohn's disease, a chronic inflammation either of the lower small intestine or the colon, or of both simultaneously, was

first described and identified as a specific pathology by Crohn and colleagues (1932). The symptoms include diarrhea, abdominal pains, rectal bleeding, fever, and loss of appetite and weight, all varying in severity from mild to disabling. Sometimes the whole body can be affected. Disease evolution can be either very slow or quite rapid; the condition may lead to a narrowing and eventual obstruction of the intestinal wall. On occasion, the inflammation may spread to bladder, skin, or other organ surfaces, producing ulcerations often associated with the formation of fissures called fistulas. Banks and colleagues (1983) reported that poor nutrient absorption and reduced food intake due to Crohn's-related abdominal cramps may cause growth failure and slowed sexual maturation (e.g., delayed onset of menstruation or even temporary cessation of menses) in adolescents.

Incidence and etiology. Months or even years may be necessary to diagnose Crohn's disease correctly, because its slow insidious onset and vague symptoms are so similar to those of other illnesses. This inflammatory bowel disease is rarely diagnosed in infancy; it may be identified at five to seven years of age but is more frequently discovered at 10 to 18 years (Banks et al., 1983). The disease reaches its peak incidence among those aged 15 to 35. Both sexes are affected equally (Latimer, 1978). The past 20 years have seen a large increase in the number of adolescents with Crohn's disease. In the United States alone, 200,000 children under age 18 are victims of inflammatory bowel diseases (National Foundation for Ileitis and Colitis, 1985); the death rate from Crohn's disease ranges from 5% to 18%.

The cause and cure of Crohn's disease are still unknown, although etiologic factors have been identified. These include genetic makeup (15% to 30% of patients have a close or distant family member with Crohn's disease or ulcerative colitis), bacterial or viral infection, immunologic deficit, reaction to an irritant (coffee, spicy food, alcohol) and psychogenesis (Mendeloff, 1974).

Medical management and prognosis. The most common Crohn's disease treatment combines a balanced high-protein, high-calorie diet, anti-inflammatory drugs (sulfasalazine, corticosteroids), and symptomatic surgery for existing bowel obstruction, hemorrhage, or fistulas. These measures are impermanent, however, and some carry additional complications of their own. Anti-inflammatory medications, for instance, have systemic side effects with both physical and psychological impact: headaches, growth impairment, delayed sexual maturation, adrenal suppression, facial rounding, acne, increased appetite/weight gain, red marks on the skin, and increased body/facial hair for both sexes.

Crohn's disease patients can never consider themselves completely cured; even after 30 years of remission, symptoms may suddenly reappear (Strauch et al., 1980). Steinhauser and Kies (1982) state that emotional stress may aggravate the symptoms, precede exacerbation, and influence the evolution of the illness. This claim is based on the assumption that disruptive psychosocial events precipitate illness in a vulnerable and predisposed organ. However, it is important to acknowledge that the disability, physical and psychological discomfort, and psychosocial impact of such illnesses as Crohn's disease generate stress that can prompt recurrence.

Normal adolescent development

Developmental issues in adolescence. Adolescence begins with puberty and ends (generally 6 to 10 years later) with the emergence of a mature and self-sufficient adult. Chronologically, it may last from 12 to 22 years of age. Blumberg and colleagues (1984) and Hofman and colleagues (1976) have identified some of the main characteristics of this transitional period:

• Preoccupation with body image/physical appearance
• Development of new social (peer) relationships, greater involvement in educational, religious, and community institutions
• Attempts to define one's own sexual role, increased desire to be accepted by peers of both sexes and to explore relationships with the opposite sex
• Independence conflicts (ambivalence over individuation versus necessary dependence on parents)
• Development of self-esteem and inner controls.

Adolescence and family development. Parents may be confused by their adolescent's increasing need to function independently. As parents, they feel rejected when their child rebels, or feel they have failed if the child shows signs of increased family dependence (Chilman, 1968).

Families must balance the challenge of raising an adolescent with their own normal developmental tasks, such as midlife marital and career issues, and increasing concern for the older generation (Wright & Leahey, 1984). Parents and adolescents alike must adjust to new communication patterns and to increasing separation. This transition period is tremendously complicated by an illness as serious as Crohn's disease.

The chronically ill adolescent

Impact on the family. There have been many studies of the effects of chronic illness on family dynamics (Sabbeth, 1984; Venters, 1981; Bruhn, 1977). Both instrumental and emotional family functioning are seriously disrupted and require reorganization and adjustment. Shifting roles and the sharing of duties, domestic tasks, and caretaking responsibilities are among the most important potential instrumental changes. Family members can accomplish and adjust to these changes successfully if roles, rules, and relationships are flexible.

The sick adolescent consumes not only a great deal of time, energy, and money but also the family's emotional resources. Family members experience anger and resentment toward the illness and treatment; their fear and anxiety regarding the disease's course and prognosis are often compounded by the perceived need to hold those feelings in and protect the ill adolescent.

Families of adolescents with Crohn's disease find it difficult to adjust to their child's illness. Feelings of guilt arise from the possibility of genetic transmission, and may result in denial of disease seriousness and chronicity; indeed, many parents believe their child will outgrow the condition (Banks et al., 1983). Guilt regarding family members' anger and resentment are often masked by overprotectiveness toward the patient, which prevents the adolescent from utilizing existing strengths and instead fosters dependence (Malone, 1977; Abrams and Kaslow, 1976).

The adolescent may use his illness to manipulate other family members and obtain special privileges and attention; this can create additional stress. "Well" siblings can develop feelings of jealousy, frustration, anger, and underappreciation.

Seligman (1983) summarized the effects of handicapped children on their "normal" siblings:
• Anger, resentment, and guilt may develop among siblings given excessive responsibility for the sick child. Insensitive parents may reinforce these feelings.
• Poor intrafamily communication about the affected child's illness can contribute to loneliness among siblings. Family secrets and implicit rules force the members to avoid discussion, conflict resolution, and ventilation of negative feelings.
• Siblings may respond with warmth toward their sick brother or sister and gain from the experience.

Venters (1981) reported that chronic illness may encourage "togetherness" among family members. Sharing the burdens of illness, he found, sometimes serves as a coping strategy against the stress and hardship imposed by the illness.

Chronic illness may have an important impact on family interactive patterns:
• Hindering communication between the married couple (Kulczycki, 1969)
• Accentuating preexisting marital problems (Allan et al., 1974)
• Creating "close dyads" on the basis of dependence/responsibility
• Isolating some family members from each other (Cleveland, 1980).

For example, a mother often becomes overly involved with her sick child's care and decreases her investment in her marriage. Left on the periphery, the father feels ambiguous, confused about his family role and position.

Berdie (1981) proposes another role for the sick adolescent within an already troubled family. In this scenario, parents focus on the vulnerable third person to avoid dealing with marital conflict. The sick adolescent thus becomes a scapegoat; all family problems are blamed on the illness so that the family unit can be maintained by avoidance of direct confrontation over other conflicts (Vogel and Bell, 1960).

Sabbeth (1984) suggests that marital distress is more frequent in couples with chronically ill children than in couples with well children. Bruhn (1977) confirms the high breakdown rate in families facing chronic illness. Cleveland (1980), on the other hand, quoted parents of children with a chronic illness who did not feel their marriage was adversely affected by their child's health problem; they stated, however, that, because their plans would always depend on the child's life situation, they would never feel free of parenthood. In general, studies of families afflicted by chronic illness emphasize the psychosocial problems imposed by the hardship of the illness.

Family assessment model. Nurses can ease the impact of chronic illness on adolescent and family by conducting a thorough family assessment and facilitating the development of coping strategies. Wright and Leahey's (1984) family assessment framework, the Calgary Family Assessment Model (CFAM), helps nurses identify major family strengths and serious problems associated with chronic illness by assessing structural, developmental, and functional dimensions. Leahey and Wright (1984) also describe nine basic assumptions about families with chronic illness which may be useful in assessing such families (e.g., "Where there is a chronic illness, families must adjust to changes in expectation for each other" and "A family's perception of the illness event has the most influence upon their ability to cope").

Nurses should meet as many family members as possible and complete a family assessment. Clients and accompanying family members can be questioned during either medical treatment or short interviews following medical visits (see Table 9.1).

Table 9.1 Sample Questions for Assessing Families Managing an Adolescent's Crohn's Disease

- What is the greatest difference you have noticed in your family since your child was diagnosed as having Crohn's disease?
- Who in your family is most affected by your child's illness?
- How was the illness explained to you? (Ask each family member individually.)
- What is your understanding of how your child has Crohn's disease?

Planning

Families of adolescents with Crohn's disease must be assessed regularly because of the child's rapid physical and emotional development and its reciprocal effect on the rest of the household. Once strengths and problems have been delineated, the nurse should plan interventions at several levels (Leahey and Wright, 1984):

• Cognitive (e.g., educating about adolescence and/or Crohn's disease)
• Affective (facilitating expression of feelings)
• Behavioral (suggesting how to answer questions from peers or family members on certain aspects of the illness).

If a psychosocial problem beyond the nurse's expertise is identified, a family clinical nurse specialist (FCNS) might be called in. If no FCNS is available, clients should be referred to another health care professional skilled in working with families facing chronic illness.

CASE STUDY

Family Assessment

Structural. Rita Johnson, 14 years of age, was diagnosed at the age of 10 years as having Crohn's disease. Rita lives in an upper-middle-class family consisting of father, Claude, a 41-year-old businessman; mother, Mary, 40-year-old homemaker; oldest child, Joan, aged 16; and the two youngest children, Sandra and Mark, 12-year-old twins. A few months after the diagnosis, Rita underwent surgery to remove a bowel obstruction and she is currently taking anti-inflammatory medication. Because of growth failure Rita has the appearance of a 9- to 10-year-old child.

During one of Rita's visits to the outpatient Inflammatory Bowel Disease Clinic, a nurse met with the child's family members to assess the impact of Crohn's disease on all of them; the CFAM enabled the nurse to identify family strengths and problems and to plan nursing care. The structural assessment included questions aimed at clarifying the family's internal and external structures. (See Figures 9.1, 9.2, and 9.3.)

As the ecomap (Figure 9.2) indicates, the nurse identified positive relationships between health care professionals, both parents, and Rita. All of the children acknowledged doing well academically in school. Joan, Sandra, and Mark had also developed strong peer relationships; Rita had distanced herself from her friends. All family members seemed to get along well with both sets of grandparents. Rita was very close to her maternal grandparents, who also had inflammatory bowel diseases.

Developmental. Developmentally, the Johnsons had reached the "families with teenagers" stage (Wright and Leahey, 1984), and the nurse assessed how the family was accomplishing the appropriate developmental tasks.

Establishment of increased autonomy. Joan, the eldest child, was described by her parents as very responsible and becoming more and more independent because of strong peer affiliations. Nevertheless, she displayed some childish behaviors, often quarreling with Rita. Both parents acknowledged that Sandra and Mark were starting to rebel against family rules but respected their parents' discipline. Rita was described by her siblings as very dependent on her mother and often childish.

Refocusing on midlife marital and career issues. Claude and Mary Johnson appeared quite satisfied with their work and supported one another when confronting family issues.

Increasing concern for the older generation. Paternal and maternal grandparents alike were self-sufficient and visited the family regularly. Mary was a little concerned about her parents' health but acknowledged that both were managing their health care very well.

The attachment diagram (Figure 9.3) illustrates family members' emotional bonds.

Functional. Nurses must understand the effects of Crohn's disease on adolescent growth and development, and consider the mutual influence of the adolescent and the social network (family and peers). "In their search for competence and balance, adolescents are responsive to the shaping influences and demands of their social environment at the same time as they are a vital shaping part of their environment" (Solnit, 1983). Consequently, the interactions between the ill adolescent and his family can significantly influence disease evolution.

Figure 9.1   Genogram—The Johnson Family

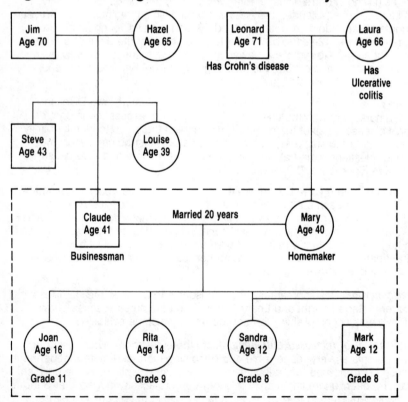

Figure 9.2 Ecomap—The Johnson Family

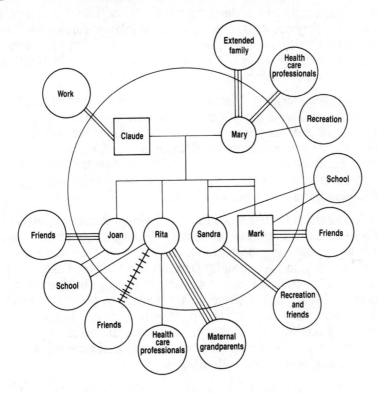

Figure 9.3 Attachment Diagram—The Johnson Family

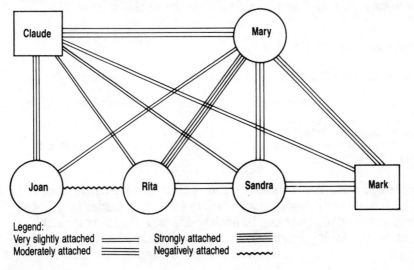

Legend:
Very slightly attached ══════ Strongly attached ═══
Moderately attached ══════ Negatively attached ～～～

The Impact of Crohn's Disease on Adolescents and Families

Illness and disability are better integrated into individual and family routines when they are congenital or begin in infancy. Adolescence is a traumatic time for a major illness to appear. Disability interferes with the acquisition of a positive body image, with sexual maturation, and with peer acceptance.

Body image. Adolescents are fearful about any bodily disruption or change. They tend to be hypersensitive, overreacting to any threat to the integrity of their body image, and display exaggerated perceptions of anatomical and biophysical insults (Hofman et al., 1976). Adolescent patients conceptualize illness in terms of its affect on their body image, rather than of what they have learned about the disease through educational programs (Hofman et al., 1976).

Any illness that affects an adolescent's feelings of physical attractiveness generates a great deal of anxiety. A comparative study revealed that a visibly disfiguring disability with a slight physical handicap was more socially and vocationally devastating to afflicted adolescents than an invisible congenital defect causing severe physical limitation (Goldberg, 1984). Crohn's disease delays adolescent physical growth, interfering with the acquisition of a positive body image. In the case example, Rita was fearful of being different from her peers, especially of retaining a child's bodily appearance. Her sense of personal worth and her self-confidence were both affected.

Some nurses find it helpful to avoid eye contact when asking adolescents questions. Also, when an adolescent refuses to answer a family interviewer's question, it may help to ask other family members how the adolescent might answer. It is interesting and informative to observe the adolescent's verbal and nonverbal reaction to this interviewing tactic.

Assessment questions:
(To the family)
• How do you think Crohn's disease affects Rita? How do you think she copes with it?
• What differences do you notice in Rita's personality since her diagnosis?
(To Rita)
• Who worries the most about your growth failure?
• What was explained to you about your growth failure and what it means to you now and in the future?

Sexual maturation. An adolescent's poor self-image may derive from lack of sexual identity, which can promote feelings of inadequacy. These feelings could intensify among ill adolescents who realize that their interest in developing heterosexual relationships is less than that of their peers. The adolescent patient's sense of dignity may also be affected if those in the environment (e.g., family, peers, health professionals), treat her like a child, or if bodily privacy is violated by health care professionals at a time of increased modesty (McCallum, 1981).

Family members acknowledged that Rita displayed childlike behaviors and that she avoided opportunities to meet peers of both sexes. Rita complained that a lot of people treated her like a 10-year-old because of her growth failure.

Assessment questions:
(To Rita)
• Do any of your friends have a boyfriend? Are they interested in having boyfriends? What about you?
• Do you prefer friends of your own age, or older, or younger?

Independence. Like any illness, Crohn's disease interferes with an adolescent's striving for independence, which is the most challenging task of that life stage. Medical treatment, parental overprotectiveness, and physical disability all reinforce dependence while diminishing any sense of self-control over health. Intense parental or professional supervision of the medical regimen (diet, lifestyle, medication) may be interpreted as "nagging" or as a lack of trust in the adolescent's judgment; this may arouse feelings of resentment and chronic anxiety about personal safety (McCallum, 1981). The sick adolescent may often face the need for autonomy with ambivalence and be tempted to abdicate responsibilities, regressing to a state of infantile dependence (Hofman et al., 1976). Parents may even promote their child's dependence to maintain meaning and identity in their family roles.

The chronically ill adolescent may also increase personal dependence and craving for the family's emotional support because of social isolation and/or discomfort arising from low self-esteem, poorly defined sexual identity and lack of confidence. Consequently the parents may experience frustration or exaggerated anxiety regarding the adolescent's future vocational, social, and emotional functioning (Todd and Satz, 1980).

Interactions between parents and their ill adolescent may exhibit a maladaptive circular communication pattern (Wright and Leahey, 1984). Often, it is difficult for parents to distinguish normal adolescent behaviors from those related to illness or treatment. The uncertainty prevents them from determining an appropriate degree of autonomy for their child, ultimately inhibiting the adolescent's knowledge of adult roles and responsibilities.

While some adolescents use a health problem as an excuse to return to childlike dependence, most want to share responsibility for their care (Schowalter, 1983). Success in independent self-care requires social support (e.g., parents willing to relinquish their responsibility) and the adolescent's physical and emotional readiness to assume care management. The adolescent who successfully assumes this responsibility will regain feelings of adequacy and competence (Gwinn, 1984).

Nurses should consider adolescent attitudes of experimentation with treatment, rebellion, or independence as necessary aspects of development and striving for identity and autonomy.

Assessment questions:

(To the family)
● How does your daughter get along with the health professionals handling her case? Do you think she should be making decisions about her care with the health care professionals, with you as parents, or both?
● Do you think you should do more or less for Rita because of her illness?
● What does your mother do or say when your sister Rita behaves like a child?
● Who feels the most responsible for Rita's medication? Who calls to make doctor's appointments?
● What do you think your sister Rita says to herself when your mother nags her about her medication?
(To Rita)
● Do you think that your parents should do more for you or less because of your illness?
● How are your parents involved in your medical treatment?

Figure 9.4 illustrates the maladaptive pattern that developed between Rita and her parents.

Figure 9.4 Maladaptive Parent-Child Communication— Rita and Mary Johnson

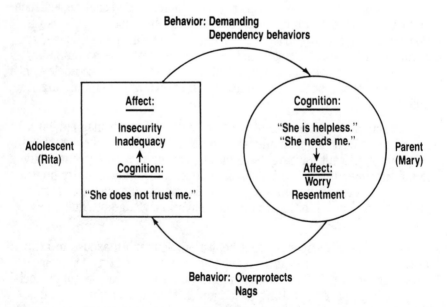

Need for peer acceptance. Peer relationships are significant in adolescent management of dependence-independence conflicts with parents. To facilitate individuation and separation, the adolescent needs a sense of belonging to a supportive peer group. A chronic illness may jeopardize this developmental stage. As noted earlier in the structural assessment, Rita neither belonged to a peer group nor had any close friends.

Growth failure in Crohn's disease can be particularly stressful for the adolescent, who may fear being ridiculed or rejected by taller age mates. Often the peer group shows discomfort and has difficulty relating to anyone who appears different or abnormal (Hofman et al., 1976).

Crohn's disease patients also often require hospitalization, resulting in school absenteeism and further isolation from peers. This may produce fear, anxiety, and withdrawal.

Assessment questions:
(To the family)
• How does Rita handle her illness with her friends?
(To Rita)
• Who explained your illness to your friends? How did they react?
• How does your illness affect your friends' behavior toward you now?
• Do you feel accepted by your friends?
• How do you think you would react if one of your friends had a chronic illness? How would you have reacted if you were not ill yourself?

Chronic illness may be devastating to the adolescent's sense of bodily integrity and personal worth. Fears of rejection, of dependence, and of pain and death generate tremendous anxiety, and delay adjustment to illness; social support can facilitate effective coping and attainment of positive health status (Janis, 1983).

The Impact of Family Dynamics on the Adolescent's Chronic Illness

Parents' reactions to an adolescent's illness, as well as their beliefs and expectations, influence all their children, but especially the sick teenager. As Daniel (1977, p. 116) has said, "How parents meet the demand for care, emotional and financial support, and alteration of their own lifestyle may be crucial in the recovery or adaptation of the adolescent to the disability."

Parental and sibling reactions (e.g., overprotectiveness or minimization of the ailment's seriousness) may generate anger and dependence in the sick adolescent. Manipulative behaviors or signs of depression may appear in response. This interaction impedes physical and emotional adjustment to illness.

The family can also covertly or overtly affect the adolescent's interest in treatment (Berdie, 1981). Parent-child conflict for instance, might discourage adherence to the treatment regimen or even impede metabolic control. On the other hand, positive family and peer support can raise the adolescent's self-esteem, facilitating compliance (Schowalter, 1983).

A nurse should understand how family interaction patterns can perpetuate an adolescent's chronic symptoms. The illness may serve to maintain homeostasis in a family challenged by a covert dysfunctional relationship or by stressful change—including the normal changes associated with adolescence. For example, the separation anxiety that accompanies adolescent tasks of seeking independence and leaving home can be powerful enough to exacerbate chronic symptoms (Schowalter, 1983).

In Rita's case, the following questions were asked to help clarify family dynamics.

Table 9.2 Results of the Johnson Family Assessment and Proposed Interventions

Systems	Strengths	Problems
Professional and whole family systems	Very good rapport between the family and health care professionals.	
Whole family system	Ability of most family members to adjust to the impact of their adolescent's illness.	
Marital system	Emotional support between both spouses in regard to their daughter's illness.	
Parent-child system		Mother is overresponsible for Rita's treatment; encourages Rita's overdependency. In turn, mother assumes more responsibility (see Figure 9.4).
Sibling sub-system		A maladaptive circular communication pattern between Rita and her oldest sister Joan (see Figure 9.5).
Individual		Rita's low self-esteem

Assessment questions:

(To the family)
- Is there anything that seems to aggravate Rita's symptoms? Do you think stress could be a contributing factor? If so, what seems to cause her particular stress or anxiety?
- Who worries most about Rita's condition? How do they show it?
- When there is a sick child in the family, parents are usually more attentive to this child. How does it work in your family? Does Rita get more attention than her siblings? What happens when one of the siblings is ill?
- Is anyone jealous of Rita because her parents are sometimes easier on her?
- Among all of the children, who is the most patient with Rita? Who is the least? How do you show it?
- How different is your family from other families who do not have a member with Crohn's disease?
- Has Crohn's disease had a positive impact on your family? Negative? What are the most positive and negative aspects of Rita's disease for the family as a whole?

(To Rita)
- How does each family member react to you when your symptoms are worse than usual?

Interventions
Normalize the different difficulties that the family may have presented adjusting to Rita's illness. Praise each family member for their coping abilities.
Praise the couple for their sensitivity to each other's emotional needs and the support they provide each other.
Reduce dependence between Rita and her mother, thereby allowing Rita more autonomy and independence in assuming her health care management.
Give Joan specific responsibilities in Rita's care; encourage Rita to ask her sister's advice regarding peer relationships and different ways to appear older despite her growth failure.
Identify and praise Rita's strengths: e.g., successful school performance despite her illness. Assist Rita in developing her potential abilities and some of her outside interests, involving her peers and family members.

The Johnson Family's Strengths and Problems

Following family assessment, the nurse scheduled a family interview during which identified strengths, problems, and interventions were discussed (see Table 9.2).

The nurse planned to reassess the family within a few weeks, and at regular intervals thereafter.

Figure 9.5   Maladaptive Sibling Communication—Rita and Joan Johnson

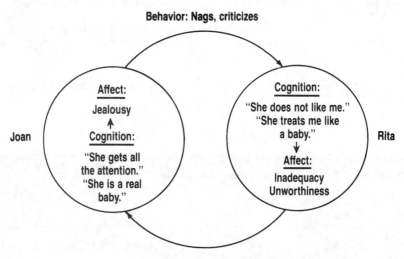

CONCLUSIONS

Illness threatens the adolescent's independence, body image, sexual identity, and social and vocational goals. It compounds the normal family challenges of establishing the young person's independence and sense of belonging. Progress toward adjustment and potential achievement depends on the complex interrelationship between adolescent, family, peers, and health care professionals:

• Parental understanding and support are required to help the adolescent acquire a sense of self-worth and feelings of mastery and control.
• Nurses should help parents encourage independence and maximize the adolescent's strengths and skills.
• Parents and professionals should acknowledge the teenager's emergent sexuality and discuss with the adolescent the hopes, fears, and problems which make them uncomfortable with the expression of that sexuality.

Assessing nurses should be aware that families can minimize the impact of chronic illness and the distress it causes them; on the other hand, coping patterns may be maladaptive, jeopardizing clinical management of the illness. Therefore it is imperative that nurses assess all families facing chronic illness in order to identify their coping strategies and understand the dynamics that exist between the illness, the adolescent, her family, peers, and the health care system.

REFERENCES

Abrams, J., and Kaslow, F. "Learning Disability and Family Dynamics: A Mutual Interaction," *Journal of Clinical Child Psychology* 5:35-40, 1976.

Allan, J., et al. "Family Response to Cystic Fibrosis," *Australian Paediatrics Journal* 10:136, 1974.

Banks, P.A., et al., eds. *The Crohn's Disease and Ulcerative Colitis Fact Book.* New York: Charles Scribner's Sons, 1983.

Berdie, J. "Family Functioning in Families with Children Who Have Handicapping Conditions," *Family Therapy,* 3(3):187-95, 1981.

Blumberg, B.D., et al. "Adolescence: A Time of Transition," in *Chronic Illness and Disability Through the Life Span.* Edited by Eisenberg, M.G., et al. New York: Springer Publishing Co., 1984.

Bruhn, G. "Impact of Chronic Illness on the Family," *The Journal of Family Practice* 4(6):1057-60, 1977.

Chilman, C.S. "Families in Development at Mid-Stage of the Family Life Cycle," *The Family Coordinator* 17:297-313, 1968.

Cleveland, M. "Family Adaptation to Traumatic Spinal Cord Injury: Response to Crisis," *Family Relations* 29(4):558-65, 1980.

Crohn, B.B., et al. "Regional Ileitis," *Journal of the American Medical Association* 99:1323, 1932.

Daniel, W.A. *Adolescents in Health and Disease.* St. Louis: C.V. Mosby Co., 1977.

Goldberg, R.S. "Toward an Understanding of the Rehabilitation of the Disabled Adolescent," in *The Psychological and Social Impact of Physical Disability.* Edited by Merinelli, R.P., et al. New York: Springer Publishing Co., 1984.

Gwinn, R., et al. "Management Problems in Dealing with an Adolescent Diabetic," *Journal of Family Practice* 18(2):207-22, 1984.

Hofman, A., et al. *The Hospitalized Adolescent.* New York: Free Press, 1976.

Janis, I. "The Role of Social Support in Adherence to Stressful Decisions," *American Psychologist* 38:143-60, 1983.

Kulczycki, L. "Somatic and Psychosocial Factors Relative to Management of Patients with Cystic Fibrosis," *Clinical Process* 25:320, 1969.

Latimer, P.R. "Crohn's Disease: A Review of the Psychological and Social Outcome," *Psychological Medicine* 8:649-56, 1978.

Leahey, M., and Wright, L.M. "Intervening with Families with Chronic Illness," *Family Systems Medicine* 3(1):60-69, 1985.

Malone, R.L. "Expressed Attitudes of Families of Aphasics," in *Social and Pathological Aspects of Disability: A Handbook for Practitioners.* Edited by Stubbins, J. Baltimore: University Park Press, 1977.

McCallum, A.T. *The Chronically Ill Child.* New Haven, Conn.: Yale University Press, 1981.

Mendeloff, A.I. "Disease of the Small Intestine," in *Principles of Internal Medicine.* Edited by Wintrobe, M.W., et al. New York: McGraw-Hill Book Co., 1974.

National Foundation for Ileitis and Colitis. Personal communication, 1985.

Sabbeth, B. "Understanding the Impact of Chronic Childhood Illness on Families," *Pediatric Clinics of North America* 31(1):47-57, 1984.

Schowalter, J.E. "Psyche and Soma of Physical Illness During Adolescence," *Psychosomatics* 24(5):453-61, 1983.

Seligman, M. "Sources of Psychological Disturbance Among Siblings of Handicapped Children," *Personnel & Guidance Journal* 4(3):529-31, 1983.

Solnit, A. "Obstacles and Pathways in the Journey from Adolescence to Parenthood," in *Adolescent Psychiatry.* Edited by Sugar, M. Chicago: University of Chicago Press, 1983.

Steinhauser, H.C., and Kies, H. "Comparative Studies of Ulcerative Colitis and Crohn's Disease in Children and Adolescents," *Journal of Child Psychology and Psychiatry* 23(1):33-42, 1982.

Strauch, B., et al. "Caring Enough to Give Your Patient Control," *Nursing80,* 24(1):54-59, 1980.

Todd, J., and Satz, P. "The Effects of Long-Term Verbal Memory Deficit: A Case Study of an Adolescent and His Family," *Journal of Marital and Family Therapy* 6(4):431-38, 1980.

Venters, M. "Familial Coping with Chronic and Severe Childhood Illness: The Case of Cystic Fibrosis," *Social Sciences and Medicine* 15A(3):289-97, 1981.

Vogel, E., and Bell, N. "The Emotionally Disturbed Child as the Family Scapegoat," in *A Modern Introduction to the Family.* Edited by Vogel, E., and Bell, N. New York: Free Press, 1960.

Wright, L.M., and Leahey, M. *Nurses and Families: A Guide to Family Assessment and Intervention.* Philadelphia: F.A. Davis Co., 1984.

10 Assessing families of the chronically ill aged in their homes

Jean R. Miller, RN, PhD
Professor and Associate Dean for Research
College of Nursing
University of Utah
Salt Lake City, Utah

Leslie L. Feinauer, RN, PhD
Associate Professor
College of Nursing
University of Utah
Salt Lake City, Utah

Dale A. Lund, PhD
Associate Director for Research
College of Nursing
University of Utah
Salt Lake City, Utah

OVERVIEW

This chapter discusses the assessment of and planning for nursing families who care for chronically ill aging parents in the home. A theoretical assessment model encompassing family environment, functional impairment, perceived support, self-worth, and well-being is presented. Planning relies on the assessment; however, several general interventional goals are presented, and the importance of a strong therapeutic alliance in both assessment and planning phases emphasized.

NURSING PROCESS

Assessment

The health problem: Chronic illness in an aging family member. Caring for an aging parent at home has become so common that it has been described as a "normative family stress" (Brody et al., 1985). This source also estimates that more than five million people are involved in parent care at any given time. Although exact figures are not available, two or more impaired elderly are estimated to be living with their families for every one residing in a nursing home (Comptroller General of the United States, 1977).

Numerous sources cite families as the major source of emotional, financial, and physical support for most elderly persons (Brody, 1977; Carter and McGoldrick, 1980; Johnson and Bursk, 1977; Pinkston and Linsk, 1984). This support enables many of the elderly to avoid institutionalization, maintain their own homes, or live in their children's homes (Branch and Jette, 1983; Brody, 1978, 1981; Brody et al., 1978; Cantor, 1975, 1980a, b; Comptroller General of the United States, 1977; Shanas, 1979a, b).

For adult children, however, having elderly parents live in their homes can be problematic. Some families tire in the face of overwhelming burdens, and there is increased potential for abuses, neglect, and inadequate care of the elderly person. Such problems often arise from unresolved past family and emotional conflicts. Indeed, dysfunctional relationships often go unnoted until a health crisis occurs. Limited interpersonal communication in maladaptive families makes it difficult to change counterproductive behavior, thus resulting in a cycle of ineffective interaction.

Even adaptive family organization can be disrupted by unsuccessful attempts to maintain supportive relationships under stressful circumstances (Brody, 1977; Brody et al., 1985; Lund et al., 1985; Robinson and Thurnher, 1979; Treas, 1977). The resulting stress is augmented by perceived deterioration of the elderly parents' mental and physical capacities and the confining nature of the caretaking situation (Bowen, 1978; Brody et al., 1985; Headley, 1977; Pinkston and Linsk, 1984; Power and DellOrto, 1980).

Intergenerational communication is a common problem (Lund et al., 1985). Cantor (1983) and Circirelli (1983), for instance, found evidence that relatives who were closely responsible for the elderly felt stress from poor communication, but lacked a medium to improve the situation. Disparity between the expectations and realities of interaction between the generations was magnified by close familial bonds and intergenerational differences.

As Gibson (1982, p. 11) points out, "family members caring for ill older relatives are a very vulnerable group," because the psychological burden of caregiving can be as difficult as the physical burden. Disruptions in a young family's personal life and the elderly person's need for constant supervision are the most often cited stressors (Gibson, 1982). Cantor (1983) found that the closer the bond between adult children and their parents, the more stressful the caregiving role. Intergenerational differences compounded the normal strains of children caring for an older person. According to Cantor (p. 603), spouses and children "appear to be priority targets for interventions to strengthen the capacity of informal supports to assist the frail elderly."

Most studies of interaction between the chronically ill elderly and their adult children focus on the family impact of dementia. Bergmann et al. (1978) interviewed 87 families of elderly victims of a dementing disorder, and concluded that family support was the most important factor in preventing institutionalization. More than half of these families, however, reported emotional upset related to their elderly parents' behavior and restrictions in their social and leisure activities. Physical effects were also noted.

Zarit and colleagues (1980) concluded that, in caregivers of elderly persons with senile dementia, the degree of perceived burden was influenced less by illness-related behavior than by the availability of social supports. In other words, the more family and friends visiting the caregivers' household, the less the perceived burden. The authors suggested that a supportive counseling relationship with a health professional would decrease stress in caregiving families and could contribute to the development of informal support networks among family members and friends.

By studying the primary caregivers of 55 patients suffering irreversible dementia, Rabins and colleagues (1982) identified several problems (see Table 10.1) shared by adult families caring for chronically ill elderly parents.

Theoretical model. The authors of this chapter are currently testing the Elderly Family Environment Model (EFEM), which guides nurses in the assessment of elderly families in their homes. The EFEM combines family and individual (elderly member) variables to predict the subjective well-being of chronically ill elderly persons. Factors considered include family environment, perceived support, self-worth, degree of impairment, and subjective well-being; their relationship is depicted in Figure 10.1.

Table 10.1 Major Problems Associated with Irreversible Dementing Disorders

Elderly Patient	Family Caretakers
• Memory disturbance	• Chronic fatigue, anger, depression
• Catastrophic reactions	• Family conflict
• Demanding/critical behavior	• Loss of friends, hobbies, free time
• Communication disorders	• Worry about own (or other healthy family member's) possible illness
	• Difficulty assuming new roles/responsibilities
	• Guilt

Source: Rabins et al., 1982.

Family environment refers to family relationships, personal growth, and maintenance of the unit. It is further defined through Olson and colleagues' (1979) Circumplex Model, which uses the structural dimensions of cohesion and adaptability as clinical tools to predict family and individual responses to change and stress. Cohesion and adaptability are defined as follows (Olson et al., 1979):

• Cohesion: Emotional bonding between family and the degree of individual autonomy within a family system.

• Adaptability: A family system's ability to change its power structure, role relationships, and relationship rules in response to situational and developmental stress.

The impact of cohesion and adaptability are evident at all life-cycle stages, but are most obvious during the final family transition—aging. At this time, when elderly persons need assistance and nurturance from their adult children and grandchildren, adult children perpetuate and modify patterns of involvement (intimacy, dependence, accountability, closeness, roles, and rules) taught by the parents for whom they are now caring.

Impairment refers to the elderly patient's limitations in performing such activities of daily living (ADLs) as bathing, dressing, toileting, feeding, moving in and out of bed, and controlling bladder and bowels. Mental status is also considered, since many common physical activities cannot be done if the elderly person has trouble remembering.

Perceived support is defined by Cobb (1976, p. 300) as "information leading the subject to mutual obligations." This information is classified as a knowledge that one is cared for and loved; is esteemed and valued; and belongs to a network of communication and mutual obligation. The social support leading to development of this awareness may come from community services, friends, and/or family members, and can enhance adaptation to stress and illness (Blau, 1973; Dimond and Jones, 1983; Lowenthall and Haven, 1968; Mueller, 1980).

Figure 10.1   Elderly Family Environment Model

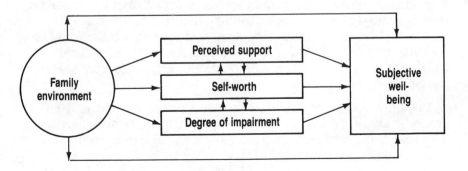

Self-worth, acceptance of or positive feelings about one's self, is an important variable in the well-being of the elderly (McClelland, 1982). In older persons, as in all age groups, feelings of self-worth influence overall life satisfaction (Kalish, 1982). Many investigators have noted that feelings of self-worth and a positive self-image are related to positive social integration, interactional patterns (Longino et al., 1980), morale (Lee and Tallman-Shinger, 1980), and effective psychological functioning (Linn and Hunter, 1979). Research by one of this chapter's coauthors revealed self-worth as one of the most significant buffers against depression during conjugal bereavement among the elderly (Lund, 1982). Positive self-worth enhances perceived well-being and can be considered a personal coping resource during crisis.

In light of the relationship between self-worth and measures of well-being, it is important to realize how perceived social supports, particularly relationships with family and significant others, can affect self-worth (Lindenthal et al., 1971; Linn and Hunter, 1979; Mutran and Burke, 1979). Family relationships, for instance, can positively or negatively affect self-worth (Eckels, 1981).

Subjective well-being, self-perceived positive feeling or state, arises from gratification of an appropriate proportion of one's major life desires. It can also be defined as the level of avowed happiness, regardless of health or other problems. The chronically ill elderly can have very positive feelings of well-being.

Assessment instruments. There are four basic tools for assessing elderly families and/or the caregiving family members: the nurses' reports, self-reports, behavioral self-reports, and behavioral methods (Olson, 1985), all of which are employed either by an insider (family member) or an outsider (nurse). The information obtained can be viewed as either subjective (feelings, attitudes, or beliefs) or objective, more easily quantified.

Nurses can use all of the aforementioned methods, although self-reporting through interviews or questionnaires is most common. Behavioral self-reports require individuals to count or record specific behavior(s) in themselves or other family members The reliability of these reports is suspect, since people making them tend to emphasize the positive and downplay the negative aspects of their own behavior. Many clinicians rely on observation of family behavior during structured tasks such as card-sort procedures for more objective and more quantifiable data.

Any of the above methods can help assess elderly families in their homes. It should be kept in mind, though, that consistent differences have been found between family self-reports and behaviors observed by health professionals (Olson, 1977).

Home assessment of EFEM variables

Family environment. Family environment can be assessed by using FACES III (Olson et al., 1985), a self-reporting instrument that provides an "insider's" perspective on family functioning. The Circumplex Model, on which FACES III is based, describes family types and classifies forms of effective family functioning (Olson and McCubbin, 1983); FACES III allows the nurse to rate family cohesion, adaptability, and communication.

FACES III consists of 40 one-sentence descriptions of family characteristics. Family members rate each characteristic on a one-to-five scale according to their perception of the family at that time and how they would like their family to be, ideally. By comparing perceptions and ideals, the nurse can assess each individual's satisfaction with the family system. She can then devise a family discrepancy score indicating how far individual family members deviate from the group mean on the dimensions of cohesion and adaptability. The score obtained during clinical assessments can be compared to developmental norms; cultural differences can be explained by the hypothesis that "families will function well as long as all family members are satisfied with these expectations" (Olson et al., 1985).

Assessment of family cohesion, adaptability, and communication is especially important to families caring for elderly relatives, because of the dramatic difference that may exist between the elderly person's perception of family cohesion and that of younger family members. As people age, they tend to desire more emotional bonding than the younger generation does. The resultant discrepancies in family members' perceptions of cohesion could erode the elderly person's sense of well-being. All members must adapt if a family is to weather the situational stress of having an elderly family member in the home; the situation requires major changes in family power structure, role relationships, and relationship rules.

FACES III can be introduced to the elderly and their families by establishing rapport with the family and then asking all those above 12 years of age to answer the questions. Although each person should answer individually, the activity can be done by several family members in the same or different rooms, and either at once or at different times, depending on the family's wishes. Sometimes elderly persons prefer to have questions asked verbally and to have someone else write their answers down. Whenever possible, FACES III should be administered twice in order to determine family members' perceptions of its functioning and ideal descriptions of the family system.

Functional impairment. Nurses usually assess functional impairment through observation; those who desire a general measurement instrument for recording functional impairment can use the Katz Index of Activities of Daily Living (Katz et al., 1963). To assess the elderly person's independence/dependence in performing the daily activities, the Katz Index asks such questions as: Does the elderly person need help in eating, getting dressed, or going to the toilet? How far is the elderly person able to walk? Can the elderly person use public transportation? This inventory can be adapted easily to a variety of data collection methods.

An instrument commonly used to assess mental status is the Mental Status Questionnaire (Kahn et al., 1960). This 10-question scale assesses short- and long-term memory; it asks questions relating to the date (day, month, week, year); the subject's age and date of birth; and where the person is at the time of the test. This inventory has been used extensively in geriatric research and practice.

Perceived support. Elderly persons' perception of support can be evaluated through questions about valued relationships, especially about people whom subjects feel they can trust and to whom they can go for help/advise or to socialize. To obtain specific information about the elderly person's perceived degree of social support, the nurse can ask for the specific number of daily/regular contacts (with family, friends, neighbors, health professionals, etc.) and if there is one person with whom they feel especially confident or secure. Other assessible support systems are: access to respite, day-care, and financial assistance.

"Confidants, Neighbors, and Friends" (CNF) (Bultena et al., 1982) is an effective tool for measuring support. This 16-item inventory addresses the elderly person's present and past relationships, including interpersonal losses and gains. CNF determines the number of the elderly person's interpersonal contacts, as well as the amount of physical support, advice, problem-solving help, or social time he expects to receive from each.

Self-worth. The elderly person's self-worth is best assessed through his statements regarding self-acceptance and positive feelings about self; the Rosenberg Self-Worth Inventory (Rosenberg, 1962) provides the necessary framework and has gained wide acceptance. Ten statements are weighted along a four-point continuum from strongly agree to strongly disagree. A typical one is, "I certainly feel useless at times."

Subjective well-being. Because subjective well-being is a global construct encompassing both stable and transitory dimensions, it requires subjective assessment at different levels. One useful tool is the Life Satisfaction Scale (Wood et al., 1969), a 13-item questionnaire that measures gratification of major life desires. It deals primarily with the stable dimension of subjective well-being; clients are asked to state their agreement or disagreement with such statements as "These are the best years of my life."

The transitory dimension of well-being can be assessed through the Affect Balance Scale (Mangen and Peterson, 1982). This scale measures the level of avowed happiness using two sets of questions to measure positive and negative affect. The client is asked to answer yes or no to such questions as, "Do you feel that things are going your way?" or "Do you feel bored?"

Planning

Therapeutic alliance. Accurate assessments of families and elderly clients are the bases for planning home care in geriatric chronic illness. During the assessment and planning phases, the nurse and family should try to achieve a strong therapeutic alliance characterized by trust and respect.

When a nurse is called to the home of adult children caring for an elderly parent, the entire family will usually be in difficulty. Problems may vary from extreme fatigue to severe interpersonal conflict. Because families rely on habitual transactional patterns that are affirmed by years of use, each member will view his behavior as appropriate in the current situation. Therefore, family members may be frightened of making the changes necessary to relieve their difficulties. The planning phase may be threatening, since this is the period when family members must accept the inadequacy of established patterns and affirm their need for assistance; they must also be willing to expose their feelings at this time.

An emotional alliance between the nurse and each family member can reduce this fear of change. This bond can be established through the use of structure, emotional accommodation, symptom acceptance, and mimicking (Lantz, 1978). The nurse provides structure by explaining how the nursing role functions, what the family will be doing, and how the family can help achieve its goals. Clarification of these issues provides treatment with direction and helps families meet their needs for order and productivity.

To achieve emotional accommodation during the planning phase, the nurse must develop empathy with the family as a group and with its members. This fosters trust in the nurse, and only through trust will the family risk changing its ways.

Symptom acceptance also promotes a therapeutic alliance. The nurse can openly accept family members' symptoms by listening to each person's viewpoint and displaying an understanding of his perception of the problem. This conveys warmth and develops trust.

Sometimes nurses feel so much concern for client families that they assume family members' characteristics—voice tone, word choice, gestures. Most mimicking behaviors are nonverbal, and provide yet another basis for beginning trust.

Goals. The treatment goals developed during the planning phase will depend on the findings in the assessment phase; several goals, however, are common among most families caring for elderly parents. For instance:

• Helping each person retain, regain, or develop a positive sense of self within their family.

• Helping family members maintain or assume control of their lives and protect what they feel is theirs, be it physical, psychological, or social.

• Establishing or encouraging an appropriate family role structure, allowing members to meet personal needs within the family framework.

• Resolving specific family problems arising from strained relationship(s) or unresolved conflict(s).

• Teaching problem-solving skills.

• Exploring institutionalization or continuing intergenerational living arrangements as alternative life-styles.

• Focusing on the future; developing the perspective and direction required to continue positive interaction despite physical or mental deterioration.

Intervention. The means by which the objectives can be met will vary according to family financial resources and desires. The nurse might schedule visits to the home, or arrange for the family to meet other caretaker families for group support. In a recent report on education/support groups for families of patients with Alzheimer's disease and other dementias (Glosser and Wexler, 1985), family members spoke positively of this method. The supportive aspects of the group and the information provided about medical and behavioral patient management were most highly rated. The same families spoke less positively about the group's value in resolving intrafamilial conflict or in obtaining information about specific legal, financial, and social problems.

Both individual and group programs have proven successful with compliant families whose members can and do follow advice and use educational resources, and who have a history of successful stress adaptation. In noncompliant families, whose members cannot agree, who rebel against information or alternative actions, and who refuse to follow through on suggestions, a less conventional and often more complicated approach may be used; some nurses have successfully used paradoxical or strategic interventions in such cases.

CASE STUDY

Emma Jones is an 83-year-old grandmother who lives in her own home. Health professionals were called after a neighbor reported concern about Mrs. Jones' health and lack of care; the nurse contacted the family and assessed the environment. Assessment revealed that Mrs. Jones had divorced 20 years earlier and had spent little time with her family in recent years, preferring instead the company of friends. In fact, her three children felt that several of the men with whom she had been involved were undesirable. On the infrequent occasions when Mrs. Jones' children visited her, she refused to listen to them or allow them to make any decisions for her, especially regarding her financial situation. In their own lives, the children saw themselves as independent, active people with autonomous relationships and marriages in which both spouses pursued independent projects or careers.

Although Mrs. Jones usually appeared passive, she "exploded" if things did not go her way. Her personality often overwhelmed her children, who tended to be passive. They did not listen to one another and allowed problems to remain unresolved.

Most members of the Jones family, including Emma, believed it was inadequate and weak to want their relatives to be near them. The children were unaware of needing other people in their lives; Emma's greatest fear was loneliness, yet she wanted to be with people only on her own terms. She saw life as meaningless and believed people should take care of themselves because no one else would take care of them.

Emma attempted to obtain care through manipulation. Her approach was very indirect; often she altered her value or belief system to fit the circumstances of the moment. She blamed crises of unpleasant experiences on others and always viewed herself as a victim of unfairness. She maintained no long-term committed relationships except with her children, whom she characterized as ungrateful and unwilling to meet their obligations to her. At the same time, she emphasized that she didn't need them or anyone else.

The nurse asked three questions to ascertain what Emma and the children wanted from their relationship and how Emma's care would be provided:
• What would be the least that family members would be willing to do to help their mother?
• What would be the most that they would be willing to do?
• What would be the least and most that Emma would expect from her children?

Discussion of the above questions resulted in more flexible, yet independent family relations. Because the change was not radical, the family was more likely to comply with the new care arrangements. The new situation encouraged the kind of respectful interaction that would maintain family goals and direction throughout Emma's care.

Several short-term goals were established to help the family remain autonomous. They hired private nurses and a housekeeper to meet Mrs. Jones's health and domestic needs. Each member scheduled one short biweekly visit with Mrs. Jones in her home. Emma and her family agreed to cooperate in determining where she would be invited for the holidays, how her financial affairs would be managed, and how decisions regarding future medical care would be made if her condition continued to deteriorate.

These changes not only assured that Mrs. Jones would receive whatever future care she might require, but it also helped her and her family to review their relationship; the legitimacy of their intimacy and dependency needs; the quality of life they might achieve; the benefits of their past experiences; their need for privacy and autonomy; and alternative ways of attaining their life's desires. They became closer, assumed increased responsibility for one another and felt more connected to others outside the family unit. The family agreed that they felt better about themselves and were less fearful of aging and/or loneliness.

Ultimately, Emma's feelings of self-worth and well-being improved, largely because the nurse enabled the family to modify its interactional style.

This example illustrates briefly how astute nursing intervention can facilitate family change and enhance the well-being of an elderly individual. This intervention requires respect for the family's goals, values, beliefs, and life-style, as well as awareness of the elderly person's perceptions of support, and realistic planning for the satisfaction of identified needs.

CONCLUSIONS

Family roles and relationships often need modification when the frail elderly come to live in the homes of their adult children. This chapter presented a model for assessing such families and their elderly members; the model uses such variables as family environment, functional impairment, perceived support, self-worth, and well-being. Each of these variables could be evaluated through nurse observations and interviews or through family members' self-reports. Proven instruments for measuring each of the model's five variables were also identified.

The importance of establishing a strong therapeutic alliance between nurse and family was emphasized, and its development (through use of structure, emotional accommodation, symptom acceptance, and mimicking behaviors) explained. The chapter demonstrated that treatment goals and methods depend on the assessment of each variable in the model, and general goals for situations involving family care of the elderly were listed. Goals can be implemented through individual family counseling or through education/support groups.

REFERENCES

Bergmann, K., et al. "Management of the Demented Elderly Patient in the Community," *British Journal of Psychiatry* 132:441-49, 1978.

Blau, Z. *Old Age in a Changing Society.* New York: Viewpoints, 1973.

Bowen, M. *Family Therapy in Clinical Practice.* New York: Jason Aronson, 1978.

Bowen, M. "Use of Family Theory in Clinical Practices," in *Changing Families.* Edited by Haley, J. New York: Grune & Stratton, 1971.

Branch, L., and Jette, A. "Elders' Use of Informal Long-Term Care Assistance," *Gerontologist* 23:51-56, 1983.

Brody, E. "The Aging Family," *Annuals of the American Academy of Political and Social Science* 438:13-27, 1978.

Brody, E., et. al. "The Family Caring Unit: A Major Consideration in the Long-Term Support System," *Gerontologist* 18:556-61, 1978.

Brody, E.M. *Long-Term Care of Older People: A Practical Guide.* New York: Human Science Press, 1977.

Brody, E.M., et al. "Parent Care as a Normative Family Stress," *Gerontologist* 25:19-29, 1985.

Brody, E. "Women in the Middle and Family Help to Older People," *Gerontologist* 21:471-80, 1981.

Bultena, G. L., et al. "Confidants, Neighbors, and Friends Scale," in *Research Instruments in Social Gerontology,* vol. 2. Minneapolis: University of Minnesota Press, 1982.

Cantor, M. "Caring for the Frail Elderly: Impact on Family, Friends, and Neighbors," Paper presented at the 33rd Annual Scientific Meeting, Gerontological Society of America. San Diego, 1980a.

Cantor, M. "The Informal Support System: Its Relevance in the Lives of the Elderly," in *Aging and Society.* Edited by Borgotta, E., and McCluskey N. Beverly Hills, Calif.: Sage Publications, 1980b.

Cantor, M. "Life Space and the Social Support System of the Inner-City Elderly of New York," *Gerontologist* 15:23-27, 1975.

Cantor, M. "Strain Among Caregivers: A Study of Experience in the United States," *Gerontologist* 23:597-604, 1983.

Carter, E., and McGoldrick, M. *The Family Life Cycle.* New York: Gardner Press, 1980.

Cicirelli, V. "A Comparison of Helping Behavior to Elderly Parents of Adult Children with Intact and Disrupted Marriages," *Gerontologist* 23:619-25, 1983.

Cobb, S. "Social Support as a Moderator of Stress," *Psychosomatic Medicine* 3:300-14, 1976.

Comptroller General of the United States. *The Well-Being of Older People in Cleveland, Ohio.* Washington, D.C.: U.S. General Accounting Office, 1977.

Dimond, M., and Jones, S.L. "Social Support: A Review and Theoretical Integration," in *Advances in Nursing Theories.* Edited by Chinn, P. Rockville, Md.: Aspen Systems Corp., 1983.

Eckels, E.T. "Negative Aspects of Family Relationships for Older Women," Paper presented at the Joint Annual Meeting of the Gerontological Society of America and the Canadian Association on Gerontology. Toronto, 1981.

Gibson, M.J. "An International Update on Family Care for the Ill Elderly," *Aging International* 11:14, 1982.

Glosser, G., and Wexler, D. "Participants' Evaluation of Educational/Support Groups for Families of Patients with Alzheimer's Disease and Other Dementias," *Gerontologist* 25:232-36, 1985.

Headley, L. *Adults and Their Families in Family Therapy.* New York: Plenum Press, 1977.

Johnson, E.S., and Bursk, B.J. "Relationships Between the Elderly and Their Adult Children," *Gerontologist* 17:90-96, 1977.

Kahn, R.L., et al. "Brief Objective Measures for the Determination of Mental Status in the Aged," *American Journal of Psychiatry,* 117:326-28, 1960.

Kalish, R.A. *Late Adulthood: Perspectives on Human Development.* Monterey, Calif.: Brooks/Cole Publishing Co., 1982.

Kane, R.A., and Kane, R.L. *Assessing the Elderly: A Practical Guide to Measurement.* Lexington, Ky.: Lexington Books, 1984.

Katz, S., et al. "Studies of Illness in the Aged—The Index of ADL: A Standardized Measure of Biological and Psychosocial Function," *Journal of the American Medical Association* 185:94, 1963.

Kenny, D.A. *Correlation and Causality.* New York: John Wiley & Sons, 1979.

Lantz, J.E. *Family and Marital Therapy: A Transactional Approach.* East Norwalk, Conn.: Appleton-Century-Crofts, 1978.

Lee, G.R., and Tallman-Shinger, M. "Sibling Interactional and Morale: The Effects of Family Relations on Older People," *Research on Aging, 2:367-91, 1980.*

Lindenthal, J.J., et al. "Psychological Status and the Perception of Primary and Secondary Support from the Social Milieu in Time of Crisis," *Journal of Nervous and Mental Disease* 153:92-98, 1971.

Linn, M.W., and Hunter, K. "Perception of Age in the Elderly," *Journal of Gerontology* 34:46-52, 1979.

Longino, C.F., Jr., et al. "The Aged Subculture Hypothesis: Social Integration Gerontophilia and Self-Conception," *Journal of Gerontology* 35:758-67, 1980.

Lowenthal, M., and Haven, C. "Interaction and Adaptation: Intimacy as a Critical Variable," *American Sociological Review* 33:20-30, 1968.

Lund, D.A. "Depression During the First Six Months of Conjugal Bereavement Among the Elderly," Paper presented at the Veterans' Administration District Conference on Disturbances in Cognitive Functioning in the Elderly. Denver, 1982.

Lund, D.A., et al. "Multigenerational Family Households: Problems and Solutions from Three Points of View," *Journal of Gerontological Nursing* 11:11, 29-33, 1985.

Mangen, D.J., and Peterson, W.A. "Social Conflicts (Neighbors and Friends) Scale and Attitudes About Support in Adult Children Scale," *Research Instruments in Social Gerontology,* vol. 2. Minneapolis: University of Minnesota Press, 1982.

McClelland, K.A. "Self-Conception and Life Satisfaction: Integrating Aged Subculture and Activity Theory," *Journal of Gerontology* 37:723-32, 1982.

Mueller, D. "Social Networks: A Promising Direction for Research on the Relationship of the Social Environment to Psychiatric Disorder," *Social Science and Medicine,* 14:147-61, 1980.

Mutran, E., and Burke, P.J. "Feeling 'Useless': A Common Component of Young and Old Adult Identities," *Research on Aging* 1:187-212, 1979.

Olson, D.H., "Commentary: Struggling with Congruence Across Theoretical Models and Methods," *Family Process* 24:203-07, 1985.

Olson, D.H. "Insiders' and Outsiders' View of Relationships: Research Stratgies," in *Close Relationships*. Edited by Levinger, G., and Ransh, H. Amherst, Mass.: University of Massachusetts Press, 1977.

Olson, D.H., and McCubbin, H.I. *Families: What Makes Them Work*. Beverly Hills, Calif.: Sage Publications, 1983.

Olson, D.H., et al. "Circumplex Model of Marital and Family Systems: 1. Cohesion and Adaptability Dimensions, Family Types, and Clinical Applications," *Family Process* 18:3-28, 1979.

Olson, D.H., et al. "FACES III," Unpublished manuscript. University of Minnesota, Department of Family Social Science, St. Paul, 1985.

Pinkston, E.M., and Linsk, N.L. "Behavioral Family Intervention with the Impaired Elderly," *Gerontologist,* 24(6):576-83, 1984.

Power, P.W., and DellOrto, D.A. *Role of the Family in Rehabilitation of the Physically Disabled*. Baltimore: University Park Press, 1980.

Rabins, P.V., et al. "The Impact of Dementia on the Family," *Journal of the American Medical Association* 248:333-35, 1982.

Robinson, B., and Thurnher, M. "Taking Care of Aged Parents: A Family Cycle Transition," *Gerontologist* 19:586-93, 1979.

Rosenberg, M. "The Association Between Self-Esteem and Anxiety," *Journal of Psychiatric Research* 1:135-52, 1962.

Shanas, E. "The Family as a Social Support System in Old Age," *Gerontologist* 19:169-74, 1979a.

Shanas, E. "Social Myth as Hypothesis: The Case of the Family Relations of Old People," *Gerontologist* 19:3-9, 1979b.

Treas, J. "Family Support Systems for the Aged: Some Social and Demographic Considerations," *Gerontologist,* 17:486-91, 1977.

Wood, V., et al. "An Analysis of a Short Self-Report Measure of Life Satisfaction: Correlation with Rater Judgments,"*Journal of Gerontology* 24:465-69, 1969.

Zarit, S.H., et al."Relatives of the Impaired Elderly: Correlates of Feelings of Burden," *Gerontologist* 20:649-55, 1980.

11 Assessing aging families and their caretakers

Shirley A. Smoyak, RN, PhD, FAAN
Professor II and Geropsychiatric Nursing Graduate
  Director
College of Nursing
Rutgers—The State University of New Jersey
New Brunswick, New Jersey

OVERVIEW

This chapter outlines medical, social, and related factors that have changed the role of the elderly in contemporary family life. It corrects some long-standing misconceptions about aging; it shows, for instance, with the use of statistics, that stereotypes of three-generational families are based on nostalgia for what never was, and that only in the last half of this century have grandparents been alive to participate in extended family relationships. Attitudes and norms for caring for the elderly are also discussed.

The genogram, as shown here, can be effective in clarifying family organizational rules, and thus in helping nurses intervene effectively with aging families who are in the process of managing an identified problem. Its applications to two families, the Rosens and the Antonios, are briefly described.

The unique stresses and demands of caring for an ill elderly person at home, and the dangers that those stresses can pose to the caretaker, the caretaker's family, and the patient himself, are also explored; appropriate nursing assessment and intervention strategies are suggested.

THE AGING AND SOCIETY

Changing Family Structures and Functions

Today there are more elderly people, proportionately and in actual numbers, than ever before in history. This trend has created unprecedented family structures and relationships. For the first time, four or five generations may be alive to share such events as births, religious rites (bar mitzvahs, first communions, confirmations), marriages, graduations, separations, successes, losses, and family crises. Where the "typical" three-generation family of the past was largely mythical, today more grandparents are alive to participate in the ongoing family life. In 1920, the chance of a 10-year-old having two living grandparents was 40%; today it is 75%. In 1920, the chance of a 10-year-old having four living grandparents was 1.7%; today, it is 8% (National Institute on Aging [NIA], 1972; American Association of Retired Persons [AARP], 1984).

Until recently, married couples could expect to live together for only one or two years after their last child left home. Today, this post-child-rearing period constitutes almost a third of the average couple's married life (13 years) and requires a readjustment of life patterns. Most of these families enjoy comparative economic well-being, even in the face of inflation, fixed incomes, and retirement. Longer parental life expectancies have created the development of new family patterns, including having the first child later in life, having fewer children, coping with the return of adult children and grandchildren (because of divorce or separation) to the parental home, and caring for aging parents.

Between the years 2020 and 2030, when the children of the post–World War II baby boom reach old age, it is projected that 20% of Americans will be over age 65. By 2030, there will be about 65 million Americans over age 65, 2.5 times the present number (AARP, 1984). Future families will be forced to reshift and rethink living arrangements; ever-increasing family mobility will require increasingly complex travel arrangements at times of crisis or holidays, thus taxing public transportation systems.

The aging process. Obviously, the need will increase for practicing nurses to understand fully the biophysical and psychosocial dimensions of aging. Aging is best understood when the following major points are kept in mind: people age in different ways because they belong to different social (ethnic, racial, religious, economic) groups whose structure and norms constantly change; and the aging process itself is never fixed or immutable, but varies greatly among individuals.

Neither genetic disposition nor childhood experience fully "programs" the aging process. Rather, aging is continually subject to modification by complex interplays of physical and social circumstances and situations; social factors appear to have the greatest influence.

The adage, "the *definition* of the situation *is* the situation," is increasingly true in the area of aging. Since the way in which individuals and families respond to physiological change largely determines their well-being, the infirmity of aging or age-related physical illness will affect different people in different ways. Some people will consider it a cause for total despair; others will view such developments as challenges or "tests" to be passed.

The elderly in the community. Research currently reported in journals and handbooks on aging leaves little doubt that most of today's older people live independent and productive lives. Indeed, only 5% of today's elderly are institutionalized; the rest function in some capacity within the community (Smoyak, 1985).

Fiske (1980), summarizing social and behavioral studies on aging, reported that, despite their increased risk of organic brain damage, older persons are no more susceptible to psychiatric impairment than younger people; the one exception seems to be in depressive illness. The reason why people in their sixties and seventies do not develop more psychiatric problems might simply be that the fittest have survived, or that some psychogenic disorders, including schizophrenia, "burn themselves out" over time.

Attitudes about aging. Persons who place the highest value on individual productivity and power are likely to view aging and the aged negatively; on the other hand, those who regard interpersonal warmth and tenderness as the primary human resources are likely to accept the aged more readily. Regarding their own situations, people tend to become more philosophical and religious as they age. They rethink their priorities and often wish that they had spent more time nurturing human relationships and less time worrying about money or "doing the right thing." They also may experience the sexism and agism that color social and familial views of marriage among the elderly. Since women commonly outlive men, there are three times as many widows as widowers in the 65 and older category. Older men who do outlive their wives have more options regarding remarriage. On the whole, society tolerates the marriage of an older man and a younger woman much better than the marriage of an older woman to a younger man. More and more families struggle with devising new "rules of organization" as they confront the fact that dad's new wife is the same age as his daughter, or that dad's new stepchildren decide to court his daughter's children.

Family attitudes and home care of the elderly. Despite the individualism of contemporary American society, few children abandon their elderly parents in order to pursue their own life goals. Although much of the care that was once performed by families in the home, from education to health care and welfare, is now performed by institutions, families still feel responsible for their individual members. Recent studies by Shanas (1979), Brody (1981), and Sussman (1982) show that families prefer not to send members outside for treatment or care, but rather to provide physical care, service, aid, and social attention at home. Sussman's (1982) use of a projective attitude test revealed that families are willing to take care of their relatives, especially parents, even when it involves long-term physical care in their own homes. Cicirelli (1983, 1984) found that highly attached adult children monitor the conditions of their aging parents so closely that at the first signs of deteriorating health, they provide help, including home health care.

While researchers have documented the concern and caring that families have for their elderly members, less is known about the burden such care places on families. Adult children who assume full-time care of an aging parent or parents and elderly spouses who are caring for their equally old or older spouses often experience intolerable stress. These caretakers may find themselves so overwhelmed by physical, emotional, and financial demands that they themselves become physically or psychologically ill. Steinmetz and Ansden (1983) have shown that such stress may even lead to psychological or physical abuse of the elderly relative.

Throughout history, women have been the primary family caregivers or caretakers, and this remains true today. Even with vast numbers of women in the work force, they are still the ones called upon for the most difficult home tasks. It is not unusual, therefore, for "nearly elderly" working women to rush home to caretaking duties; their free time is devoted to desperate efforts to catch up on undone tasks, leaving little time for individual needs.

Extended family relationships. Grandparents and grandchildren can be wonderful resources for each other, simply because they can exchange ideas and feelings unencumbered by the worries so characteristic of middle-generation parents. A retired grandparent may be available to his grandchildren more often and for longer intervals than can the parent who is distracted by the demands of work, housekeeping, money management, and social obligations. The grandparent may listen more patiently to a toddler's explanation of what happened at nursery school, or to an adolescent's worries about the transmissibility of AIDS in gym class. A grandmother recently said in a family session where four generations were present, "I see now that I sure wasted a lot of time worrying and yelling about things that I didn't have to—like toilet-training and eating carrots. I think I made things harder for all of us by making an issue out of it, instead of just letting it be." The grandmother was gently urging her son and daughter-in-law to rethink the way they spent their parenting energies.

Many families are also finding the need to invent new names for "layers" of surviving grandparents. "Granny" or "grandpop" served well enough when there was only one generation beyond the parents, but now there might be two or three. Many families solve the problem by adding a last name, such as "Grandma Smith" or "Grandad Jones." Others are more inventive, coming up with terms like "Grandpop-pop" for great-grandfather.

The Family Life Cycle: Aging Families

Butler and Lewis (1982, pp. 25-26) define the major developmental task of old age as learning to "clarify, deepen, and find use for what one has already attained in a lifetime of learning and adapting. Older people must teach themselves to conserve their strength and resources when necessary and to adjust in the best sense to those changes and losses that occur as part of the aging experience." Aging is more likely to be a positive experience for individuals who enjoy relatively good physical health, a social support network, financial security, and a personality which engages others rather than puts them at a distance. Old age alone does not change an established personality; it does, however, sharpen both good and poor features of interpersonal styles and habits. Warm and friendly people become more so, as do the distant and crotchety.

As life expectancies increase and health care improves, chronological age becomes an increasingly poor predictor of how people live and what they do for work or pleasure. Patterns and activities traditionally reserved for or associated with younger people are being tried and mastered by the elderly. For instance, cohabitation without marriage is now relatively common among retired as well as college-aged populations, much to the amazement of the generation in between. Older people are going back to school and pursuing certificates and degrees; some are embarking on second or third careers. People in their fifties are starting new families with adopted children, often children of different ethnic origins.

THE NURSING PROCESS

Assessment

The genogram: A family assessment tool. Aging is both an individual and a family process. Changes in the structure, composition, organization, and values of families provide useful perspectives from which to understand the aged, their caretakers, and the aging process. Those changes are perhaps most accurately assessed through the genogram (Smoyak, 1982).

The genogram provides a succinct picture of family relationships that encompasses all family members in a generational context (Smoyak, 1982). Nurses in many specialties have found it very useful in family assessment and intervention. For instance, psychiatric nurses conducting family therapy can begin by constructing a genogram; community health nurses coordinating hospice arrangements in terminal illness can use it to identify caretaker resources and respite alternatives; nurses working in the area of substance abuse can, with the genogram, identify a family alcohol or drug history and reveal the vulnerability of succeeding generations; and acute care nurses have used the genogram in discharge planning to identify resources and areas of possible strain.

Construction. A three-generation genogram (see Figure 11.1) can be constructed on one 8½-by-11-inch sheet of paper. Four- or five-generation families will require a second sheet. If, in order to identify potential caretaking or respite resources, the nurse includes siblings' families in the genogram, additional pages might be necessary.

Males are identified on the genogram by boxes, and females by circles. Husbands are placed on the left and wives on the right, with symbols connected by a straight, horizontal line; dotted horizontal lines indicate cohabitation without marriage. Pregnancies are represented by triangles at the end of a child line, and abortions as triangles in the child line. Adoptions are indicated by a two-line break in the line perpendicular to the marriage line; biological birth lines are solid. Divorces and separations are noted by drawing a squiggle in the middle of the marriage line, above where the child perpendicular line would begin. The marriage date is shown on the marriage line, preceded by "m." Divorce is "d," and a separation, legal or otherwise, is "s."

People who are not family members, but are closely involved in family life, can also be included in the genogram. Their boxes or circles should be connected by dotted lines to the family member or members to whom they are closest. A long-time housekeeper might be so pictured, or a paid companion, home health aide, or visitor.

For most purposes, the following data should be noted for each person on the genogram:
• Birthdate, shown as "b" and date (e.g., b. 1935).
• Present age, noted under the birthdate.
• Education, noted by whatever shorthand system is convenient (e.g., BS, hs, 4th gr.).
• Occupation, noted by whatever shorthand system is convenient (e.g., stud., mgr., bus., acc't., ret.).
• Ethnic/religious origin, noted for the oldest generation level included in the genogram, above the oldest parent in the generation. A shorthand system, again, can be used (e.g., Irish RC, Polish Jew, WASP, Bl. South Bapt.).
• Existing (serious) health problem(s); if needed, these can be noted by

Figure 11.1 Genogram—The Rosen Family

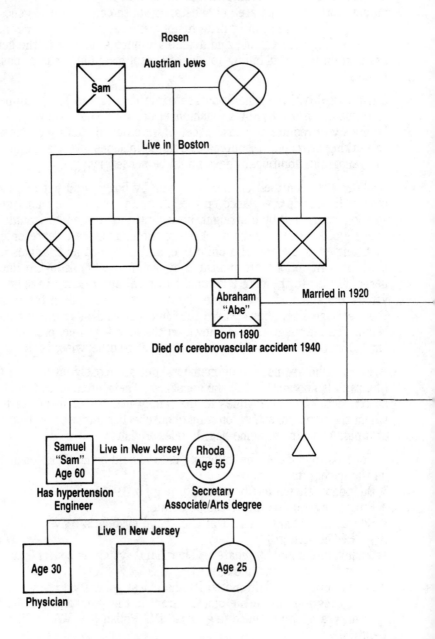

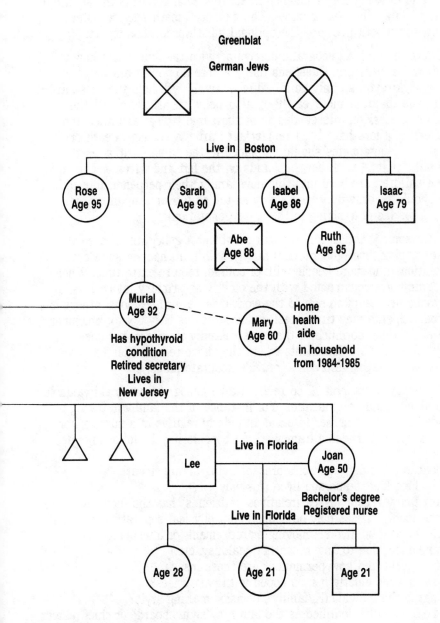

Greenblat

German Jews

Live in Boston

Rose
Age 95

Sarah
Age 90

Isabel
Age 86

Isaac
Age 79

Abe
Age 88

Ruth
Age 85

Murial
Age 92

Has hypothyroid
condition
Retired secretary
Lives in
New Jersey

Mary
Age 60

Home
health
aide
in household
from 1984-1985

Live in Florida

Lee

Joan
Age 50

Bachelor's degree
Registered nurse

Live in Florida

Age 28

Age 21

Age 21

a symbol at the left bottom of the person's box or circle (e.g., BP, mi, cva, alc.).
• Death, noted by placing a small "d," with the date, under the birth-date, and drawing four shortened lines from each corner of the square or circle through the box or circle. The cause of death may be noted under—or substituted for—the optional health problem category.

Before drawing a genogram, determine with the family just how to position the members. Questions like, "Where do you fit among your siblings? Are you an only child? Number two?" will help the nurse ar-range the diagram more easily. It also helps to ask, "Are all the brothers and sisters descended from the same biological father and mother?" If there have been remarriages after a spouse's death or divorce, the new mates should be placed in the same position as the originals, that is, with new husbands on the left and wives on the right. When children are born into this new family, their perpendicular child line should be drawn in such a way as to "skip over" any other mar-riage lines (as of a sibling in the same generation).

After some practice, a nurse can construct a genogram of even the most complex three-generational family within an hour or so. More generations and more people will, of course, require extra time. When genograms are constructed with the elderly as primary informants, it may be necessary to spread the work over several sessions; otherwise, the participants may tire or feel undue stress as they try to remember, in a short time, so much of their past. Family members can check their Bible or other documents where they have recorded births, mar-riages, and deaths, in order to provide accurate dates.

Use in family assessment. A correctly drawn genogram can yield valuable data about family organization. For instance, if the family is trying to decide how to or whether to place an elderly relative in a nursing home, the genogram provides a framework for considering the following ques-tions:
• What is the elderly person's present living arrangement?
• How long has the person lived this way?
• How many recent losses (relatives or friends) has the individual experienced? ("Loss" may be defined as a physical separation, such as death, separation/divorce, moving or retirement, or interpersonal estrangement due to anger, conflict, jealousy, etc.)
• How recent and how permanent are these losses?
• How has the elderly person coped with past crises?
• What is the individual's/family's decision-making style?
• Who is usually identified as the family's "switchboard" or chief relayer of information?
• How willing is the family to allow or to seek out non-family members' assistance?

• Throughout life, how self-sufficient or independent has the elderly member been?

By providing direction for questioning in a crisis, the genogram prevents reactivity and emotionalism from disrupting the decision-making process. Both nurse and family must name the problem, lay out its various definitions, specify alternatives, and choose a decision-making method before trying to make decisions. This approach usually prevents blame-placing and scapegoating. It is a thoughtful, "no-fault" approach to solving family problems.

CASE STUDY

The genogram in Figure 11.1 illustrates the Rosens, who are considering what to do about the elder Mrs. Rosen (Murial), who has recently become disoriented. The genogram notes the geographical locations of key family members, because place of residence is a central issue in this case.

Murial Rosen has lived alone, by choice, since the death of her husband 45 years ago. For the past five years, she has resided in a senior citizens' apartment one mile from her son's home. On weekends, she visits her son's family and sleeps in a room designated as hers; it is furnished with her possessions and with changes of clothing. Before this was arranged, she had lived in Boston, near most of her siblings, in the apartment she and her husband had shared.

Her son, Sam, says a bit defensively, "She had to be moved down here with me. I just couldn't put up any more with the back-and-forth stuff if she needed me." The genogram clarified circumstances and practical issues for family members as they struggled to balance Murial's needs for independence and family support with her children's own work, social, and family obligations. Mrs. Rosen's disorientation may be due to a physical thyroid problem. She is on medication and is watched carefully by a nurse for cognitive changes.

With holidays approaching, Sam, his wife, and some of Murial's Boston siblings hope to gather and decide upon a workable resolution to the problem. Nieces or nephews may be identified as caretakers or respite staff, thus enabling Mrs. Rosen to return to a setting she prefers.

This case illustrates how a genogram can be modified to isolate particular family concerns, such as geographical distance. New data can be added as it comes to light, and new connections between people and events can be made throughout the assessment process. For instance, as the anniversary of a spouse's death approaches, the widow may develop chest pains or depression. If the psychological connection is made through the genogram, overmedication can be avoided.

Caretakers' cushion. Advances in science and medicine allow the successful management of illnesses and other health crises that previously led to almost certain death. Furthermore, many of these crises are now managed at home rather than in professional health care settings. Home caretakers today have access to equipment that 10 years ago was available only in acute care hospitals; it is no longer unusual, for instance, for oxygen and intravenous therapy to be maintained at home. At the same time, there has been renewed interest in home care for dying children and other relatives.

This increase in home-care technology has also raised the psychological expectations of both patients and families. Thirty-five years ago, Parsons and Fox (1952) argued that the "sick role" carried with it several benefits, such as excusing the victim from normal work responsibilities and condoning dependence or poor humor. Today the ill individual is expected to assume a "coping" rather than a "sick" role. Even when dying, or when suffering from a degenerative disease process, the patient is expected to function as normally as possible—to adapt to limitations rather than to give in to them. Some complaining is still acceptable, but it should be kept to a discrete level.

A patient's ability to cope with any life crisis, including increasing age and/or disability, usually depends on the presence of a caretaker. Caretakers function not only as social supports, but also as medical advisors, nurses, advocates, financial managers, and adjunct decision-makers. For instance, when a family chooses to enroll in a hospice program, the agency carefully considers the caretaker's nature and ability to care for the patient at home.

While the literature mentions the caretakers' dilemma, descriptions and analyses of the role tend to be global, anecdotal, or superficial. The nurse should regard the caretakers' situation as a kind of "cushion"— the caretaker cushions the impact of illness on the elderly (but also requires a cushion of support in order to cope with the extraordinary demands of the caretaking role). The concept of a "cushion" can help caretakers understand, rationally and cognitively, the dimensions of their commitment to their elderly relative.

Soon after becoming caretakers, many well-meaning persons experience an array of unanticipated and frightening symptoms, ranging from fatigue and disorganization to physical illness, and even to depression, alienation, or "burn-out." They are not aware that their own "cushion" has been removed. Caretaker roles usurp so much time and energy that the usual "repair time" that is needed in normal, daily living to re-charge one's batteries is eroded or gone entirely.

Cushions are not frivolous; they are necessary for the daily repair processes to occur. For instance, many people use the time before falling asleep to assess the day's events and to plan for the next day. When, after assuming a caretaker role, they fall into bed and drop right off to sleep, this important reorganizing time is lost. Other people use a leisurely shower, or a long walk to reflect. Such activities are among the first to go when a caretaking function is taken on. The second cup of morning coffee may seem trivial, but it is another necessary "cushion" that quickly gets pushed aside.

When cushions are removed, pain results. Too many caretakers blame their painful fatigue symptoms on their own aging, on an illness, or a lack of willpower, when all they really need are cushions. Often they do not even mention these symptoms, because they assume that the patient or others will think they are weak.

Of course, in many instances, patient care alone requires almost constant vigilance, as it does in the later stages of Alzheimer's disease. When caretaking clearly demands a high expenditure of physical energy and resources, others are more likely to sympathize and offer help. What is less obvious, but just as demanding, is the chore of acquiring facts—about medications, costs, insurance, power of attorney, wills, alternatives to the present treatment, and so on. Explaining the elderly patient's problem to others, or grappling with the meaning for the situation (Why did this happen to me? to him? Why did God allow this?) also absorb endless hours. Finally, finding a philosophy that is not only adequate, but growth-producing, takes time.

Many caretakers and families struggle to decide who should be told what about the patient's condition—and when. Some families use a newscast system of communication, requiring all major announcements to be made at a specified time. Information disseminated through such a system must be weighed carefully when the caretaker has both good and bad news to tell.

Caretakers must also allow time to rework priorities. Often, a beginning caretaker fails to realize just how time-consuming or disruptive the new responsibilities will be. Schlag (1984) found instances where a caretaker had taken a leave of absence from work that was scheduled to end with the anticipated death of the ill relative, only to have the patient live much longer than expected. On the other hand, caretakers may turn down new jobs or transfers, only to find that the patient no longer needs them.

Caretakers themselves need caretakers—someone who can maintain normal family and home routines. In some families, the caretakers' siblings, spouse, or children provide help. In other families, a health professional may have to identify this need.

Nurses can provide useful preventive services to caretaking families by alerting them to the realities of their new responsibilities. Armed with a realistic picture of their dilemma, caretakers can plan more wisely to meet the patient's—and their own—support needs.

Figure 11.2 Genogram—The Antonio Family

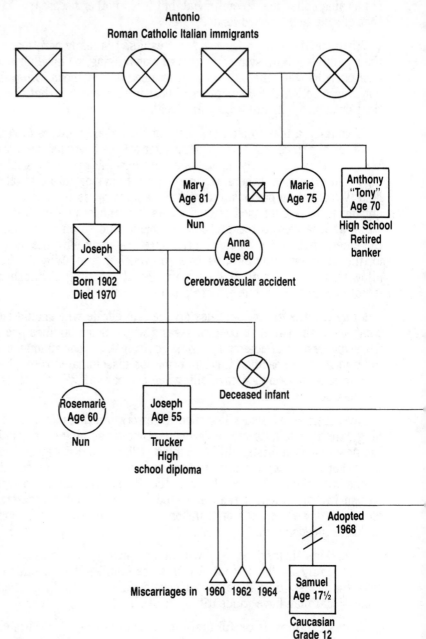

Antonio
Roman Catholic Italian immigrants

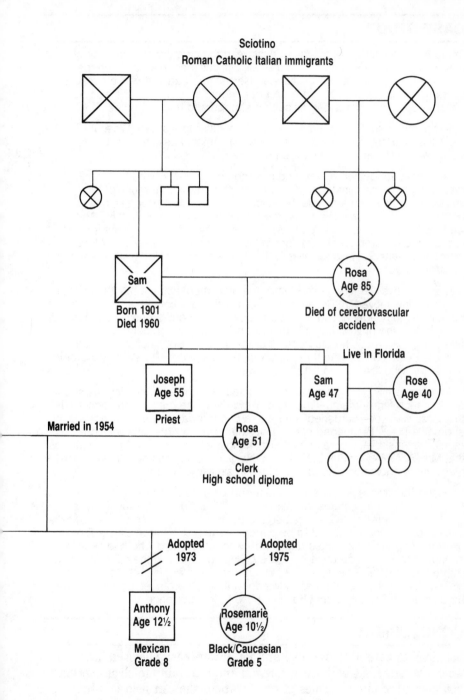

Sciotino
Roman Catholic Italian immigrants

Sam
Born 1901
Died 1960

Rosa
Age 85
Died of cerebrovascular
accident

Joseph
Age 55
Priest

Rosa
Age 51
Clerk
High school diploma

Live in Florida

Sam
Age 47

Rose
Age 40

Married in 1954

Adopted
1973

Adopted
1975

Anthony
Age 12½
Mexican
Grade 8

Rosemarie
Age 10½
Black/Caucasian
Grade 5

CASE STUDY

In the Antonio family, Rosa had not only been the caretaker for her elderly mother, but also wife, mother of three (all "difficult") adopted children, part-time sales clerk, and church volunteer. Her mother had suffered a stroke 10 years before and remained weak and dependent on a walker; she also had difficulty speaking, making it difficult for strangers to understand her.

Six months ago, Rosa's mother-in-law also suffered a stroke. When it became clear that she could no longer live alone, Mr. Antonio assumed that Rosa would welcome her into their large house.

The nurse suggested a family counseling session, at which Mr. Antonio reaffirmed his determination to bring his mother into the household. With a smile and arms extended wide, he said "Well, we're all Americans, now, right? [Both sides of the family had emigrated from the same town in Italy.] And we take in the tired and the poor. See, we already did it many times [pointing to the three children and his mother-in-law]. So what's different now? Rosa, what's the matter?" Rosa sat silently, twisting a handkerchief, tears streaming down her face.

A family physician suggested family therapy when, about a month after her mother-in-law moved in, Rosa developed a series of ailments ranging from backaches to headaches to a rash that covered her entire body. Her husband, Joseph, told the physican that "Rosa just has to adjust—to get used to this new thing." However, he did consent to the session. Both mothers were there, as were Rosa, Joseph, the three children, and the elder Mrs. Antonio's brother and sister, who lived a short distance away.

After the family genogram was constructed, the nurse conducting the session elicited each family member's point of view. Everyone but Joseph conceded that Rosa was "overburdened" and that a change was needed. Joseph's aunt and uncle finally persuaded him to help the family explore new solutions, rather than insist that Rosa should just "handle it." One of their arguments was that Mrs. Antonio's mother had come down with "consumption" (tuberculosis) many years ago when placed in a situation similar to Rosa's.

During the discussion, the family referred often to the genogram. They pointed and made gestures to "this side," or "that side" of the family. When Uncle Tony wanted to make notes on the genogram, the nurse offered to make copies for everyone and to distribute them at the next session. Uncle Tony used his copy to make notes about who was retired, and who had "a little, enough, and more than enough" money. Placing himself in the third category, "more than enough," he asked for help in arranging for his sister to live with him. A life-long bachelor, he acknowledged that this arrangement would surely be different, but affirmed that he would rise to the challenge.

CONCLUSIONS

Solutions to caretaker overload are not always easily devised. However, when the nurse has both the genogram and the ability to elicit information about the family's rules of organization, she can help families find workable alternatives. As one aged gentleman succinctly put it, "I'll vote for that—a new way is better than a new pill!!"

REFERENCES

American Association of Retired Persons. *A Profile of Older Americans.* Washington, D.C.: AARP, 1984.

Brody, E.M. "'Women in the Middle' and Family Help to Older People," *Gerontologist* 21(5):471-80. 1981.

Butler, R. and Lewis, M. *Aging and Mental Health: Positive Psychological and Biomedical Approaches,* 3rd ed. St. Louis: C.V. Mosby Co., 1982.

Cicirelli, V.G. "Adult Children's Attachment and Helping Behavior to Elderly Parents: A Path Model," *Journal of Marriage and the Family* 45:815-25, 1983.

Cicirelli, V.G. "Adult Children's Helping Behavior to Elderly Parents," *Journal of Family Issues* 5(3):419-40, 1984.

Fiske, M. "Tasks and Crises of the Second Half of Life: The Inter-Relationship of Commitment, Coping Adaptation," in *Handbook of Mental Health and Aging.* Edited by Birren, J., and Sloane, R.B. Englewood Cliffs, N.J.: Prentice-Hall, 1980.

Hareven, T. "American Families in Transition: Historical Perspectives on Change," In *Normal Family Processes.* Edited by Walsh, F. New York: The Guilford Press. 1982.

National Institute on Aging. *Metropolitan Life Statistical Bulletin,* 1972.

Parsons, T., and Fox, R. "Illness, Therapy and the Modern Urban Family," *Journal of Social Issues* (8):31-44, 1952.

Schlag, M. "Ethnomethodological Study of a Hospice," Unpublished doctoral dissertation. New Brunswick, N.J.: Rutgers State University, 1984.

Shanas, E. "The Family As a Social Support System in Old Age," *Gerontologist* 19(2):169-74, 1979.

Smoyak, S.A. "The Genogram," in *Family Therapy.* Edited by Clements, I. New York: John Wiley & Sons, 1982.

Smoyak, S.A. "Old Age," in *The Clinical Specialist in Psychiatric Mental Health Nursing.* Edited by Critchley, D., and Maurin, J. New York: John Wiley & Sons, 1985.

Steinmetz, S.K., and Ansden, D.J. "Dependent Elders, Family Stress and Abuse," in *Family Relationships in Later Life.* Edited by Brubaker, T.H. Beverly Hills, Calif.: Sage Publications, 1983.

Sussman, M.B. "Willingness to Assist One's Elderly Parents: Responses from United States and Japanese Families," *Human Organization* 41(3):614-18, 1982.

12 Assessing families and chronic pain

Kathleen M. Rowat, RN, PhD
Associate Professor and Associate Director
(Graduate Program)
School of Nursing, McGill University
Montreal, Quebec, Canada

OVERVIEW

This chapter offers two perspectives on families of chronic pain patients and discusses how these perspectives may be implemented in nursing assessment. Critical issues within the assessment process are identified, and a case study is presented to illustrate the model "family as the unit of concern."

NURSING PROCESS

Assessment

The health problem: Chronic pain. Four out of every 10 Americans will be treated for pain at some time in their lives (Bonica, 1984). Chronic pain in particular is thought to be approaching epidemic proportions, (Brena, 1978) with an estimated cost to American taxpayers of 60 billion dollars annually for health services and lost work productivity (Bonica, 1980).

Chronic pain presents a major challenge to the health care field. It is a disease state in its own right and must be differentiated from acute pain (Bonica, 1973). Unlike acute pain, chronic pain cannot be explained on the basis of tissue damage or pathophysiology (Pinsky and Crue, 1984; Sternbach, 1984). Response patterns typically associated with acute pain may be absent in the chronic pain patient, and physiological changes indicating autonomic nervous system activity may not be present (Jeans et al., 1979). With pain that persists for months or years, sympathetic responses become habituated and vegetative signs, especially sleep disturbance and irritability, emerge (Sternbach, 1984). Failure to recognize the differences between acute and chronic pain has historically been a major stumbling block in accurate nursing assessment (Benoliel and Crowley, 1977).

Need for family involvement. Long-term illnesses such as chronic pain are a major contemporary health concern, not only because of their rising incidence but also because of their complexity and far-reaching effects. The family has assumed particular importance in models of chronic illness (Cogswell and Weir, 1964; Gerson and Strauss, 1975; Pratt, 1973). Increasingly, both clinical and research evidence suggests that chronic illness impinges on the lives not only of the ill individual but of the family as a whole (Bruhn, 1977; Klein et al., 1967; Strauss, 1975).

The importance of the family in chronic illness management has also been acknowledged; indeed, it has been proposed that the major responsibility for managing such conditions rests with patients and their families rather than with health professionals (Benoliel, 1970; Cogswell and Weir, 1964; Pratt, 1973; Strauss, 1975).

Although Reeder (1974) argued that the critical variables in family response to chronic illness were the presence and intrusiveness of pain, only recently have writings in the field of pain addressed the family issue (Block, 1981; Bonica, 1978; Crowley, 1975; Mohamed et al., 1978; Rowat, 1983, 1985; Swanson and Maruta, 1980).

Family assessment models. As our awareness of the significance of the family in chronic pain expands, the necessity of a family data assessment appears self-evident. Although the literature offers a number of models through which the chronic pain family may be viewed, two perspectives appear to dominate. The first one views the "family as context" for the individual in pain; the second establishes the "family as the unit of concern."

The family as context. Jeans and colleagues (1979) suggest that the person in pain lives in a complex system of others, the most important of whom may be the family. Litman (1974) proposed that the family is the most important context within which illness occurs and is resolved.

"Family as context" models focus primarily on the individual sufferer; the family helps illuminate the pain etiology and the pattern and improves care and patient outcome. The family's role in predisposing, precipitating, or perpetuating behaviors in the chronic pain patient may be analyzed (Mohamed, 1982). Family health histories and family environment are prominent assessment considerations.

Family pain history. A family's past experiences with pain have been cited as possible influences on present situations. A number of authors have pointed out that individuals may actually learn pain behaviors by observing how other family members deal with pain (Craig, 1978; Craig and Prkachin, 1981; Crook et al., 1984; Mohamed et al., 1978; Violon and Giurgea, 1984).

Associations have been found between the location of a family member's pain (Mohamed et al., 1978), the number and gender of pain models available to the patient, and the patient's current pain experiences (Christensen and Mortenson, 1975; Craig, 1978; Edwards et al., 1985; Gentry et al., 1974; Turkat et al., 1983; Violon and Gurigea, 1984) thus pointing to the importance of including these variables in a family history.

Such questions as "Has anyone else in your family experienced a problem with pain?" and "What did they do when they were in pain— that is, how did they handle their pain?" can elicit important information about a patient's prior experiences with pain. Asking clients to compare their pain to that of their family members (e.g., "How do you think your pain compares with [x's] pain?") also makes the nurse more aware of patients' interpretations of their health problems.

Family environment. Factors within the family environment have been identified as critical in the development of chronic pain. One such factor is the marital relationship. Studies of marital maladjustment within families of chronic pain sufferers suggest that family dynamics play an important "predisposing role" in individual pain tolerance and pain behavior (Merskey and Boyd, 1978; Merskey and Spear, 1967; Mohamed et al., 1978; Waring, 1977; Waring et al., 1978). Various measures are available for assessing marital adjustment; the Locke-Wallace Marital Adjustment Scale is especially popular among those studying chronic pain families (Block, 1981; Block and Boyer, 1984; Mohamed et al., 1978).

When the family is viewed as a context for chronic pain, the effect of family dynamics on the patient's response to treatment becomes evident. Members' responses to or attitudes toward the patient are known to be crucial determinants of the ill individual's response and ability to cope with the illness (Bruhn, 1977).

According to Hudgens (1979), a strong family support system is a major predictor of treatment outcomes for the chronic pain patient. Studies of such patients and their spouses have revealed a significant correlation between marital adjustment, spousal health, personality characteristics, and treatment outcomes (Block, 1980, 1981; Mohamed et al., 1978; Roberts and Reinhardt, 1980). Roberts and Reinhardt (1980), for example, noted that spouses of unsuccessfully treated patients recorded higher Minnesota Multiphasic Personality Inventory (MMPI) scores for hypochondriasis and hysteria than those of successfully treated patients. Such evidence argues for the inclusion of these variables within a family assessment.

The family also may provide an arena for testing and maintaining pain behaviors. A link between family members' responses and patients' displays of functional ability receives considerable support in the literature (Block, 1981; Block and Boyer, 1984; Block et al., 1980; Fordyce, 1976, 1978; Khatami and Rush, 1978; Shanfield and Killingsworth, 1977; Sternbach, 1974). Block and his colleagues (1980), for instance, demonstrated that patients' pain behaviors can be encouraged and perpetuated by the spouse's solicitous and attentive responses. According to Maruta and colleagues (1981, p. 307), a spouse's "interaction with the patient is the most powerful reinforcer of illness (pain) behaviors of the patient."

Such findings indicate the value, to a nurse, of family members' descriptions of the way they react to the sight of their relative in pain. The use of open-ended questions, for instance, "What do you do when you see your husband in pain?" and "How do you respond when your wife begins to talk about her pain?", help the nurse identify possible links between patient behaviors and family responses.

The family as the unit of care. The "family as context" perspective focuses on ill individuals and their needs. Families are included because of their association with identified patients rather than as entities in their own rights (Stevens, 1979).

In contrast, health care professionals who view the family as the unit of care acknowledge not only that the family shapes patient experience, but also that the family may be affected by the illness. Schwenk and Hughes (1983) argued that the family must be the fundamental unit of medical care delivery. This reorientation toward the family necessitates a major shift in a nurse's thinking. To quote Livsey (1972, p. 248), "It is essential to keep in mind the conceptual framework of the family as a whole when evaluating the family when one of its members is ill."

Living with chronic pain, therefore, is a "family affair," not merely the burden of the designated patient. A recent study (Rowat, 1983) of families of chronic pain sufferers supports this assumption and suggests four main avenues of investigation for the assessing nurse:
• The meaning assigned by family members to the pain problem and their understanding of it
• The impact of chronic pain on all family members' health
• Pain's effect on family roles and responsibilities
• Family members' efforts to manage pain.

By stressing the interactive features of chronic pain and focusing on the family as the unit of care, this assessment model yields a broad data base from which the nurse may operate.

Defining the problem. Perhaps the most critical aspect of any chronic illness is the definition process (Stewart and Sullivan, 1982). Following a review of several studies dealing with the impact of an illness on family function and stability, Schwenk and Hughes (1983, p. 9) concluded that "the way in which the family perceived the illness or accident...was directly related to the eventual level of family stability and coping."

Block and Boyer (1984), in a study of spouses' adjustment to chronic pain, hypothesized that spouses' cognitive interpretation of the illness and of the meaning of its symptoms helped explain their response to their mate's pain. This study demonstrated that the meanings spouses ascribe to the chronic pain syndrome reflect their own emotional adjustment and marital satisfaction. Spouses' perceptions were elicited through an original questionnaire, The Spouse's Perception of Disease (SPOD). This questionnaire, although still at a preliminary stage of development, shows promise for future clinical use.

Other approaches to ascertaining spouses' perceptions and understanding of the pain problem have also been described. Swanson and Maruta (1980) gave identical lists of 21 checklist inquiries covering pain duration, location, severity, aggravating or relieving factors, and effects on sleep, emotions, sexual life, work, and medication use to chronic pain patients and their next of kin. This tool not only illuminated family members' perceptions but also allowed the clinician to compare these impressions with the client's view. Their studies led to the observation that treatment outcome was related to the congruence of patient and family members' perceptions of the pain problem. Indeed, a number of authors have noted that congruence or incongruence in family perceptions of a health problem may be critical in that family's health experience (Kaplan et al., 1976; Llewellyn-Thomas, 1982; Rowat, 1983; Swanson and Maruta, 1980).

Rowat (1983) suggested two other avenues of insight into family members' perceptions of pain. Such questions as "Can you describe for me what your husband/wife's pain is like?"; "What do *you* think has caused the pain?"; "Why do *you* think the pain has lasted so long?"; and "How serious do *you* think the problem is?" elicited rich data reflecting family members' understanding. This study revealed considerable family confusion and uncertainty concerning chronic pain. In trying to understand the pain situation, family members often compared chronic pain with more familiar acute pain experiences; when such a match could not be found, uncertainties arose, producing anxiety and distress. As one spouse states, "I've never heard of people having pain such that there's no apparent cure...people that have pains that can't be explained." Without a clear understanding of chronic pain, family members developed their own explanations. One spouse, for instance, commented, "It's really serious; it's like cancer or something like that." It was hypothesized that the distress engendered by such uncertainties determined family responses to this health problem.

Rowat (1983) also used a second approach to obtain family members' views of chronic pain. The McGill Pain Questionnaire (MPQ) was administered to spouses, and each spouse's ratings were compared to the patient's. Spouses who reported high levels of distress rated their mate's pain significantly higher than did low-distress spouses, even though the patients' self-reported pain levels were comparable in each group. This finding suggests the usefulness of the MPQ in assessing the chronic pain family. However, since this family application has not yet been validated, results must be interpreted cautiously. In assessing spouses of chronic pain patients, Mohamed et al. (1978) also found the Personal and Family History portion of the MPQ useful.

Ascertaining the family's understanding of the pain problem and its meanings should be considered central to family assessment; it enables the nurse to correct misunderstandings and to supply needed information.

Impact on family members' health. When the family is the unit of care, assessment must address the health of all family members. Numerous studies (Block and Boyer, 1984; Rowat, 1983; Shanfield et al., 1979) reveal both physical and psychological health problems in the spouses and children of chronic pain patients. Waring (1982) noted that depression was often more severe in family members than in the chronic pain patients themselves. In one study (Rowat, 1983), 83% of chronic pain spouses reported health disturbances that they attributed to the presence of chronic pain in their lives. Although such spouses claimed that their mates' pain had disrupted their physical, emotional, and "social" health, emotional health was seen to have suffered the most; this same study indicated that children's health was also in jeopardy.

An array of instruments for assessing chronic pain's impact on family health is described in the literature. One widely used measure of psychologic symptom distress is the SCL-90 (Hopkins Symptom Distress Checklist). This self-reported clinical rating scale offers insights into specific areas of psychological disturbance; Shanfield and colleagues (1979) demonstrated its use with a group of spouses of chronic pain sufferers. Block and Boyer (1984) used the Global Symptom Index in a study of spouse's adjustment to chronic pain in order to obtain an overall measure of emotional disturbance.

Although such assessment tools as these are available to help nurses determine family members' health status, the more traditional interview format also has demonstrated value (Rowat, 1983). Such questions as "Do you think your health has been affected by your partner's illness?" reveal spouses' perceptions of the effects that a mate's health problem has on them. Indeed, knowledge of the individual's perception of his or her situation may be more valuable than data from more structured questionnaires.

Effect on family roles, responsibilities, and relationships. An individual's chronic illness may require major shifts in existing family roles and responsibilities (Bruhn, 1977; Power, 1976; Reeder, 1974), and tension may arise as family members search for new ways of relating and behaving. Within the family perspective under discussion, marital problems may be seen as secondary to chronic pain problems rather than contributing to it (Turk & Flor, 1984). A study by Maruta and colleagues (1981) supports such a hypothesis by showing consistent deterioration in sexual activity after the onset of pain complaints.

"What has it been like in your family since your husband/wife developed this pain?"; "Have there been any changes in the family in terms of what each of you do or how you feel since the pain began?" and similar questions can help the nurse explore the effects of chronic pain on family life. Not only can roles/responsibility changes be identified but, more importantly, the nurse can ascertain whether or not such changes have led to family disruption and stress.

Roy (1984) demonstrated the use of another assessment tool based on a model of family functioning. This instrument addresses six distinct dimensions of family functioning:
- roles
- communication
- affective involvement
- affective responsiveness
- problem-solving
- behavior control.

The author noted that the model goes beyond the strictly behavior focus on only one aspect of family functioning, i.e., pain-reinforcing behaviors.

Role in pain management. One member's chronic pain requires the entire family to live with and manage the pain. The perspective here suggests that, even though family members try to cope with the pain, many are uncertain how to proceed (Rowat, 1983). As one spouse said, "I'm not sure how to act; to be strong and tell him that he has to cope? Or to baby him?"

The nurse assessing the family's role in pain management might begin by asking, "What kinds of things seem to make your wife/husband/parent's pain worse/better?" Often, factors that augment or reduce chronic pain go unrecognized by family members; therefore family efforts to manage pain are haphazard and ill conceived (Jeans and Rowat, 1984). Further, family members' perceptions that their actions or approaches are ineffective lead to feelings of helplessness and distress (Rowat, 1983).

These and similar observations underscore the importance of assessing both the family's perceived role in pain control and individual members' responses to the pain. Such questions as "Have you tried anything to help with the pain?" and "Did it make any difference?" give the nurse information necessary to help families learn new coping skills which will benefit not only the pain sufferer but also the family as a whole.

For most families, chronic pain is the first stop on a long-term health care journey. Previously effective coping skills may now be inappropriate. To quote one spouse, "He's had other illnesses which we've coped with as crises, but this is not a crisis, this is a chronic situation and I have to learn to live with it."

Planning

Implementation of a family nursing assessment requires careful planning. The first step is one of definition. What exactly is family assessment and how is it conducted? Because the current American health care system is geared to short, intensive patient (family) encounters (Aiken, 1976), the word "assessment" is equated often with a single scheduled appointment, usually at the onset of the nurse-client relationship. Chronic illnesses, however, demand prolonged nursing involvement with client and family, and a view of assessment as an ongoing process rather than an isolated event.

Second, who should be involved in assessment? Must all members of the family be involved directly in the assessment process, or can family data be obtained from the patient? According to Maruta and colleagues (1981), clinical information obtained from only the patient gives a skewed view of the family environment.

This issue raises another question—should family members be seen without the patient or should assessment meetings be joint efforts? Clinical and research findings suggest that both forums are needed. Families need an opportunity to air concerns and vent frustrations without the restraining effect of the patient's presence. As Maruta and colleagues (1981) note, such opportunities can markedly reduce family stress. On the other hand, joint sessions allow the nurse to identify family communication patterns, as well as areas of agreement or disagreement.

The benefits of a family evaluation conducted within an atmosphere of trust and collaboration are well documented (Jeans and Rowat, 1984); the assessment process in itself serves a therapeutic purpose.

Schwenk and Hughes (1983) point out that the diagnostic tools required to provide care for entire family units are still primitive; considerable work remains to be done in this area. Although, as noted earlier, numerous assessment tools are available to nurses working with chronic pain families, the choice of assessment model can be a significant planning issue. What measurements will be clinically appropriate? Is the information from a particular assessment relevant to the individual nurse's practice?

CASE STUDY

Mr. L., age 67, was referred to the Multidisciplinary Pain Center of a large general hospital with severe phantom limb pain secondary to the loss of a leg. He was retired and lived with his 66-year-old wife in a one bedroom apartment. Their two sons, both of whom were married with young families, lived in a nearby city.

Mr. L.'s pain has persisted for years and had been unresponsive to treatment. Like many chronic pain sufferers, Mr. L. had consulted one specialist after another in hope of finding some relief. He considered the Pain Center his "last resort."

Although Mr. L. first visited the Center alone, arrangements were made for an additional assessment session including his wife. Because, in addition to his severe pain, Mr. L. lacked a properly fitting prosthesis, his trips to the Pain Center posed considerable physical and financial (he had to come via ambulance) hardship. Therefore, it was determined that the nurse's family assessment would be carried out in the home. As will be seen later, this particular decision proved valuable.

Before the home session, the couple was informed that the nurse would like to talk to them together but would also like time alone with Mrs. L. The request came as no surprise, since the Center's "family as the focus of care" orientation had already been explained to Mr. L.

The centrality of pain in his family's life was apparent as soon as the nurse entered their home. At the center of the living room was Mr. L.'s hospital bed. All other objects in the room, such as the television, faced the bed.

In order to convey the message that the entire family is involved in the pain problem, the nurse began her visit by interviewing the couple together. Following the opening question, "How have things been going for you both?," the couple launched into a detailed discussion of their shared distress at Mr. L.'s unrelieved pain; frustration with a health care system that had provided no answers; uncertainty about what phantom limb pain was all about; and fears about their ability to manage in the future. The picture that emerged showed a couple struggling to understand and manage their problem and feeling very much alone in their "fight." This discussion also showed that Mrs. L. was not revealing her personal feelings or experiences. All of her comments or inquiries dealt with her husband.

Mrs. L. went into the kitchen to prepare a cup of tea, giving the nurse a moment to talk with her alone. When the nurse asked, "How has it been for you?", Mrs. L.'s eyes filled with tears and she began to reveal health problems of her own. She attributed these problems directly to the stress of her husband's persistent pain. Another stressor was also revealed: social isolation that was enforced by Mr. L.'s fear of being left alone. Her potentially rewarding activities, such as assisting with a catering service, had been abandoned. Mrs. L. also expressed a sense of helplessness, saying that "all my efforts to help seem in vain."

The conversation with Mrs. L. enabled the nurse to validate a "hunch" that she had developed while talking to the couple together: that Mrs. L. did not want her husband to know how upset she was or how much his illness affected her. "He's got enough to cope with without worrying about me," was her explanation.

As a result of this assessment, the nurse hypothesized that much of this couple's distress resulted from a feeling that the health care system had abandoned them, leaving them with no options. The nurse determined that one of the first things Mr. and Mrs. L. needed was the assurance that they were not "fighting" alone, but would be joined by the Pain Center team (Jeans and Rowat, 1984), and that a team member, in this case the nurse, would be available to them by phone at any time.

It was also clear that the family had designated some issues as "family" issues and others as "personal"; the Pain Center team considered it important to respect the couple's way of handling their situation. Defining phantom limb pain and assuring Mr. L. that he was not "crazy"; helping the couple find community resources that would facilitate travel to the Center; and discussing pain management strategies were some of the interventions planned after the initial family assessment.

Although couple-oriented issues were given priority, the nurse also urged Mrs. L. to attend to her own health. Arrangements were made for her to seek treatment for her physical symptoms. Mrs. L. also needed to devise new coping strategies, since her past adaptations (i.e., giving up all outside activities) had only heightened her stress. It was agreed that ongoing "problem-solving" sessions with the nurse would be helpful.

CONCLUSIONS

A major challenge faces the nurse caring for a chronic pain family, particularly in the area of assessment. Roy (1984, p. 32) states that "Without the benefit of a careful family assessment, the clinical picture of the pain patient has to be considered incomplete." Those nurses whose assessment regards the family as the unit of care aspire to an even broader goal—"complete" assessment can be achieved only when the nurse has a clinical picture of the entire client family.

REFERENCES

Aiken, L. "Chronic Illness and Responsive Ambulatory Care," in *The Growth of Bureaucratic Medicine*. Edited by Mechanic, D. New York: John Wiley & Sons, 1976.

Benoliel, J. "The Developing Diabetic Identity: A Study of Family Influence," in *Communicating Nursing Research: Methodological Issues,* vol. 3. Edited by Batey, M. Boulder, Co.: Western Interstate Commission for Higher Education, 1970.

Benoliel, J., and Crowley, D. "The Patient in Pain: New Concepts," *Nursing Digest* 41–48, 1977.

Block, A. "A Trimodal Assessment of Spousal Response to Pain Behavior," Paper presented at the Second Annual Meeting of the Society of Behavioral Medicine. New York, 1980.

Block, A. "An Investigation of the Response of the Spouse to Chronic Pain Behavior," *Psychosomatic Medicine* 43:415–22, 1981.

Block, A., and Boyer, S. "The Spouse's Adjustment to Chronic Pain: Cognitive and Emotional Factors," *Social Science and Medicine* 19:1313–17, 1984.

Block, A.R., et al. "Behavioral Treatment of Chronic Pain: The Spouse as a Discriminative Cue for Pain Behavior,"*Pain* 9:243–52, 1980.

Bonica, J. "Conclusion," in *Pain Research Publications, Association for Research on Nervous and Mental Disease,* 58. Edited by Bonica, J. New York: Raven Press, 1980.

Bonica, J. "Introduction," in *Chronic Pain: America's Hidden Epidemic.* Edited by Brena, S. New York: Atheneum/SMI, 1978.

Bonica, J. "Management of Pain," *Post-Graduate Medicine* 53:56–57, 1973.

Bonica, J. "Pain Research and Therapy: Recent Advances and Future Needs," in *Advances in Pain Research and Therapy.* Edited by Kruger, L., and Liebeskind, J.C. New York: Raven Press, 1984.

Brena, S. "The Staggering Cost of Chronic Pain," in *Chronic Pain: America's Hidden Epidemic.* Edited by Brena, S. New York: Atheneum/SMI, 1978.

Bruhn, J. "Effects of Chronic Illness on the Family," *Journal of Family Practice* 4:1057–60, 1977.

Christensen, M.F., and Mortenson, D. "Long-Term Prognosis in Children with Recurrent Abdominal Pain," *Archives of Disease in Childhood* 50:110–14, 1975.

Cogswell, B., and Weir, D. "A Role in Process: The Development of Medical Professionals' Role in Long Term Care of Chronically Diseased Patients," *Journal of Health and Human Behavior* 5:95–103, 1964.

Craig, K. "Social Modeling Influences on Pain," in *The Psychology of Pain.* Edited by Sternbach, R.A. New York: Raven Press, 1978.

Craig, K.D., and Prkachin, K.M. "Social Influences on Public and Private Components of Pain," in *Stress and Anxiety,* vol. 7. Edited by Sarason, I.C., and Spielberger, C.D. Washington, D.C.: Hemisphere Publishing Corp., 1981.

Crook, J., et al. "The Prevalence of Pain Complaints in a General Population," *Pain* 18:299–314, 1984.

Crowley, D. "Chronic Pain: Social Aspects," in *ANA Clinical Sessions, American Nurses' Association.* East Norwalk, Conn.: Appleton-Century-Crofts, 1975.

Edwards, P.W., et al. "Familial Pain Models: The Relationship Between Family History of Pain and Current Pain Experience," *Pain* 21:379–84, 1985.

Fordyce, W. "Behavioral Concepts in Chronic Pain and Illness," in *The Behavioral Management of Anxiety, Depression, and Pain.* Edited by Davidson, P. New York: Brunner-Mazel, 1976.

Fordyce, W. "Learning Processes in Pain," in *The Psychology of Pain.* Edited by Sternbach, R. New York: Raven Press, 1978.

Gentry, W.D., et al. "Chronic Low Back Pain: A Psychological Profile," *Psychosomatics* 15:174–77, 1974.

Gerson, E., and Strauss, A. "Time for Living: Problems in Chronic Illness Care," *Social Policy* 6:12–18, 1975.

Hudgens, A.J. "Family Oriented Treatment of Chronic Pain," *Journal of Marital & Family Therapy* 5(4):67–78, 1979.

Jeans, M.E., and Rowat, K.M. "Counselling the Patient and Family," in *Textbook of Pain.* Edited by Wall, P.D., and Malzack, R. Edinburgh: Churchill Livingstone, 1984.

Jeans, M.E., et al. "Assessment of Pain," *Canadian Family Physician* 25:159–62, 1979.

Kaplan, D., et al. "Predicting the Impact of Severe Illness in Families," *Health and Social Work* 1(3):71–82, 1976.

Khatami, M., and Rush, J. "A Pilot Study of the Treatment of Out-Patients with Chronic Pain: Symptom Control, Stimulus Control and Social System Intervention," *Pain* 5:163–72, 1978.

Klein, R., et al. "The Impact of Illness Upon the Spouse," *Journal of Chronic Disease* 20:241–48, 1967.

Litman, T.J. "The Family as a Basic Unit in Health and Medical Care: A Social-Behavioral Overview," *Social Science and Medicine* 8:495–519, 1974.

Livsey, C. "Physical Illness and Family Dynamics," *Advances in Psychosomatic Medicine* 8:237–51, 1972.

Llewellyn-Thomas, H. "Patient and Spouse Perceptions in Malignant Lymphoma: A Research Proposal," in *Recent Advances in Nursing 3. Cancer Nursing.* Edited by Cahoon, M. Edinburgh: Churchill Livingstone, 1982.

Maruta, T., et al. "Chronic Pain Patients and Spouses: Marital and Sexual Adjustment," *Mayo Clinic Proceedings* 56:307–10, 1981.

Merskey, H., and Boyd, D. "Emotional Adjustment and Chronic Pain," *Pain* 5:173–78, 1978.

Merskey, H., and Spear, F.G. *Pain: Psychological and Psychiatric Aspects.* London: Bailliere, Tindall and Cassell, 1967.

Mohamed, S. "The Patient and His Family," in *Chronic Pain: Psychosocial Factors in Rehabilitation.* Edited by Roy, R., and Tunks, E. Baltimore: Williams & Wilkins Co., 1982.

Mohamed, S.N., et al. "The Relationship of Chronic Pain to Depression, Marital Adjustment, and Family Dynamics," *Pain* 5:285–92, 1978.

Pinsky, J., and Crue, B. "Intensive Group Psychotherapy," in *Textbook of Pain.* Edited by Wall, P.D., and Melzack, R. Edinburgh: Churchill Livingstone, 1984.

Power, P. "Family Behaviors in Chronic Illness: A Perspective for Rehabilitation" (Doctoral dissertation, Boston University, 1975), *Dissertations Abstracts International* 36:8300A–01A, 1976.

Pratt, L. "The Significance of the Family in Medication," *Journal of Comparative Family Studies* 4:13–35, 1973.

Reeder, S. "The Impact of Disabling Health Conditions on Family Interaction," Doctoral dissertation. University of California, 1974.

Roberts, A.H., and Reinhardt, L. "The Behavioral Management of Chronic Pain: Long-Term Follow-up with Comparison Groups," *Pain* 8:151–62, 1980.

Rowat, K. "Chronic Pain: A Family Affair," in *Recent Advances in Nursing: Long-Term Care.* Edited by King, K. Edinburgh: Churchill Livingstone, 1985.

Rowat, K. "The Meaning and Management of Chronic Pain: The Family's Perspective" (Doctoral dissertation, University of Illinois at the Medical Center, 1983), *Dissertation Abstracts International* 44:1414B, 1983.

Roy, R. "Chronic Pain: A Family Perspective," *International Journal of Family Therapy* 6(1):31–43, 1984.

Schwenk, T., and Hughes, C. "The Family as Patient in Family Medicine," *Social Science in Medicine* 17:1–16, 1983.

Shanfield, S., et al. "Pain and the Marital Relationship: Psychiatric Distress," *Pain* 7:343–51, 1979.

Shanfield, S., and Killingsworth, R. "The Psychiatric Aspect of Pain," *Psychiatric Annals* 7:24–35, 1977.

Sternbach, R. *Pain Patients: Traits and Treatment.* New York: Academic Press, 1974.

Sternbach, R. "Acute Versus Chronic Pain," in *Textbook of Pain.* Edited by Wall, P.D., and Melzack, R. Edinburgh: Churchill Livingstone, 1984.

Stevens, B. *Nursing Theory: Analysis, Application, Evaluation.* Boston: Little, Brown & Co., 1979.

Stewart, D., and Sullivan, T. "Illness Behavior and the Sick Role in Chronic Disease: The Case of Multiple Sclerosis," *Social Science in Medicine* 16:1397–404, 1982.

Strauss, A. *Chronic Illness and the Quality of Life.* St. Louis: C.V. Mosby Co., 1975.

Swanson, D., and Maruta, T. "The Family's Viewpoint of Chronic Pain," *Pain* 8:163–66, 1980.

Turk, D., and Flor, H. "Etiological Theories and Treatments for Chronic Back Pain II: Psychological Models and Interventions," *Pain* 19:209–33, 1984.

Turkat, I.D., et al. "The Effects of Vicarious Experience on Pain Termination and Work Avoidance: A Replication," *Behavior Research and Therapy* 21:491–93, 1983.

Violon, A., and Giurgea, D. "Familial Models for Chronic Pain," *Pain* 18:199–203, 1984.

Waring, E.M. "The Role of the Family in Symptom Selection and Perpetuation in Psychosomatic Illness," *Psychotherapy and Psychosomatics* 28:253–59, 1977.

Waring, E.M. "Conjoint Marital and Family Therapy," in *Chronic Pain: Psychosocial Factors in Rehabilitation.* Edited by Roy, R., and Tunks, E. Baltimore: Williams & Wilkins Co., 1982.

Waring, E.M., et al. "Chronic Pain and the Family," Paper presented at the Second World Congress of the International Association for the Study of Pain. Montreal, 1978.

Yelin, E., et al. "Toward an Epidemiology of Work Disability," *Health and Society* 58:386, 1980.

13 Assessing families and end stage renal disease

Rosalie C. Starzomski RN, MN, CDP
Nephrology Clinical Nurse Specialist
Vancouver General Hospital
Clinical Assistant Professor
University of British Columbia
Vancouver, British Columbia, Canada

OVERVIEW

End stage renal disease (ESRD), or irreversible kidney disease, affects thousands of persons in North America each year. With the aid of modern science and technology, persons with ESRD can now live productive lives on dialysis or following kidney transplantation. Life as an ESRD patient, however, requires numerous life-style changes not only on the part of the patient, but also on the part of the family. This chapter briefly discusses ESRD treatments and reviews the value of comprehensive patient/family assessment in ESRD. A case example is presented to illustrate the use of a self-care model in ESRD.

Technological developments in diagnosis and treatment have resulted in an overall increase in human life expectancy. However, age-adjusted death rates have declined, and chronic illness in the population has increased, causing a shift in the focus of health care from disease elimination to functional maintenance and symptom management (Cluff, 1981; Craig, 1983). In North America today, most health care resources are devoted to chronic disease, and many persons have dysfunction directly related to chronic illness (Cluff, 1981; Craig, 1983). Health care personnel alone cannot provide all of the long-term care required by persons with chronic illness, however; increased responsibility for symptom management and long-term treatment has been placed on patients and their families (Cluff, 1981; McCarthy and Millard, 1979; O'Brien, 1983).

NURSING PROCESS

Assessment

The health problem—End stage renal disease. Because many of the problems experienced by the patient in end stage renal disease *and its treatment* resemble those of other chronic diseases (Levy, 1979; Rettig, 1980), ESRD is considered a paradigm for chronic illness in general. The stressors identified by the ESRD patient and family—enforced adherence to special diets and regimens; dependence on medical equipment and personnel; loss of financial security; uncertain prognosis; changed body image, reduced freedom of movement; and the ongoing challenge of dealing with physical limitations—are common to all chronic illnesses (Dzaczkes and Kaplan De-Nour, 1978; Devins et al., 1981; Lewis, 1985; Miller, 1983).

End stage renal disease is defined as irreversible kidney disease that causes chronic abnormalities in the patient's internal environment and results in a variety of biophysical and psychosocial problems (Lancaster, 1984). The rate of kidney deterioration resulting from underlying renal disease varies; early ESRD usually produces overt biophysical or psychological symptoms. As the disease progresses, however, a constellation of symptoms known as uremic syndrome develops. These include fatigue, nausea, vomiting, weight loss, insomnia, confusion, difficulties in concentration, and emotional lability. At this point, without dialysis or kidney transplantation, patient death is inevitable (Brundage, 1980; Lancaster, 1984).

The primary treatment alternatives in ESRD are hemodialysis, peritoneal dialysis, and kidney transplantation. Each has advantages and disadvantages which should be well understood by both patient and family before the treatment decision is made.

Hemodialysis is performed two to three times weekly. Each session lasts three to five hours, depending on specific needs. During hemodialysis, the patient's blood circulates outside of the body through an artificial kidney where it is cleansed of excess toxins and fluid. Such treatments can be done in the hospital, in a limited care/self-care unit, or in the patient's own home. Home hemodialysis involves a helper, most often the patient's spouse, and requires extensive training for both patient and helper in machine set-up and dialysis maintenance (Peterson, 1985). One advantage of hemodialysis is that the patient undergoes treatment for only 12 hours a week, leaving the rest of the week for other activities.

In peritoneal dialysis, the patient's own peritoneum is used as a dialyzing membrane. Dialysis fluid is introduced into the peritoneal cavity through a permanent indwelling abdominal catheter, and toxins and excess fluid are filtered from the blood. In-hospital treatments may take 36-48 hours per week, or the patient may choose continuous at-home dialysis (continuous ambulatory peritoneal dialysis, or CAPD). On CAPD, dialysis fluid is exchanged three to four times per day; the equipment required is simpler than that for hemodialysis, and the procedure allows greater patient mobility, since supplies are easily transported.

Kidney transplantation requires the donation of a kidney from a living relative or from a compatible donor. It is a treatment rather than a cure for ESRD. Improved matching techniques and immunosuppressive medications have made the transplant more successful over the years, but rejection is still possible.

The incidence of ESRD in the U.S. population has been estimated at 40-60 new cases per million per year, varying with population charac-teristics. As with other chronic illnesses, improved treatment and greater patient longevity have increased the numbers of diagnosed ESRD patients. In Canada, among a population of approximately 25 million, 4,053 patients were under treatment with chronic dialysis and 3,166 patients were alive with functioning kidney transplants in 1984 (*Cana-dian Renal Failure Registry,* 1985). United States statistics suggest that by the year 1995, 90,000 patients will be undergoing treatment for ESRD (Rettig, 1980). Obviously, increases in these numbers puts pres-sure on health care providers to find alternative ways to offer efficient, quality care. Home and limited/self-care treatment of ESRD patients can reduce health care costs and allow greater patient control over both treatment and environment. In addition, it prevents adoption of the "sick role." Home dialysis patients can also adjust treatment schedules to suit their lifestyle (Blagg and Scribner, 1980; Lindsay, 1982).

Family involvement in end stage renal disease

ESRD treatment confronts patient and family with a variety of new stressors. Predictably, some patients cope with ESRD better than others. Many have active and fulfilling family, professional, and personal lives; others stop work, neglect themselves, and become angry and depressed. The literature suggests that depression and negative morale in chronic illness may, in part, indicate a lack of social support (Hobfoil and Walfisch, 1984; Schaeffer et al., 1981). Researchers point to the impor-tance of emotional or social support systems in successful adjustment to life on dialysis (O'Brien, 1983; Richmond et al., 1982).

The family is the major source of emotional support for most ESRD patients; it helps cushion the many stresses associated with chronic disease. On the one hand, a critical illness can strengthen a family unit by enhancing the sharing and giving aspects of its relationship. On the other hand, living with a family member who is receiving ESRD treatment can impose such great strains that the unit may even dissolve. Further complicating the clinical picture is Dzaczkes and Kaplan De-Nour's (1978) suggestion that the same family reaction that helps one patient can hurt another. For example, the diagnosis of ESRD will spur some families not only to support the patient emotionally but also to assume his responsibilities. If the patient fails to understand the reason for this, resentment and breakdown of interfamily communication can occur. Other patients, however, require this extra support until they have adjusted to the diagnosis. Needless to say, this variability in family/patient response and attitude influences the treatment course; comprehensive family assessment acquaints the nurse with the family's characteristics and predictable reactions, thereby allowing development of an effective plan of action.

The strength of the family network also influences patient attitudes and responses to ESRD treatment and outcome. Family members' participation in ESRD care and assistance in choosing a treatment method also have an impact. As ESRD treatment alternatives improve, lifestyle considerations become a larger factor in the development of a care plan. For example, a woman with young children at home may choose CAPD over hemodialysis, since that treatment requires no complex equipment or frequent hospital/self-care unit visits, and allows maximum time at home in the wife and mother role. For her, CAPD would cause minimal change within the family system, and would reinforce the stability of the unit as a support system.

Dialysis greatly increases the stress and demands on all family members. Time schedules are disrupted, financial problems may develop, and communication among members may be strained as anxiety escalates (O'Brien, 1983; Schoeneman and Reznikoff, 1983; Stamek, 1981). The mere presence of the patient's dialysis equipment in the home can be a constant stressful reminder of the problem (Peterson, 1985; Stamek, 1981). A parent's dialysis can force children to confront the unknown; children often fantasize about dialysis and think that their parent is dying. The word *dialysis* itself can trigger such fantasies. Children in dialysis families often relieve anxiety by "acting out," and their behavior can be mistakenly labeled a discipline problem (Kossoris, 1970).

Theories and models of family assessment. In-depth family assessments can provide valuable structural and functional information to the health care team; such data can, in conjunction with other biophysical and psychosocial findings, help team members enhance patient/family adaptation to ESRD. The nurse plays an integral role in postdialysis patient and family assessment and follow-up throughout the patient's life.

Various models facilitate data collection and ongoing assessment of ESRD patients and their families. The author's eclectic model (Figure 13.1) shows how diverse concepts and theories can be used to adapt the nursing process to comprehensive assessment.

Figure 13.1 Model for End Stage Renal Disease Assessment

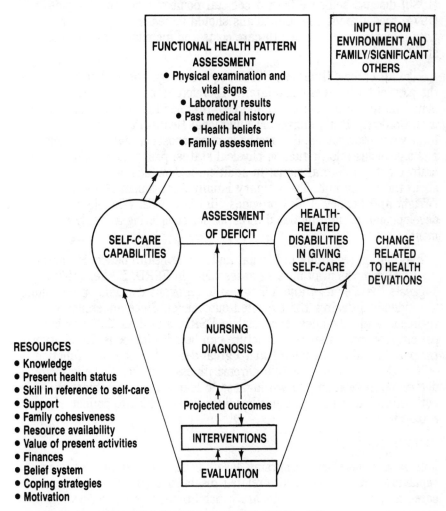

Adapted from: Crashaw and Wong, 1980; Gordon, 1982; Levin, 1978; Norris, 1979; Orem, 1980; Miller, 1983.

The model is derived from self-care theory. Self-care may be defined as activities performed by an individual on his own behalf to maintain life, health, and well-being (Henderson, 1966; Orem, 1980). As such, individuals have practiced self-care since the beginning of mankind. It is not a difficult concept to understand or put into operation. Orem (1980) has devised a nursing model for self-care while Levin (1978) discusses the topic from a medical perspective. Crawshaw and Wong (1980) discuss self-care from a societal point of view and Lalonde (1974) recommends that Canadians should increase their self-care practices in order to reduce health care costs and increase personal responsibility for health.

Like all chronic illnesses, ESRD requires large doses of self-care on the part of both patient and family. Therefore, a patient/family care plan requires data from many sources. It is helpful to collect information with Gordon's (1982) suggested Functional Health Patterns. This framework provides explicit methods of psychosocial data collection, and assembles information on physical status, past medical history, laboratory data, and vital signs. In addition, it demands detailed data about the family unit. The Calgary Family Assessment Model (CFAM) (Wright and Leahey, 1984) provides clinicians with valuable structural, developmental, and functional direction for completing a family assessment.

Information regarding individual and family health beliefs is another essential component of nursing assessment in ESRD. Becker (1978) suggests that behavior and adherence to regimens depends on how much the individual desires the expected outcome(s). Since adherence to regimens and schedules is crucial in ESRD, any data that predicts patient response to such a structure can be advantageous. In addition, the patient and family must learn a great deal before they can function within the constraints of this chronic illness, and health beliefs often determine motivation and willingness to learn. The assessment tool outlined in Table 13.1 provides headings under which to collect appropriate data.

Planning

Following comprehensive nursing assessment, patient/family self-care capabilities (SCC) and health-related disabilities (HRD) affecting self-care can be determined. Self-care capabilities can be described as resources; family cohesiveness, physical energy, self-esteem, coping strategies, beliefs, and motivation level are all resources that can enhance the patient/family's ability to perform maximal self-care (Miller, 1983). Health-related disabilities are factors that limit the patient/family ability to perform self-care.

Table 13.1   Summary of Assessment Data to Be Collected

- Demographic Information
    Name
    Birth date
    Age
    Sex
    Ethnic background
    First language
    Contact person
- Past Medical History (patient and family)
- Medical Diagnosis
- Physical Examination
- Laboratory Values
- Medications
- General Health Pattern and Family Assessment
    Health perception/health management pattern (degree of control desired in reference to health care)
    Nutrition-metabolic pattern (appetite, eating habits, uremic symptoms)
    Elimination pattern (urinary output)
    Activity—exercise pattern (energy level)
    Cognitive—perceptual pattern
    Sleep—rest pattern
    Self-perception—self-concept pattern (body image, externally/internally motivated)
    Role—relationship pattern (family structure [genogram], family functioning)
    Sexuality—reproductive pattern
    Coping—stress tolerance pattern (coping patterns, impact of illness on lifestyle)
    Values—belief pattern (health beliefs)
- Patient Education Assessment
    Readiness to learn (physical [visual/hearing] limitations, stress level, emotional limitations, cognitive problems, interest level)
    Ability to learn (active/passive seeker of information, vocabulary, reading habits, education)
    Preferred methods of learning (reading [posters/pictures], TV, lectures, demonstrations, doing by self, alone, with a group)

If, after thorough assessment, an SCC or HRD deficit is calculated, the nurse may prepare a nursing diagnosis and begin to plan appropriate interventions. The model represented in Figure 13.1 provides an ongoing open feedback system for assessment, diagnosis, and intervention, as well as follow-up.

Miller (1983) suggests that medical over-management of chronically ill patients can make them powerless to care for themselves. Health care providers must be careful not to remove control from the patient/family, but to foster group decision-making and treatment participation. Seligman (1975) also addresses this situation. In his learned helplessness theory, individuals become more helpless as others take on tasks and roles for them. By including the patient and family in care plan development, as well as in the formulation of teaching plans and overall treatment course (Figure 13.1), the patients/families should feel more power and control within the health care situation, thus improving both adherence to treatment and quality of life.

Marked changes in health care policy and efforts to balance quality health care with reduced costs have encouraged patient/family and nursing participation in long-term illness management. This trend has already produced cost savings within the health care system (Campbell and Campbell, 1978; Evans et al., 1985; Lindsay, 1982).

CASE STUDY

Mrs. H. is a 49-year-old chartered accountant, a partner in a local firm. On a routine visit to her physician, she is told that she has polycystic kidney disease. Her serum creatinine is now 8 mg/100 mls and the physician tells her that ESRD treatment will soon be necessary. She and her family are referred to the Nephrology Clinical Nurse Specialist (NCNS) for predialysis education and orientation.

The NCNS contacts Mrs. H. and her family and arranges an initial family interview at the local hospital's renal unit. All agree to attend an evening session. The nurse explains to the family that the interview is intended to gain information about the family impact of the diagnosis and to determine what members need to know in order to incorporate ESRD and its treatment into their lives. The initial family interview and assessment provide valuable data from which the nurse can structure an individual orientation and education program, identify potential areas of concern, and assess the family impact of the ESRD diagnosis (Mazzuca, 1982; Whitson, 1982).

Setting
The interview is conducted in a patient lounge area within the renal unit. The room is equipped with posters, educational material, and a video playback unit. Members are seated in a circular array of comfortable chairs.

Physical assessment
Physical assessment, laboratory values, and vital signs confirm that Mrs. H. is experiencing uremic syndrome. She is slightly volume overloaded and hypertensive; her appetite is diminished and she is losing weight. The family medical history reveals that Mrs. H.'s mother died from kidney disease in 1950, before dialysis was available. Mrs. H. remembers the death quite clearly.

Except for her kidney disease, Mrs. H. appears quite healthy. All other family members are in good health.

Family assessment
The family consists of Mrs. H., her 52-year-old husband, and four children (ages 21, 19, and 17 [twins]). The two older daughters attend a university in the city and have their own apartment. The twin boys attend a local high school. The family owns a four-bedroom home and has lived there for 15 years.

Mr. and Mrs. H. have been married for 25 years and have been partners for 10 years in a chartered accounting firm. Their goal has been to retire and travel when Mr. H. reaches 55 (in 3 years) and the children become more independent.

This family is at stage six of the developmental life cycle: the Family as Launching Center. "This stage begins with the actual departure of the first child from the home and continues until the youngest child has left home" (Wright and Leahey, 1984, p. 47). Presently, the family appears to be adapting to the changes associated with the children leaving home. Mrs. H. has expressed a desire to retain as much independence as possible and to continue in her home and work roles. Although the oldest daughter offers to return home to assist her mother, Mrs. H. says that the children must go on with their own lives and that if she requires help she will let them know.

Functional health pattern assessment

Functional health pattern assessment reveals that Mrs. H. and her family want to learn as much as possible about ESRD and its treatment. Since Mrs. H.'s mother died before dialysis was available, it is important to educate the family about modern treatment and its effect on ESRD prognosis. In addition, since polycystic kidney disease is an inherited condition, it is important to address the possibility that the children might develop the condition.

The family enjoys sports and visits a mountain cabin frequently. Mrs. H. enjoys swimming and attends weekly aerobic classes. She has a university education, but has noticed recently that her memory is deteriorating. This concerns her since her job requires clear, accurate thinking. She is experiencing some insomnia and "restless legs" at night.

There appear to be sexual problems, though the subject is not explored in detail in front of the entire family. Mrs. H. expresses some concern about changes in her body image and ability to continue present activities.

Mrs. H. describes herself as a happy, outgoing person who likes to be in control of any situation. She believes in following medical advice as much as possible, and she believes she knows when something is wrong with her physical functioning.

Educational assessment

Patient/family educational assessment reveals the H.'s as active seekers of information who wish to learn more about Mrs. H.'s condition and treatment. Because of Mrs. H.'s concentration problems (a sign of progressing uremia), all educational sessions are kept short (two to three hours) and a variety of teaching aids are used.

Assessment summary

Various concerns are identified during the total family interview. Many were identified through such direct questions as:
• What do you know about ESRD and its treatment? What would you like to know?
• What do you worry most about now that you/your wife/your mother has ESRD and you/she will soon need dialysis?
• How do you see your life/lives changing as a result of the introduction of dialysis treatments?

As a result of the interview, the following list of concerns/problems are generated by the CNS and family:

Mrs. H.
• concern about loss of independence and potential inability to control her situation, increasing dependence on others

- anxiety and fear of the unknown and of necessary lifestyle changes
- fear of death
- anxiety about changes in body image
- fear that wife/mother/work roles will be affected by illness

Mr. H.
- fear of wife dying
- anxiety and fear of the unknown and of necessary lifestyle changes
- lack of knowledge about what to expect with treatment
- fear that role of wife in home and office may change
- uncertainty about possible new responsibilities

Children
- fear of developing polycystic kidney disease
- fear of mother dying
- lack of knowledge about what to expect with treatment
- anxiety and fear of the unknown and of necessary lifestyle changes
- fear that mother's role may change
- uncertainty about new family responsibilities

The family's identified self-care capabilities include strong bonds and mutual concern, considerable resources, and open internal communications.

Health-related disabilities include lack of information about ESRD and its treatment, uncertainty about the future and the possible treatment plan, and increasing deterioration in Mrs. H.'s mental abilities and overall health.

Several deficits relative to maintaining or increasing Mrs. H.'s self-care level can be identified. At this time, however, the primary nursing diagnosis is the knowledge deficit related to lack of information about:
- uremia signs and symptoms
- ESRD and available treatment options
- life-style changes necessary for both Mrs. H. and family members
- nutritional requirements in ESRD
- what to expect in regard to life on dialysis or with a kidney transplant.

The care plan developed with the family includes education in regard to topics identified above; the plan is individualized and all family members are encouraged to participate. As a result of the patient/family assessment and the subsequent care plan, the H.'s make a smoother transition to life with ESRD.

This case study outlines one way in which patient/family assessment and subsequent use of the nursing process can enhance adjustment to chronic illness. Lewis (1985, p. 15) describes adapting to chronic illness as follows:

> Terminal illness involves dying...the breathing out of the spirit. Daily ongoing illness, where you neither die or get well, involves the challenge of grieving one's losses, of absorbing the illness as just another part of the self, of letting go of the past and not focusing on the future and of turning to face living and its difficulties, while rejoicing and celebrating the spirit for the daily gift of that life.

CONCLUSIONS

All family members are affected when one member is diagnosed as having ESRD. Living with ESRD presents a challenge to both patient and family, who must learn to incorporate new treatments, schedules, and roles into their existing system. Moreover, patient and family must cope with a variety of long-term biophysical and psychosocial stressors throughout the term of the illness (O'Brien, 1983).

As a member of the nephrology team, the nurse is in an ideal position to develop patient/family assessment skills. The self-care model illustrated in Figure 13.1 provides one way for the nurse to conduct comprehensive patient/family assessment and determine each family's ability to adapt and live with this chronic illness.

Many persons are now living for 20 or 30 years on dialysis; as technology and treatment methods advance, this length of time will probably increase. As health care professionals, nurses must use their skills to help patients and families adjust to life through all stages of ESRD.

When dealing with persons with chronic illness, it is imperative that health professionals never lose sight of the fact that the *patient is the family.*

REFERENCES

Becker, M.H. "The Health Belief Model and Sick Role Behavior," *Nursing Digest* 6(1):35–40, 1978.

Blagg, C.R., and Scribner, B.H. "Long-term Dialysis: Current Problems and Future Prospects," *American Journal of Medicine* 68:633–35, 1980.

Brundage, D.J. *Nursing Management of Renal Problems.* St. Louis: C.V. Mosby Co., 1980.

Campbell, J.D., and Campbell, A.R. "The Social and Economic Costs of End Stage Renal Disease," *New England Journal of Medicine* 299(8):386–92, 1978.

Canadian Renal Failure Registry. Montreal: Kidney Foundation of Canada, 1985.

Cluff, L.E. "Chronic Disease, Function and the Quality of Care," *Journal of Chronic Disease* 34(7):299–304, 1981.

Craig, H.M. "Adaptation in Chronic Illness: An Eclectic Model for Nurses," *Journal of Advanced Nursing* 8(5):397–404, 1983.

Crawshaw, P., and Wong, B. *Achieving an Attitude of Self-Care.* Vancouver, B.C.: Health and Welfare Canada, 1980.

Devins, G.M., et al. "Helplessness and Depression in End Stage Renal Disease," *Journal of Abnormal Psychology* 90(6):537–45, 1981.

Dzaczkes, J.W., and Kaplan De-Nour, A. *Chronic Hemodialysis as a Way of Life.* New York: Brunner-Mazel, 1978.

Evans, R.W., et al. "The Quality of Life of Patients With End Stage Renal Disease," *New England Journal of Medicine* 312(9):553–59, 1985.

Gordon, M. *Nursing Diagnosis: Process and Application.* New York: McGraw-Hill Book Co., 1982.

Henderson, V. *The Nature of Nursing.* New York: MacMillan Publishing Co., 1966.

Hobfoil, S.E., and Walfisch, S. "Coping with a Threat to Life: A Longitudinal Study of Self-Concept, Social Support, and Psychological Distress," *American Journal of Community Psychology* 12(1):87–100, 1984.

Kossoris, P. "Family Therapy—an Adjunct to Hemodialysis and Transplantation," *American Journal of Nursing* 70(8):1730–33, 1970.

Lalonde, M. *A New Perspective on the Health of Canadians.* Ottawa: Government of Canada, 1974.

Lancaster, L.E., ed. *The Patient with End Stage Renal Disease.* New York: John Wiley & Sons, 1984.

Levin, L. "Self-Care: An Emerging Component of the Health Care System," *Hospital and Health Services Administration* 23(1):17–25, 1978.

Levy, N. "Psychological Factors in Rehabilitation of the Patient Undergoing Maintenance Hemodialysis," in *Rehabilitation in Chronic Renal Failure.* Edited by Chyatte, S. Baltimore: Williams & Wilkins Publishing Co., 1979.

Lewis, K. "Death and Rebirth in Chronic Illness," *Humane Medicine* 1(1):11–15, 1985.

Lindsay, R. "Adaptation to Home Dialysis: The Use of Hemodialysis and Peritoneal Dialysis," *AANNT Journal* 9(5):49–51, 74, 1982.

Mazzuca, S.A. "Does Patient Education in Chronic Disease Have Therapeutic Value?" *Journal of Chronic Disease* 35:521–29, 1982.

McCarthy, M., and Millard, P., eds. *Management of Chronic Illness.* London: Pittman Medical Publishing Co., 1979.

Miller, F.M. *Coping with Chronic Illness: Overcoming Powerlessness.* Philadelphia: F.A. Davis Co., 1983.

Norris, D.P. "Self-Care," *American Journal of Nursing* 79(3):486–89, 1979.

O'Brien, M.E. *The Courage to Survive: The Life Career of the Chronic Dialysis Patient.* New York: Grune & Stratton, 1983.

Orem, D. *Nursing: Concepts of Practice.* New York: McGraw-Hill Book Co., 1980.

Peterson, K.J. "Psychosocial Adjustment of the Family Caregiver: Home Hemodialysis as an Example," *Social Work in Health Care* 10(3):15–31, 1985.

Rettig, R.A. *Implementing the End Stage Renal Disease Program of Medicare.* Santa Monica: The End Corporation, 1980.

Richmond, J.M., et al. "Psychological and Physiological Factors Predicting the Outcome of Home Hemodialysis," *Clinical Nephrology* 17(3):109–13, 1982.

Schoeneman, S., and Reznikoff, M. "Personality Variables in Coping with the Stress of a Spouse's Chronic Illness," *Journal of Clinical Psychology* 39(3):430–36, 1983.

Seligman, M.E.P. *Helplessness: On Depression, Development, and Death.* San Francisco: Freeman, 1975.

Shaeffer, C., et al. "The Health-Related Functions of Social Support," *Journal of Behavioral Medicine* 4(4):381–405, 1981.

Stamek, J.K. "Psycho-Social Care for the Home Dialysand and Partner," *Nephrology Nurse* 3(1):37–41, 1981.

Whitson, S.E. "Individualized Instruction for the Chronic Renal Failure Client," *Nephrology Nurse* 4(2):12–18, 1982.

Wright, L.M., and Leahey, M. *Nurses and Families: A Guide to Family Assessment and Intervention.* Philadelphia: F.A. Davis Co., 1984.

SECTION III

Intervening with Families with Chronic Illness

14 Intervening with families of infants with cleft lip and palate

Ruth Kramer Young, RN, MS, MA
Associate Professor
College of Nursing
University of Oklahoma Health Sciences Center
Oklahoma City, Oklahoma

OVERVIEW

This chapter focuses on the dynamics of nursing care for a family that has an infant with a congenital defect. The family's initial acute grief and chronic sorrow responses are discussed, as are appropriate nursing interventions at different stages in the family's experience. A case study demonstrates how a family might be assessed, what family dynamics the nurse might identify, and appropriate intervention.

CASE STUDY

John and Marie Klein had been married six years when Marie became pregnant. Both are now 33 years old. John has a doctoral degree and teaches history at a state college; Marie completed her master's degree in accounting and works for an accounting firm. The pregnancy was planned and was an exciting experience for both, since they shared many hopes and dreams for their unborn child. There were no complications with pregnancy, labor, or delivery, but the entire family's lives were changed when the infant, Mark, was diagnosed as having bilateral cleft lip and cleft palate. It shattered their world. Mark was transferred to a special care nursery in the children's hospital, and John and Marie, along with other family members, arranged to stay with him. Physicians and nurses talked with John and Marie, expressing concern and offering basic information about cleft lip and cleft palate.

Family Assessment

The Klein family was given an appointment to a clinic specializing in families who have children with cleft lip and cleft palate. The family assessment used general guidelines set forth in the Calgary Family Assessment Model (CFAM) (Wright and Leahey, 1984). The family's social network, especially its supportive capacity, was also analyzed (Young, 1982, 1985).

Structural

Internal. The Kleins' nuclear family consists of the mother, age 33; father, age 33; and their infant. John's parents live in a city 50 miles away. His brother is 35 years old, married, and lives with his family in the same city as their parents. Marie's father died of a heart attack two years before assessment; a married sister, 3 years younger than she, and the sister's husband, live in the same city as John's parents. Marie's brother, aged 29, is married, childless, and attending graduate school in an adjoining state.

Structural

External. Both John's and Marie's families are of German descent and place a high value on home, family, children, work/profession, and fulfillment of personal potential. The Kleins grew up in the Lutheran Church and continue that religion's affiliation.

Functional

Instrumental. Both John's and Marie's mothers are traditional homemakers and never pursued professional training; both fathers assumed the patriarchal provider role within their families. John's and Marie's role definitions differ. Both have been students and members of the workforce during much of their marriage. They share household responsibilities and have discussed sharing parental duties. Questioning revealed that Marie is primarily responsible for organizing the household, while John retains responsibility for house, yard, and car maintenance.

Functional

Expressive. John and Marie both report the ability to express emotions (happiness, sadness, anger) to each other, and have intentionally arranged to do things together in order to nurture their relationship. Both agree that it seems easier for Marie to initiate communication, and she usually suggests special shared activities.

Developmental

Stage/Task. John and Marie are now beginning the childbearing and childrearing stage. They have completed the developmental tasks of selecting a mate and establishing a profession; they have had time to adjust to marriage, and now they will concentrate on the parenting roles. Both have been preparing and planning for parenting, but their infant's bilateral cleft lip and cleft palate will alter their anticipated responses and role behaviors.

Attachment. John and Marie have developed adaptive family member attachments. They agree that their relationship is meaningful; their relationship with extended family members seems positive, without antagonism or overdependence.

Network analysis: Assessment of family resources

Network analysis enables the nurse to determine the family's existing network of relationship interactions and the network's existing or potential helping resources. Although network analysis ordinarily uses a macroperspective including environmental determinants, this section will focus on the micro aspect: four factors affecting the client's perceived or potential closeness to personal and institutional network resources (Young, 1985). These factors are:
- identification
- availability
- duration
- intensity.

Table 14.1 summarizes network analyses of the Klein family's personal and institutional resources. As the analysis shows, this family has a strong network system that can potentially fulfill different family needs.

Family Assessment Summary

Highest priority problems
• First child born with cleft lip and cleft palate
• Parental grief
• Infant feeding problems

Major strengths
• Parental affection and supportive relationship
• Effective social network/support system
• Adequate physical and financial resources

Nursing diagnosis
• Potential family dysfunction related to grief over birth of child with cleft lip and cleft palate.

Planning

Goals
• The family will find adequate ways to work through their grief at not having the healthy "ideal" child they had anticipated.
• The family will develop ways to cope with the chronic sorrow that follows delivery of a child with a congenital defect.

Outcome criteria
The parents will:
• describe what their son's defect means to them
• share their grief with each other, as well as with kinship and other support group members
• perform feeding and other required child care.

Interventions

In the hospital, intervention included managing the parents' shock and disbelief, often through direct and simple explanations. All questions were answered patiently and caringly. One of the first specific interventions was encouraging John and Marie to hold Mark and talk to him. The special feeding devices and procedures required by cleft lip/cleft palate infants were discussed and demonstrated. Eventually both parents were encouraged to participate by feeding Mark. When the long-range treatment plan was discussed, this couple became very interested in pictures of other infants taken before and after surgery.

Surgery to repair Mark's cleft lip would be delayed until he had gained weight following discharge from the hospital. In the interim, a nurse made a home visit, noting that John and Marie demonstrated signs of the "developing awareness" stage. Their facial expressions were strained, sad, and anxious; Mark had been fussy, and they were worried that he was not eating enough. Their comments reflected helplessness, frustration, and hopelessness. Nursing interventions included active listening and demonstrating a genuine interest in the child, the parents, and the other family relationships. The necessary feeding procedures were discussed, and some helpful suggestions made. The nurse weighed Mark and found that he had gained 8 ounces since discharge. Much of the focus was on problems and frustrations faced by most parents of new infants, and the good care John and Marie were giving Mark was positively reinforced. Scheduling the next clinic appointment and setting a date for Mark's cleft lip repair were both discussed.

Table 14.1   Network Analyses of Resources—The Klein Family

Personal Resources

Relationship Variables	Kinship	Neighborhood	Groups
Identification	Strong relationship in nuclear family Close identification with extended family	Moved into home purchased 18 months ago	Marie, choral group; John, sailing
Availability	Most family members live within 50 miles	Close, readily available	Members live in same city
Duration	Nuclear family since marriage Extended family continuous/lifelong	18 months	2 years
Intensity	Close relationship	Forming friendships, some closer than others	Good friends
Potential resources	Emotional support, time, some money	Time, emotional support	Concern, possibly time

Institutional Resources

Relationship Variables	Clinic	Church
Identification	Care for children with cleft palate and cleft lip	Attend regularly; members. Also maintain some ties with hometown church.
Availability	In same city, flexible appointment system	When need expressed or recognized
Duration	Short term, since Mark's diagnosis	Lifelong (varying degrees of participation)
Intensity	Open communication, feelings expressed	Perceive religion as an important dimension of life
Potential	Knowledge, facilities, time	Time, knowledge, facilities (counseling and child day-care)

NURSING PROCESS

Assessment

The health problem: Cleft lip and cleft palate. Cleft lip and cleft palate are part of a large heterogeneous group of congenital defects and disorders. One study (Bergsma, 1979) lists 1,005 different birth defects. Such problems are so varied in type and cause that no satisfactory classification method yet exists. Known causes of chromosomal abnormality include the intrauterine environment, gene mutation, viral infection, and/or drugs ingested during pregnancy. The causes of many congenital anomalies remain unexplained (Whaley and Wong, 1983).

Fusion of the upper lip at the midline usually takes place between the seventh and eighth weeks of gestation. Fusion of the band and soft palate is usually completed between the seventh and twelfth weeks of gestation. Congenital cleft lip and cleft palate result from failure to fuse. The incidence of both problems varies widely. For instance, the rate is 1 in 1,000 live births in Caucasians, twice that in Japanese, and less than half that in American Blacks. The risk increases to 11 in 100 live births if one parent has the defect (Waechter et al., 1985); Whaley and Wong, 1983). These facial malformations are common to all human populations and constitute severe handicaps for affected individuals. Since cleft lip is external and visible, it creates emotional trauma for new parents and, if left unrepaired, can cause emotional anguish for the child.

Treatments for cleft lip and cleft palate are surgical. The surgeon may repair the cleft lip soon after birth, or the procedure may be delayed until the infant weighs 10 pounds or more. Most surgeons prefer to close the cleft palate between one and two years of age to prevent speech impairment. The repair technique is generally quite successful. Cleft repair may require more than one surgical procedure, depending on the degree of deformity.

Feeding a cleft lip/palate infant must be the immediate nursing focus. Special devices are available to facilitate feeding. These include Lamb's and flanged nipples, a Breck feeder, and even spoons and medicine droppers (Waechter et al., 1985; Whaley and Wong, 1983). Immediate care also focuses on the parents' reactions to the defect. Any facial deformity is difficult for parents to accept.

Long-term complications of cleft lip or palate may include speech and hearing problems, orthodontic malposition, or alteration in nasal airway. More problematic complications relate to the child's social adjustment. Long-term goals involve cleft repair, complication prevention, habilitation, facilitation of normal childhood growth and development, and development of a good self-concept in the child (Waechter et al., 1985; Whaley and Wong, 1983).

Different defects vary in their degree of social and psychological impact on the infant, the family, and the entire social network. For example, the parental distress caused by an infant's syndactyly or brachydactyly would in no way compare to that associated with childhood myelomeningocele or hydrocephalus. Assessment must include the entire family system, since all members are affected by the birth of an infant with a defect. Siblings, grandparents, aunts, uncles, and other relatives and friends should all be carefully evaluated. Nursing assessment begins at the first interaction with the infant and family, and must continue after discharge and throughout ongoing specialized care. The Kleins, for instance, will need ongoing assessment as they manage special feeding procedures, cope with Mark's surgeries, and manage other problems that will arise as their son gets older.

Chronic sorrow. In some ways, the initial reaction of parents to the birth of a child with a congenital defect resembles the mourning that ensues after a child dies (Solnit and Stark, 1961); in both cases, they have lost the perfect child they hoped for. Compounding these intense feelings is the reality that the defective child who has created the family's emotional trauma also needs care and attention. Olshansky (1962) coined the term "chronic sorrow" to describe this phenomenon, contending that, although parents may pass through the period of grief over the loss of the "dream" child, their sorrow continues as long as the defective child lives. Jackson (1974) described this phenomenon as "chronic grief" and stated that, unlike acute (limited) grief, chronic grief is both prolonged and recurrent; it follows the same stages as acute grief, but without resolution.

Although chronic sorrow affects the parents most intensely, the entire family system, including siblings, grandparents, aunts, uncles, and cousins, is most definitely affected, as are close friends who function as family members.

The *process* of chronic sorrow begins with the *birth* of the defective child. An obvious external defect is usually diagnosed more quickly than an internal problem, thus hastening the onset of chronic sorrow. Soon after diagnosis, parents experience initial *acute grief* over the loss of their "dreamed for" or "idealized" child.

Denial is a common third response to a newborn infant's congenital defect. Parents are unprepared for such a traumatic event, and they bolster their denial until they can accept the reality and accompanying consequences of the situation. Other common reactions are shock, disbelief, and transient detachment.

The fourth stage is visually *developing awareness*, which is character-ized by feelings of helplessness, hopelessness, and sadness/anxiety. *Helplessness* is the sense of being overwhelmed by an uncontrollable life situation; in this case it is the birth of a defective child. Helpless persons feel they cannot do anything themselves, and that help must come from others. *Hopelessness* reflects a sense of overwhelming defeat in the face of the impossible. The hopeless person feels devastating despair and futility, and usually has an altered future orientation or none at all (Carlson and Blackwell, 1978).

During the developing awareness stage, parents often lash out at the professionals who are caring for their child. They experience self-doubt and guilt. Responses include avoidance, talking a lot, inordinate physical exercise, or excessive work. Different people find different ways to channel frustration.

The fifth, or *restitution*, phase may be conceptualized in terms of a continuum with adaptive responses at one end and maladaptive ones at the other. In an adaptive response, parents find their own ways to cope with day-to-day problems, asking for or obtaining whatever help they need. At the extreme maladaption end of the continuum lies inabil-ity to function and to meet their own and the child's day-to-day needs. Associated behavior might include such responses as child neglect, extreme overprotection, or withdrawal from existing social support systems. There is no clear-cut line between adaptive and maladaptive responses. Most parents' responses fall toward the adaptive end of the continuum. Some responses/behaviors may be misinterpreted as maladaptive by a nurse who does not understand the individual nature of adaptive response. Further complicating the matter, most parents function adaptively at some times and maladaptively at others. Occa-sional or recurrent feelings of disappointment, anger, guilt, or self-doubt should not be labeled maladaptive. Even such events as divorce or job loss may not be maladaptive responses to the birth of a child with a defect. A nurse must remember that some family changes are totally unrelated to the child or the defect.

All families experience some stresses secondary to a child's defect; most eventually discover the coping patterns that are most effective for them. Copley (1985) found that a *critical incident* may initiate progress from an inner-directed denial-grief cycle to a more external focus. One such incident might be life-threatening illness in the defective child. This experience permits grief resolution and the beginnings of accep-tance.

Chronic sorrow is ultimately resolved only with the death of the child or of the parents. The degree of chronic sorrow that parents experience depends on the severity of the defect, its long-term consequences, and how much the child's care and parents' emotional concerns alter family activities. For instance, the long-term effects of severe mental retardation on parents and family would vary greatly from those of cleft lip or cleft palate. Parents of a severely mentally retarded child know the child's limitations and potentials, and therefore worry about what might happen to the child if something were to happen to them. Also, because people differ, individual responses to the same defect will differ. All of these factors compel nurses to assess each family and consider its unique strengths and problems before planning care.

Families with infants. The birth of an infant creates a family crisis. Murray and Zentner (1985) state: "The coming of the child is a *crisis*, a turning point in the couple's life in which old patterns of living must be changed for new ways of living and new values...With the advent of parenthood, a couple is embarking on a journey from which there is no return. To put it simply, parents cannot quit."

These statements would probably not be *fully* understood by a childless couple or even a couple awaiting their first child. The changes that the birth of an infant create in a family are too numerous to list; separately and together they affect a couple's ability to cope with change.

One important predictor of parents' responses to the birth of a child is whether or not the pregnancy was planned and the baby was a wanted family addition. Other factors include parents' emotional maturity, their ability to provide for the infant's basic physical and emotional needs, their ability to adjust to change, a good relationship between the parents, and a positive personal experience of each parent in their family as a child. Many other factors relate to satisfactory adjustment to parenting, and the ones mentioned are not necessarily listed in order of importance.

An infant's birth brings financial obligations to the family, causes physical changes within the mother, and changes family dynamics by adding another member. Roles change as the couples' parents become grandparents. Lifestyles alter dramatically, as schedules begin to revolve around the infant's schedule and demands. The birth of a child may also alter the couple's sexual relationship for a short time and affect social participation with friends, especially those without children. Financial adjustments may be marked if the mother (or father) quits work to care for the infant. Such adjustments are never complete; all must be repeated with every birth. When a new infant has a congenital defect, even more profound adjustments must be made. Few new parents are prepared for all of these changes, which explains why developmental theorists define parenthood as a new stage.

The infant's first year is dominated by growth and rapid developmental changes. Sleeping, eating, and social patterns change from week to week; fortunately parents can be taught to anticipate them.

Parents can usually find ways to cope effectively with the changes that follow the birth of an infant, although many will need assistance in meeting the new demands. Fortunately, parenting also brings feelings of joy and excitement, which can be enhanced by nurses who make an effort to understand each family's dynamics and its unique developmental characteristics.

Planning

General nursing goals for families of congenitally defective infants are to:
- facilitate grief work after the defect has been diagnosed
- facilitate adjustment to chronic sorrow
- monitor the child's care plan (this often involves coordinating plans of several nurses, physicians, and other members of the health care team)
- help parents focus on their child's normal aspects and activities that correspond to parenting a "perfect" infant.

Nursing care planning for families of children with congenital defects must remain flexible. The needs of different families, even those managing the same congenital defect, will differ as will their responses to life events. Nursing goals must be continually evaluated and updated so they remain relevant to each family situation.

Interventions

Nursing interventions can be defined according to stages in the chronic sorrow process.

During acute grief a nurse must remember that parents are experiencing the *loss* of their expected perfect child. Featherstone (1980) reports on a physician who experienced anxiety prior to a family conference to discuss their infant's diagnosis. The anxiety decreased as the physician learned that the couple, like most parents, could handle the situation. Featherstone also notes that their levels of experience may set parents and professionals apart. Few parents, for instance, realize the stress experienced by the professional who has to tell them about their infant's congenital defect. Similarly, few nurses have themselves experienced the parents' anguish upon hearing that their infant has a defect. Education can show nurses how to communicate more effectively with these parents, but it seems that, ultimately, learning will require direct *personal effort*.

Useful nursing interventions for the acute grief period include listening, basic education, permitting denial, recognizing parents' emotional shock and numbness, and accepting their expressions of anxiety. Other specific interventions include providing information openly, offering basic explanations unless asked for in-depth answers, offering empathetic support, and assessing *all* family members' needs.

In an effort to make sure that the infant's needs are met, the nurse may inadvertently overlook the needs of other family members. The nurse must understand that acute grief is not static; parents eventually begin to accept the reality of their loss and experience despair and depression. Parents should be allowed to express their feelings of anger, frustration, and sadness.

As the acute grief reaction progresses, its dynamics usually shift toward the reality of the existing child and the defect. Nevertheless, *denial* remains an effective coping mechanism. Parents still have to learn about the defect and, depending on the exact nature of the problem, what immediate physical care is required. Since the family may not yet have accepted the reality of the defect, nursing care at this time requires patience and understanding. Parents must be allowed to progress at their own pace; the nurse must remember that the family's future seems very uncertain to them. They will be uncertain about the medical and/or surgical treatment that their child will need, and will wonder how their child's defect will alter total family structure and function. Simple reassurance can help such parents express their anxiety and fear. The nurse should assure parents that their response is accepted, because the "normality" of their response might be an additional concern to them. Necessary infant care procedures should be managed and explained by the nurse. Parents usually cannot participate in the care at this point, and may prefer to assume this role gradually.

Listening remains an important intervention as the parents move into the *developing awareness* stage. Couples begin to ask for more detailed and accurate information, and may repeat questions. Positive reinforcement is important, since they usually retain some degree of guilt and self-doubt; existing family strengths should be promoted. The nurse can help the family identify network strengths and how they can be nurtured.

A nurse should remember that support that is appropriate to one family may not be appropriate for another. Some families need encouragement to ask for outside help, while others may need encouragement to become independent and self-confident. The nurses must draw on every possible piece of assessed information in order to decide an appropriate supportive approach.

Reassurance and support must continue through the *restitution* stage. Even parents whose responses are adaptive may need help during the normal ups and downs. The nurse should plan specific interventions to educate parents about normal infant developmental patterns and to adjust their expectations to fit their child's specific defect. Throughout, the child's normalcy should be stressed. If the child's defects involve physical complications, appropriate preventive or care techniques should be discussed. The current trend toward home care means that parents are assuming responsibility for prevention and care of infections, decubiti, fractures, seizures, and such complicated procedures as respirator use and adaptive feeding techniques. Parents may also play a larger role in teaching the child self-help skills. Perhaps most importantly, parents can minimize future emotional complications simply by maintaining a positive attitude, which will shape the child's own outlook. For example, in the Klein family case study, John's and Marie's attitudes toward Mark's cleft lip and cleft palate will help determine his own interpretation of the defect's impact on his life.

Many parents need nursing guidance in disciplining their imperfect child, especially if mental retardation is involved. Parents should be reassured that discipline is part of their responsibility and a necessary part of their child's socialization. Realistic developmental expectations and adequate adjustment to any physical defects can help parents set standards of conduct and implement appropriate discipline.

Parents may also need help locating and arranging for child care. Finding a baby-sitter or day-care facility for a child requiring complex physical care is often problematic. The family network is one potential resource; the Klein family's network could probably help by learning and implementing the special feeding procedures required until the complete surgical repair of Mark's defects.

The birth of a child with a defect affects each member of the family system emotionally, physically, and financially. Often, parents of children with congenital defects need encouragement to plan time for themselves and for nurturing their marriage. If there are siblings, it is extremely important to meet their individual needs and to include them in the overall care plan, thus preventing regression. Regressive behavior is usually handled best by avoiding parental overreaction to the behavior and ensuring that parents spend time with each of their children. Fatigue from physical and emotional distress is also common, especially for the parents. Self-help groups for parents of children with specific congenital problems, in which parents faced with similar challenges teach and learn from each other, are often helpful.

Intervention for parents displaying maladaptive responses usually involves referral to a professional counselor. No precise description of maladaptive responses exists. The total family system must be considered; the nurse often contributes to the referral process by assessing the family's coping skills and problems. Nurses may find it necessary to make independent decisions regarding referral, in which case they must probe for existing problems and the nature of the maladaptive response.

Referrals are appropriate for families that exhibit a variety of needs and varying degrees of disruption. The nurse may help the family to arrange for day-care services, discussion of feelings with clergy (this type of referral is generally in response to family request), nutritional counseling, or sessions with a counselor experienced in the difficulties of families of infants with congenital defects. Outside professionals brought into the case may include specialty nurses, nutritionists, physicians, family support groups, special welfare agencies, or qualified family therapists.

If special needs are met satisfactorily during infancy, both child and the family will probably be able to cope with the stresses brought on by future maturational and developmental changes. The unique developmental problems of a child with a congenital defect can never be *fully* anticipated nor understood by parents during the child's infancy; they can only be faced and addressed as they arise.

As described earlier, *resolution* comes only with the death of parent or child. The focus here will be on the child's death. Parents again experience acute grief, along with possible relief and associated ambivalence or guilt. Talking with a nurse who has known and cared for the child may be helpful. Reassurance that their feelings are normal and accepted can be comforting to such parents. Since the family will have had good as well as bad times, the nurse should encourage discussion of both.

Parents need the support of a nurse who loved and respected their child as a special person and who understood the family relationships. It is important to remember that the dead child played a role in the family system, and made a unique contribution. Siblings often need support to work through this stage successfully. Follow-up clinic appointments or home visits by a professional familiar with the family's experience may be necessary. Parent groups are often helpful.

Anniversaries of the child's birth or death are often difficult for bereaved parents, as are holidays or other events where experiences with the child were meaningful. Parents sometimes need to talk about and resolve unfinished questions or feelings about something that happened to them or to their child. The nurse cannot prepare family members for all of the feelings and responses they may experience; she can, however, direct them toward available help. The family may need continued professional support, of a duration and intensity dictated by its special needs.

Evaluation

Evaluation begins with the birth of the infant with a congenital defect. Since that birth creates a highly complex family situation, comprehensive evaluation is critical. Each family member's needs, the nursing and family goals, and the results of all interventions with infant and other family members must be included; a systematic approach will allow a more thorough evaluation. For example, the Kleins' nurse stated her goals and her specific outcome criteria and conducted an initial evaluation to determine if the family could describe the personal meaning of their son's defect; share their grief with each other as well as others in their support network; and participate in Mark's care, for instance by feeding him. Mark's and his parents' ability to cope with required surgical procedures and the long-term care required for children with cleft lip and cleft palate would be monitored over time. Also to be evaluated were Mark's physical and emotional responses, as well as those of his parents and others in the family support network. Since children with cleft lip and cleft palate are at increased risk for ear infection and hearing loss, this area would require ongoing assessment, as would speech development. How the child responds to a cleft lip, cleft palate, or any congenital defect is influenced strongly by others' responses, especially those of the parents and other significant members of the network system. This makes a family approach in nurses' care planning imperative. The desired outcome is for the child to have good self-esteem and minimal physical or emotional problems related to the deformity.

CONCLUSIONS

The diagnosis of an infant's congenital defect constitutes a crisis for parents. Most experience chronic sorrow, characterized by hurt feelings, disappointment, and frustration that will persist throughout their efforts to cope with the day-to-day reality of the child's condition.

The nurse's role is to facilitate the parents' ability to manage their child's defect and control its impact on family members' lives. Conceptualizing parental responses in terms of stages helps nurses; it provides a frame of reference for family care, not a rigid guide for sequential responses. Chronic sorrow is not abnormal, but rather a normal reaction to an abnormal situation; the nurse must strive to increase positive parenting experiences and minimize the periods when chronic sorrow predominates.

REFERENCES

Bergsma, D., ed. *The March of Dimes Birth Defects Compendium.* New York: Alan R. Liss, 1979.

Bristor, M.W. "The Birth of a Handicapped Child: A Holistic Model for Grieving," *Family Relations* 33:25–32, 1984.

Carlson, C., and Blackwell, B. *Behavioral Concepts,* 2nd ed. Philadelphia: J.B. Lippincott Co., 1978.

Copley, M.F. "Chronic Sorrow in Families of Disabled Children," Unpublished manuscript, 1985.

Darling, R.B., and Darling, J. *Children Who are Different: Meeting the Challenges of Birth Defects in Society.* St. Louis: C.V. Mosby Co., 1982.

Featherstone, H. *Difference in the Family: Living with a Disabled Child.* New York: Penguin Books, 1980.

Jackson, P.L. "Chronic Grief," *American Journal of Nursing* 74:1288–91, 1974.

Kushner, H.S. *When Bad Things Happen to Good People.* New York: Schocken Books, 1981.

McKeever, P.T. "Fathering the Chronically Ill Child," *American Journal of Maternal Child Nursing* 6(2):124–28, 1981.

Moses, K. "Meeting the Child's and the Family's Needs," Keynote address presented at the Association for the Care of Children's Health 19th Annual Conference. Houston, 1983.

Murray, R.B., and Zentner, J.P. *Nursing Assessment and Health Promotion Through the Life Span.* Englewood Cliffs, N.J.: Prentice-Hall, 1985.

Olshansky, S. "Chronic Sorrow: A Response to Having a Mentally Defective Child," *Social Casework* 43:190–93, 1962.

Portier, L.M., and Wanlass, R.L. "Family Crisis Following the Diagnosis of a Handicapped Child," *Family Relations* 33:13–25, 1984.

Solnit, A.J., and Stark, M.H. "Mourning and the Birth of a Defective Child," *Psychoanalytical Study of the Child* 16:523–37, 1961.

Waechter, E.H., et al. *Nursing Care of Children.* Philadelphia: J.B. Lippincott Co., 1985.

Whaley, L.F., and Wong, D.L. *Nursing Care of Infants and Children.* St. Louis: C.V. Mosby Co., 1983.

Wikler, L., et al. "Chronic Sorrow Revisited: Parent vs. Professional Depiction of the Adjustment of Parents of Mentally Retarded Children. *American Journal of Orthopsychiatry* 51(1):63–70, 1981.

Wright, L.M., and Leahey, M. *Nurses and Families: A Guide to Family Assessment and Intervention.* Philadelphia: F.A. Davis Co., 1984.

Young, R.K. "Assessing the Client's Community Resources Through Network Analysis," *Journal of Community Health Nursing* 2(1):3–11, 1985.

Young, R.K. "Chronic Sorrow: Parents' Response to the Birth of a Child with a Defect," *American Journal of Maternal Child Nursing* 2(1):38–42, 1977.

Young, R.K. *Community Nursing Workbook: Family as Client.* East Norwalk, Conn.: Appleton-Century-Crofts, 1982.

15 Intervening with families of infants with Down syndrome

Fay F. Russell, RN, C, MN
Associate Professor, Child Development and Chief of Nursing
The University of Tennessee, Memphis
Health Sciences Center, Child Development Center

Associate Professor, Maternal Child Nursing
The University of Tennessee, Memphis
Health Sciences Center, College of Nursing
Memphis, Tennessee

OVERVIEW

This chapter provides a systematic approach for the nurse interviewing and intervening with families raising infants with genetic defects. The nursing process serves as a model for exploring some of the complex problems that families encounter. A case study highlights the emotional implications of the genetic defect and a typical parental grief reaction. Nursing strategies for a family's critical first year with a handicapped infant are discussed in the context of current theory and practice.

CASE STUDY

Clair, age 1 month, was referred to the University of Tennessee Center for the Health Sciences Child Development Center (CDC) with a diagnosis of trisomy 21 (Down syndrome). The referring physician asked for a developmental evaluation and enrollment in the CDC's Early Intervention Program.

The family consisted of Mr. Gambino, the 44-year-old father, Clair's mother, age 34 years, and Clair. They were a middle- to upper-middle-class family who lived in a small rural town. Mr. Gambino owned a tire business and had a 24-year-old child by a former marriage. Mrs. Gambino, an early childhood teacher, was on maternity leave but planned to return to her previous position. The couple had been married four years. Both parents were reported to be in good health. The pregnancy with Clair was planned and wanted.

Because of lack of cervical dilation in the birth process, Clair was delivered by cesarean section. Her birth weight was 8 pounds, 13 ounces, and Mrs. Gambino reported that her cry and respirations were immediate. Because Clair displayed physical features characteristic of trisomy 21, a tentative diagnosis was made in the delivery room, and the couple was informed by an on-call pediatrician whom, according to the parents, cited Mrs. Gambino's age as a factor in the birth defect.

Chromosomal analysis confirmed the diagnosis and the family was referred to CDC. According to the referring counselor, both parents were shocked and overwhelmed by the diagnosis. Therefore, they were placed in the Early Intervention Program, which is designed to provide group therapy for parents as well as a comprehensive developmental intervention program for developmentally delayed infants and young children. As coordinator of that program, this writer received the referral for further family assessment.

Family Assessment

The parents came to the appointment with their infant carefully dressed for the occasion. (In any initial family interview, attention should be paid to the infant's appearance and physical care.) Mr. Gambino was noted to be a handsome, rather quiet, distinguished-looking man who could easily have been mistaken for Clair's grandfather. Although he spoke little, he obviously shared in the interview by listening carefully. Mrs. Gambino was an attractive blond woman with a pleasing sense of humor. She was talkative and responsive to the nurse, but became tearful as she spoke of the events surrounding Clair's birth. Both parents responded positively to the nurse's empathy and support, and asked numerous questions related to Clair's care. Both were caring and attentive to Clair, who at 10 weeks of age exhibited many of the stigmata of Down syndrome—the wide nasal bridge, large tongue, and eyes with small white areas called Brushfield spots in the irides. Small ears and redundant tissue on the posterior portion of the neck were also present as was generalized moderate hypotonia. To her parents' relief, Clair did not have any of the heart defects or other major problems often associated with trisomy 21.

Clair had been breast-fed successfully since birth; no difficulty was observed sucking. A routine of feeding every four hours had been established. Mrs. Gambino found breast-feeding satisfying, and Clair's height and weight were within the normal range.

The parents reported that Clair had some problem with constipation, which they handled by adding one tablespoonful of corn syrup to her daily water. Clair's immunizations were up to date.

At the first appointment, Clair's parents were primarily interested in activities to enhance her development. Both parents experienced continuing difficulty in understanding why this happened to them and their daughter; they decided to forego having other children, choosing instead to devote their resources to obtaining the best possible care for Clair.

Further exploration revealed that Clair shared her parents' bed and was not sleeping through the night; the Gambinos also reported leaving her unattended.

The parents' main sources of emotional support were siblings, to whom both were close. Though the family attended church regularly, they did not consider that affiliation sufficiently supportive. For more detailed information, see the genogram (Figure 15.1).

The family assessment also included a systems list of family strengths and problems, as conceptualized in the Calgary Family Assessment Model (CFAM) (Wright and Leahey, 1984). The assessed strengths and problems are shown in Table 15.1.

Table 15.1 Identified Strengths and Problems— The Gambino Family

Systems	Strengths	Problems
Whole Family	• Adequate income	
Marital/Parental	• Concerned parents • Mutual caring • Ability to grieve together	
Parent-Child	• Strong parental attachment to Clair; breast-feeding • Willingness to learn about handicap	• Clair sharing her parents' bed—limits parents' opportunity for marital closeness and prevents optimum rest and sleep for all • Denial of extent of handicap • Lack of information about handicapping condition
Individual	• Good health • Parental maturity	• Clair's Down syndrome
Other	• Demonstrated willingness to seek appropriate care unavailable in small town and to keep appointments • Availability of adequate health care	• Lack of community understanding of and information about Clair's handicap

Developmental Assessment (Child)

Clair was assessed using the Denver Development Screening Test (DDST). The Alpern Boll Developmental Profile and informal observation results indicated possible developmental delay; Clair's functional age was estimated to be at least one month below her chronological age.

Planning

A program of individualized developmental activities was organized (see Table 15.2) and the parents taught to conduct it at home.

It was made clear that this plan was flexible, and that all objectives probably would not be met. The Gambinos called twice during the ensuing two months to report that Clair was making progress.

Interventions

Clair was five months old when the interdisciplinary developmental team evaluation was completed and the family enrolled in early intervention program sessions. During the 10 weekly interviews, the nurse offered support and empathy, as well as answers to specific questions. Mrs. Gambino reported recurring flashbacks of the moment she was told that Clair had Down syndrome, usually occurring as she showered. Several times during these sessions she recounted the circumstances of how she was told. Sharing this experience over and over seemed to be the catharsis that she needed. Again Mr. Gambino

Figure 15.1   Genogram—The Gambino Family

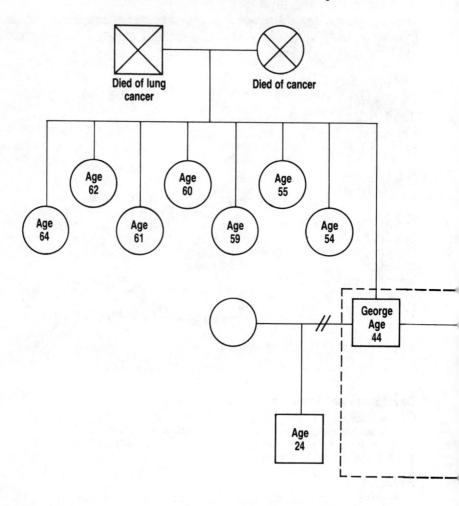

participated more by listening to and supporting his wife than by talking. Mrs. Gambino called frequently between sessions, mostly to share Clair's progress or to ask questions.

Clair's behavioral objectives were reviewed and updated periodically. New developmental interventions were added weekly, and others deleted. Physical therapy, nutrition, and speech/language therapy were part of each interventive session. Also, as an integral part of the Early Intervention Program, the Gambinos attended group therapy sessions conducted by social workers. Mr. Gambino was more reluctant to share emotional reactions with the group; his wife expressed annoyance at an article that appeared in her home town newspaper stating that the Intelligence Quotient (IQ) range of persons with Down syndrome was between 50 and 70 points. She also objected to the article's use of the term "retarded"; she preferred the term "challenged." Mrs. Gambino's feelings about Clair were ambivalent and at times overly optimistic.

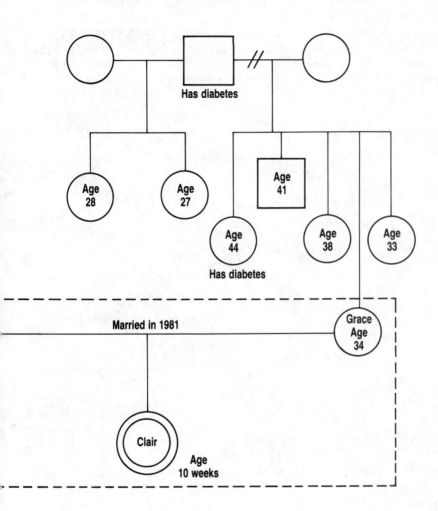

Both parents grieved realistically. Mrs. Gambino emerged as a socio-emotional leader in the group. During the group experience her ambivalence was expressed and her grief shared with others. Both parents' denial was reduced as they gained insight into the significance of Clair's developmental delay.

Clair progressed steadily; at 8 months of age, she was reaching out to other children in play and appeared to enjoy the activities and exercises. She continued to be breast-fed, but tolerated solid food well when introduced. Her feeding skill development approached the 6- to 7-month level. At the nurse's recommendation, she was placed in a crib in her own room, and the parents reported that they, too, were more comfortable with this arrangement. The parents, probably motivated by their emotional pain, followed rigidly the suggestions given for Clair. The nurse assured them that they were doing prescribed activities properly.

Table 15.2 Excerpts from the Beginning Developmental Program for the Gambino Family

Behavioral Objectives (Clair)	
Fine Motor Skills	• Follow a moving object with her eyes 180 degrees horizontally and vertically 100% of the time. • Explore both hands spontaneously in front of her face for 2 minutes during daily play. • Hold an object or toy in each hand for 15 seconds and in both hands at the same time for 15 seconds on 3 of 4 tries.
Gross Motor Skills	• Hold her head steady as she sits in the corner of the couch for 2 to 3 minutes. • Begin to roll from side to back and back to front.
Social Skills	• Maintain eye contact with someone who is talking with her for one minute, 1 of 4 tries. • Smile responsively when played with or talked to by a family member, several times daily. • Laugh aloud when she is tickled. Usually tickling on the stomach will elicit a laugh.
Language Skills	• Begin to turn eyes and/or head towards loud sounds, 50% of time. • Vocalize when talked to or happy. • Make cooing sounds ("aah," "ooo").

Evaluation

Clair, now age eight months, has been well the past six months and has received all infant immunizations. She is easily managed and responsive, with an overall developmental level estimated at six months. Although she is making progress, Clair's delays are becoming obvious. Mrs. Gambino will return to teaching this fall, and her husband will bring Clair and the sitter for weekly sessions. He will also participate in the parent therapy group. The Gambinos still find it difficult to think of Clair as mentally retarded. Limited community resources, such as an absence of preschool opportunities for retarded children and no parents' organization (i.e., an Association for Retarded Citizens), make it difficult for the family to plan for Clair's future.

Name: Clair   Age: 4 months
Projected Date of Achievement: 6-8 months

Strategies to Achieve Objectives (Parents)

- Move a brightly colored toy (red or yellow) 180 degrees both vertically and horizontally as demonstrated. Move the object slowly, vary the distance from Clair, and allow time for her to focus and follow. She will lose it, at first. Do several times daily.
- While Clair is on her back, gently push her hands into her field of vision. Direct her attention to her hands, gradually increasing your help as she "finds her hands."
- Put an object or toy in Clair's hand—use hand-on-hand guidance as demonstrated. One-inch blocks work well. Do two times per day during week.

- Place Clair in the corner of a sofa, couch, or upholstered chair in a sitting position. Her head will bob a bit to begin with, but she will gradually be able to maintain her head straight while in this position. Try this for a few seconds to begin with and work toward the goal as long as she can tolerate it.
- Do 5 to 10 sit-ups holding your hands at Clair's shoulders. Work up to 5, as she may tire with too many at first. Proceed slowly and do 3 or 4 times per day. Diaper change is also a good time for this exercise.
- Do the fast rolling (rolling Clair over and over both ways) as demonstrated before doing any of the gross motor activities.

- Talk with Clair daily, from eye level. Once a week, time her attention to such conversation. (Current duration is 10 seconds.)
- The goals of smiling and laughing are self-explanatory.
- Call Clair's attention to activities (i.e., feeding and bathing) before initiating them and await her response.
- Put a mobile over her crib, 8 to 12 inches above her head. Change objects on the mobile two or three times per week (hang another toy on it, or add a colored swatch). Occasionally using a patterned sheet on her bed will provide additional visual stimulation.

- Use a noisemaker as aural stimulation. See if she will look toward the noise.
- Continue "talking" to Clair, and reward sounds that she makes by smiling, kissing, or telling her that you are pleased.
- Imitate her own sounds to her. This gives her added feedback and helps her to learn to respond to sounds.

NURSING PROCESS

Assessment

The health problem: Down syndrome. Trisomy 21 is called Down syndrome after Dr. Langdon Down, who first described it in 1866. It results from the presence of an extra chromosome in all body cells; specifically, three chromosomes instead of the normal pair at position 21. It is the most common genetic cause of mental retardation, affecting all races and levels of society equally. The literature describes three types of trisomy 21, which result from an error in cell division and occur in over 93% of the persons diagnosed as having Down syndrome (Pueschel and Rynders, 1982).

Translocation trisomy 21 is defined as the existence of an extra chromosome 21 which has broken and become attached to another chromosome; such translocations can be identified correctly through a technique called banding (Pueschel and Rynders, 1982). When this type of Down syndrome is found, the parents' genetic makeups are studied to determine whether the disorder is familial; the results of that screening will affect the counseling necessary. Some persons can carry this type of Down syndrome because they possess the correct amount of genetic material, but with altered chromosomal placement. Four to six percent of all Down syndrome patients are of the translocation type (Pueschel and Rynders, 1982).

In mosaic Down syndrome, both normal and affected cells are present. Several variations of mosaicism are described; since there are some normal cells, the condition is less apparent physiologically. Thompson and Thompson (1980) report that approximately 0.5% to 1% of Down syndrome patients have a mosaic disorder. Inheritance is not thought to be a factor in mosaicism since the defect results from meiotic or mitotic nondisjunction in individual cells (Pueschel and Rynders, 1982).

The overall incidence of trisomy 21 averages 1 in 650 to 1 in 800 live births, with risks increasing dramatically with advancing maternal age. Approximately 50% of all spontaneously aborted fetuses display some chromosomal anomaly—and at least half of those are trisomic. A slightly higher incidence of trisomy 21 is reportedly associated with increased paternal age (Pueschel and Rynders, 1982).

Parental age might be significant in the Gambino case. At conception, Mrs. Gambino was 33 years of age, her husband 43. Pueschel and Rynders (1982) report the incidence of Down syndrome as 3.39 per 1,000 live births at maternal age 30 to 35 years.

Trisomy 21 may be diagnosed in utero. Amniocentesis, an analysis of amniotic fluids, should be done within the first 20 weeks of pregnancy, and can be used to diagnose other defects, such as neural tube defect (spina bifida or meningocele). A mother who has borne one Down syndrome child stands a 1 in 100 chance of having another infant with the same abnormality. Since trisomy 21 is a potential problem for all childbearing families, nurses should be familiar with diagnostic options and be able to share this information with at-risk families. Since parents of diagnosed Down syndrome fetuses might be asked to consider abortion, prenatal diagnosis may present ethical or legal problems;

however, most parents who agree to one have already decided to terminate the pregnancy if major abnormalities are found (Thompson and Thompson, 1980).

Trisomy's underlying cause is unknown. At-risk families with a history of trisomy 21 or those who have had one child with trisomy 21 should consider genetic counseling. Wright (1981) states that genetics has moved into the mainstream of health care and that nurses need the skills to deliver it properly.

Pueschel and Rynders (1982) describe the typical physical manifestations of trisomy 21. These include microcephaly with brachycephaly; short stature; flat nasal bridge; oblique palpebral fissures; epicanthal folds; low-set and/or rotated ear placement; short neck; loose skin on nape of neck; high, arched, and narrow palate; abnormally large tongue; muscular hypotonia; gaps between first and second toes; transverse palmar crease; and short and/or incurved fifth finger. Inexplicably, some Down syndrome patients display many of these signs, while others have only a few. Ninety-nine percent of all trisomy 21 patients are mildly to seriously mentally retarded. Morgan (1979) reported that most of the trisomy 21 patients studied display moderate mental retardation with a mean IQ of 50. Trisomic infants also experience characteristic physical problems including inadequate nutrition with inappropriate weight loss or gain, dry skin, frequent upper respiratory and other infections, otitis media, constipation, feeding difficulties, and hearing and visual problems.

Informing family of diagnosis. Trisomy is obvious to most experienced physicians and nurses at the time of delivery. The task of telling the parents becomes a major undertaking, for this event is never forgotten, and the way the diagnosis is shared with the parents affects how they will accomplish necessary family developmental tasks.

A recent retrospective study of 72 sets of parents whose trisomic infants were born between 1970 and 1982 indicated that many were not informed of their child's problem in a warm and caring way, that 37.5% of the conferences were too brief, and that 58% of the respondents received no information about additional help for themselves or their infant (Soto-Viera et al., 1984). Although nurses seldom share the diagnosis with the parents (only 2.8% of the above cases), families are in their care. Therefore, nursing care plans should reflect appropriate family developmental tasks: integrating the infants into the family unit; accommodating new parenting and grandparenting roles; and maintaining the marital bond (Wright, 1981). The case study illustrates the impact of this first encounter and underscores its lasting significance for the parents. Parental perceptions do vary in terms of the reaction to the news and how it is told.

In this writer's experience, many parents feel isolated and unable to communicate with nursing staff after the birth of a trisomic infant. They cannot remember receiving comfort, empathy, or understanding on occasions when their crying expressions of grief were observed by nursing staff.

Romney (1984) maintains that "identity" is the critical issue in managing the birth of an infant with a congenital anomaly. Families need help to classify and to form a realistic and positive identification for the new infant while they mourn the "lost" one. Romney suggests the actions listed in Table 15.3.

Family reactions to diagnosis. The birth of an infant with a genetic defect is usually unexpected—and devastating for the parents. Tooley and Rawls (1982) describe the mourning process associated with this family trauma, and maintain that families must mourn their lost dream of a healthy infant before accepting their handicapped child. Johnson (1978) identifies the nurse as a major intervener, helping parents and family members deal with typical reactions surrounding the birth of a defective child.

Solnit and Stark (1961) also describe several stages of mourning, including denial, anger, bargaining, despair, and, finally, acceptance. Accompanying these stages of mourning are fear, guilt, resentment, and sorrow.

Denial and disbelief. The grieving individuals cannot deal with the reality of their situation and maintain that no problems exist. In parents, this grief stage might be displayed by such statements as, "He will outgrow this," or, "This is a minor problem and we accepted it right away," or, "He does not look any different from other infants." Denial should not be reinforced. Such responses as "I think I hear what you are saying, however, through no fault of yours, your baby does have a genetic defect. It is true that he is more like other babies than he is different," may be helpful.

Anger. Virtually all parents of defective newborns feel anger, often at professionals. Seeking someone to blame often becomes an obsession. Most nurses have no difficulty identifying this grief stage. Appropriate therapeutic responses might include, "You seem to be angry." The nurse must be prepared to deal with the ensuing parental outburst, remembering that this opportunity for family members to share feelings may be very helpful. The nurse must also remain alert to the possibility and indications of child abuse at this stage, if parents make the child an object of their anger.

Bargaining. As parents move through the mourning and grief process, many try to "bargain" for their child's health—for instance, with God

Table 15.3 Suggested Nursing Actions in Cases of Infants with Genetic Disability

- Encourage the parents to see the infant; the longer they wait, the more distorted and fixed their concept of the child's condition may become. Ideally, the physician or nurse practitioner should examine the infant in the parents' presence, emphasizing the child's normal aspects as they delineate problems. The examiner can also model parenting behaviors by relating and responding to the infant as a person, not as an anomaly. The examination provides an opportunity for parents to ask questions, express feelings, and clarify misunderstandings.
- Provide realistic information about the infant's disability. This will emphasize and clarify the infant's "real" identity to parents.
- Encourage other hospital staff members to model positive and therapeutic caretaking behaviors toward the infant.
- Encourage the parents to explain the situation to friends and relatives. The process will help them come to terms with the situation.
- Adapt or adjust hospital routine when medically appropriate, to facilitate parent-infant bonding. The more time the parents spend with their infant, the stronger the bond will be.
- Involve hospital staff and family in care planning. Meetings can be held regularly, allowing staff and parents to ventilate concerns and feelings in a therapeutic environment.
- Progress at the parents' pace: emphasize facilitating communication, keeping the family together, and assisting and supporting the family to work toward acceptance of their disabled infant and his disability.

Reprinted with permission from Hemisphere Publications

("If I pray long and hard enough this problem will be solved"). At the same time, they may seek developmental help for their infant, admitting the possibility of mental retardation and opening the door for nurses to help parents as well as the infant. Other parents begin to shop for the "right" professional. This process may be prolonged in some families, consuming much time and energy and possibly imposing financial burdens, but it remains a positive sign of problem recognition.

Despair. When "bargaining" fails, parents can become depressed and give up, perhaps even rejecting help. Tooley and Rawls (1982) described this as the lowest point of the grief process, and suggested that the nurse recognize these behaviors, accept the rejection, and renew therapeutic efforts when parents are more accepting. However, they stress the need for the nurse to stay in touch with the parents, perhaps through occasional phone calls, and reassure them of continued interest and willingness to help. Health needs may also help keep the family in contact with the health care delivery system.

Acceptance. Most families do not reach this final stage until more than a year after the birth of the defective infant. Feelings continue to vacillate and earlier reactions reoccur unpredictably. A family achieves acceptance when all members are reconciled to the significance of the disability. Parents may reach out toward others with a child with similar disabilities and begin to participate in community efforts to obtain increased services.

Adding to the stress on parents of trisomic newborns is the fact that such infants often have other serious or even life-threatening problems, such as heart defects or gastrointestinal malformations. Also stressful are such activities as showing the infant to others, having photographs taken, naming the child, and sending birth announcements. Under these circumstances, marital stress is inevitable. Murphy (1982) maintains that stress studies in families of genetically imperfect infants have offered no meaningful solutions to these problems, and concludes that parental stress cannot be isolated from the status of the child.

Parental grief after a Down syndrome birth can be overwhelming. Mothers have reported lengthy episodes of uncontrolled crying up to several months after birth. At the same time, it is not rare for parents to report that former friends have become aloof, leaving them isolated in their pain and grief.

When and how to tell grandparents and siblings about the new baby's defect(s) are often major stumbling blocks. Grandparents often deny the infant's problem, thereby encouraging the parents to ignore it. The child's illness itself can hinder parental bonding and attachment, especially if care treatment is required or if the parents are too upset to hold and cuddle the baby. Obviously, parents whose first child has trisomy 21 or a similar handicap would have much difficulty without professional assistance.

Family assessment models. New parenthood itself is a developmental crisis; a defective infant only deepens this crisis. Conventional grief theories are useful in assessing such families and planning care for the parents. Olshansky's (1962) classic work on chronic sorrow in parents with mentally retarded children is an appropriate adjunct to the theories described earlier, and is especially useful for assessing the family over time.

The Calgary Family Assessment Model (CFAM) (Wright and Leahey, 1984) is helpful in evaluating Down syndrome families through three major categories:
• structure
• development
• function.

Structural assessment clarifies the family's internal and external components. Internal components are composition, rank order, subsystem, and boundary; while culture, religion, social class status and mobility, environment, and extended family are defined as external components. The family developmental assessment determines life-cycle stage, family tasks at that stage, and adaptive or maladaptive attachments within the family unit. The functional assessment addresses instrumental and expressive factors. The Gambino family case study illustrates how the CFAM can be implemented, and the use of a genogram provides a framework that may be used over time and amended as the family evolves.

This comprehensive holistic nursing focus is the model of choice. During that crucial first year, however, parental feelings about the infant with a genetic defect are the primary concern. For some families, even infant care is secondary to coping with grief and sadness. In such cases as this, serial assessment of the infant's physical growth and development is necessary. Community resources should be fully mobilized, since many professionals' expertise may be needed to deal with the complex lifelong problems these families and children will experience.

Planning

Ideally, prevention is the first—and only—intervention needed in genetic illness. Appropriate referral of parents at high risk of having a genetically handicapped child is crucial. Older parents and those with a history of translocation trisomy 21 need early referrals. The nurse is in a pivotal position and can offer supportive counseling and determine parental understanding of their situation. More and more prospective parents are seeking help in avoiding the birth of genetically imperfect infants. To provide the help they need, the nurse must have up-to-date information on preventive and interventive genetic practices (Cohen, 1984). By integrating structural, developmental, and functional assessments, the nurse can plan individualized interventions. The effective plan will take into account the parents' knowledge base and grief state, and the infant's genetic disability. If possible, the family should be included in the planning process; however, some families cannot tolerate the necessary responsibility and involvement at this time.

Hospital discharge planning should include advising parents of available helping resources, such as parent groups, developmental centers, health and educational facilities, and the local association for retarded citizens. If the infant has an associated defect, the parents will have been referred to the appropriate specialist. The importance of keeping appointments must be stressed. Often clear explanations will clarify unstated parental misunderstandings. The nurse must also remember that parents may not give the Down syndrome infant the same degree of care they provided to previous healthy children, simply because the infant is "different." If the handicapped child is the firstborn, then parents must be taught to care for it as they would for any "normal" child.

Both short- and long-term goals must be established, with priority given to short-term goal achievement. Often, the one-day-at-a-time attitude is the most effective short-term objective. It must be remembered that initial planning is but a small step in the lifelong process of nurturing a child with a disabling genetic defect such as trisomy 21.

Institutionalization is no longer a viable alternative for families who cannot adequately care for a defective infant. More practical options are adoption, foster care, or employment of a full-time sitter. Most families, however, prefer to care for their infant themselves, at home, seeking whatever help is recommended.

Referral to an appropriate community nurse is recommended in order to assure continuous family-centered care after discharge. The referring nurse must therefore have a thorough knowledge of available community resources and services.

Interventions

Dealing with affect. Nurses must be sensitive to parents' feelings and grief in cases of genetically defective infants. Veach (1983) writes as a nurse and as a mother of an infant with trisomy 21. She underscores such parents' need for comfort and support, and suggests that nurses remain with parents when they are told of the diagnosis, because they will need someone to repeat what was said until they can absorb it. She also advises nurses to let the parents decide if they want to be isolated from other patients on the maternity unit, and to inquire about other family members in order to gauge how their responses will influence parental reactions. The nurse should also provide time for parent-infant bonding. Veach further suggests that nurses help parents become organized and encourage them to make notes and list questions. They should also refer the parents to appropriate social and (hospital) pastoral service staff, to a public health nurse, and to a parents' organization. Finally, she cautions nurses not to be judgmental in caring for parents who decide not to keep their infant.

Nurses caring for Down syndrome families must be attuned to their own biases about mentally retarded and genetically defective infants. Negative attitudes in health professionals are obvious to parents and add to their already heavy burden. It takes time and soul searching to understand one's own feelings and attitudes, but the effort is vital for effective care. While the focus is on the family, nurses should also regard the infant as a unique individual of worth. They should hold the infant and reach out to touch the parents in some way at each interview.

Therapy. Family, group, and/or individual therapy can be effective interventions. The therapeutic group process offers support, coping strategies, and techniques to ease parents' pain and help them deal with grief. Individual counseling is less intense, but offers support, valuable information, and guidance for stress reduction. Parent-to-parent networks also provide peer support; an effective national network, the Down Syndrome Congress (Dept. N83, 1640 Roosevelt Rd., Chicago, IL 60608), is in place for parents with Down syndrome children. Along with emotional therapy, Down syndrome parents need continuing health care, perhaps with emphasis on family planning.

Interdisciplinary early intervention programs. Longitudinal studies reveal that interdisciplinary early intervention programs incorporating both parent group therapy and developmental intervention are very effective for Down syndrome infants and their families (Connolly and Russell, 1976; Connolly et al., 1980, 1984). Specialized somatosensory, gross and fine motor, social and self-help, and receptive and expressive language interventions aimed at enhancing the infant's development help to maximize functioning. Oral motor therapy and feeding skill development are particularly important. Developmental nursing specialists, physical and occupational therapists, and speech/language pathologists are therefore critical members of the early intervention team. Nutritional guidance must also be integrated into a comprehensive program, as should audiological, otolaryngological, psychological, and other specialty consultations.

Nurses' expectations of family members must be realistic if a home habilitation program is to succeed. In their efforts to accomplish all recommended infant stimulations, exercises, and activities, family members may become overburdened and develop difficulty in coping. A comprehensive, family-centered, individualized, interdisciplinary team approach, with nursing participation, is considered by some to be the most effective way to prevent this overload during the infant and early toddler stages (Russell, 1985).

Nursing contributions to health care team. Zelle and Coyner (1983) characterize nursing intervention with families of handicapped infants as action on, with, or on behalf of the infant and his family. As they state (p. 53), such activities as "counseling, administering of a therapeutic technique, routine or medication, adjustment of the physical environment, health education, assessments of physical integrity or function, referral to other health, social, or educational services, and communication with other health care providers are within the realm of the professional nurse."

In sum, the care plan for a family with a Down syndrome infant must have certain necessary features. These include attention to parent-child attachment; observation of the quantity and quality of parent-child interactions and appropriate protective parent functions; and provision of general health care, including routine immunizations. Preventive care, anticipatory guidance, and early identification and treatment help alleviate some of the distress caused by the child's physical problems, family reactions, and long-term parental adjustment.

Evaluation

Two areas must be evaluated: process and outcome. Process evaluation requires examination of how things are being done: Are the mother and father satisfied with care? With their coping abilities? With their other children's adjustment to their sibling's disability? Outcome evaluation considers whether or not established goals were achieved, and if they were not, whether the goals were appropriate, and how the family has adapted to its situation.

CONCLUSIONS

This chapter has provided a foundation for assessing, planning, intervening, and evaluating nursing care for families with infants with genetic defects. Nurses must remember, however, the complexities of such care provision; each family brings into its situation a unique set of circumstances. The nurse's challenge is to provide the most current and creative approaches available.

REFERENCES

Alpern, G.D., and Boll, T.J. *Developmental Profile Manual.* Indianapolis: Psychological Development Publications, 1972.

Cohen, F.L. *Clinical Genetics in Nursing Practice.* Philadelphia: J.B. Lippincott Co., 1984.

Connolly, B., and Russell, F. "Interdisciplinary Early Intervention Program," *Physical Therapy* 56:155-58, 1976.

Connolly, B., et al. "Early Intervention Program with Down Syndrome Children: Follow-up Report," *Physical Therapy* 60:1405-08, 1980.

Connolly, B., et al. "Evaluation of Children with Down Syndrome Who Participated in an Early Intervention Program: Second Follow-up Study," *Physical Therapy* 64:1515-19, 1984.

Frankenburg, W.K., et al. *The Denver Developmental Screening Test Reference Manual.* Denver: University of Colorado Medical Center, 1975.

Johnson, P. "Nursing Roles, Responsibilities, and Facilities," in *Current Practice in Pediatric Nursing,* vol. 2. Edited by Brandt, P.A., et al. St. Louis: C.V. Mosby Co., 1978.

Morgan, S.B. "Development and Distribution of Intelligence and Adaptive Skills in Down's Syndrome Children," *Mental Retardation* 17:247-49, 1979.

Murphy, M.A. "The Family with a Handicapped Child: A Review of the Literature," *Journal of Developmental and Behavioral Pediatrics* 3:73-82, 1982.

Olshansky, S. "Chronic Sorrow: A Response to Having a Mentally Defective Child," *Social Casework* 43:190-93, 1962.

Pueschel, S.M., and Rynders, J.E. *Down Syndrome: Advances in Biomedicine and the Behavioral Sciences.* Cambridge, Mass.: Academic Guild Publishers, 1982.

Romney, M. "Congenital Defects: Implications on Family Development and Parenting," *Issues in Comprehensive Pediatric Nursing* 7:1-15, 1984.

Russell, F.F., ed. *Interdisciplinary Early Intervention with Developmentally Delayed Infants and Young Children: A Family Oriented Approach.* Memphis: University of Tennessee Center for the Health Sciences, Child Development Center, 1985.

Solnit, A., and Stark, M. "Mourning and the Birth of a Defective Child," *Psychoanalytic Study of the Child* 16:523-37, 1961.

Soto-Viera, M.E., et al. "Initial Information Given to Parents of Children with Trisomy 21," Unpublished manuscript, 1984.

Thompson, J.S., and Thompson, M.M. *Genetics in Medicine,* 3rd ed. Philadelphia: W.B. Saunders Co., 1980.

Tooley, J.H., and Rawls, R.F. "Family Grief Reactions to Children's Handicaps," *Orthopedic Nursing* 1:27-32, 1982.

Veach, S. "Down's Syndrome: Helping the Special Parents of a Special Infant," *Nursing83* 13:42-43, 1983.

Wright, L. "Education in Genetics for Nurses," in *Education in Genetics: Nurses and Social Workers.* Edited by Forsman, I., and Bishop, K.K. Washington, D.C.: U.S. Government Printing Office, 1981.

Wright, L.M., and Leahey, M. *Nurses and Families: A Guide to Family Assessment and Intervention.* Philadelphia: F.A. Davis Co., 1984.

Zelle, R.S., and Coyner, A.B. *Developmentally Disabled Infants and Toddlers: Assessment and Intervention.* Philadephia: F.A. Davis Co., 1983.

16 Intervening with families of preschoolers with epilepsy

Patricia Buzinski Dardano, RN, MS
Clinical Instructor
College of Nursing
Northeastern University
Boston, Massachusetts

OVERVIEW

This chapter describes and defines the health problem of epilepsy and applies two developmental frameworks to life with a chronically ill child. The impact of epilepsy on the family is presented. Assessment questions that might assist the nurse in planning interventions are suggested. A case study of a preschooler with epilepsy highlights the assessment and intervention issues described in the chapter.

CASE STUDY

Ellen Jay was nearly 5 years old when she suffered her first seizure. At that time, she was attending kindergarten and living with her mother and stepfather; she has numerous older stepsiblings from both parents. The seizure occurred at 5:45 a.m. while both parents were asleep; it lasted from 30 to 60 seconds. (This and subsequent data was obtained from Mrs. Jay.)

Initial Seizure Event

Both parents were awakened by a clicking noise ("Probably Ellen trying to swallow her tongue") and found Ellen at the foot of their bed. "It appeared as if she knew something was wrong and tried to get to us." Ellen was rigid with her eyes rolled to the back of her head. With much effort the parents lifted Ellen into bed ("Because of her stiffness, it seemed like she weighed 150 pounds"), removed pillows and blankets, and then tried unsuccessfully to insert a finger in her mouth. Afterwards Ellen seemed to be "in a fog."

Ellen was examined at the local health center, and Mrs. Jay was informed that Ellen had a seizure disorder and would probably need lifelong medication. Phenobarbital was prescribed and an electroencephalogram (EEG) scheduled for the next day. Soon after, Ellen was referred to the publicly funded seizure clinic for follow-up and treatment.

Past History

From birth to age 16 months, Ellen's progress had been typical. Both the course of this unplanned pregnancy and the 1-hour labor and delivery went smoothly. Ellen weighed 7 pounds at birth and seemed in excellent health. Although certain milestones were reached a month late, Mrs. Jay considered Ellen's development to be normal.

At age 16 months, however, after a series of family difficulties, Ellen was placed in foster care where she remained until age 3. At some point during that time, Mrs. Jay was told that Ellen had cerebral palsy (mild left hemiplegia). Her initial reactions were disbelief and devastation, but they were replaced by relief when she saw that Ellen was not wheelchair bound or severely handicapped. Mrs. Jay needed to make two major adjustments when Ellen was returned to her. First, she had to discover her daughter "as a person"—an individual with her own likes, dislikes, daily patterns, and routines—and to learn basic parenting skills, such as how to balance limit-setting with privileges. Secondly, because of Ellen's cerebral palsy, Mrs. Jay had to learn how to interact with the various inpatient and outpatient facilities that would be providing treatment for her daughter. The onset of Ellen's seizure disorder represented a major family stressor.

Family-Focused Care

A team composed of a neurologist, a nurse, and a social worker manages Ellen's seizure care. Nursing contact has been made by phone, during several clinic visits, and during one home visit. Mrs. Jay also initiates contact with the nurse when problems arise. Overall, nurse-parent contact has focused mainly on teaching Mrs. Jay the nature of seizures and seizure management, acquainting her with her medication-related responsibilities, and demonstrating the correct management of Ellen at home and school.

Both Mrs. Jay and her school nurse and teacher initially feared for Ellen's safety because of the possibility of another seizure, but they soon abandoned what was obviously an overrestrictive approach to her activities.

During an early clinic visit, Mrs. Jay learned that the development of a seizure disorder was predictable because of Ellen's cerebral palsy. "But nobody told me that before," Mrs. Jay said. Since then, she has accepted the fact that Ellen has a seizure disorder, but refuses to acknowledge it is epilepsy. Mrs. Jay reiterates that the prognosis is uncertain; although she expresses dread at the thought of Ellen's having another seizure, she knows what to do if one occurs.

Family compliance with the medication regimen seems optimal. When serum phenobarbital began to exceed safe levels, the dosage schedule was modified from a total of four tablets daily to alternating four- and three-tablet daily doses. This information was passed to the Jays by phone and reiterated in a letter that included a monthly dosage calendar.

Family-staff contact was very frequent soon after Ellen's diagnosis, a result of the hyperactivity she developed (probably as a response to her medication). This condition affected the child at home ("She was bouncing off the walls") and at school, strained already-tense family interactions, and taxed Mrs. Jay's child management skills. "Then all of a sudden one day there was calm," reported Mrs. Jay. The improvement was so dramatic that she rejected the suggestion that another drug be tried; she requested that the drug not be changed unless absolutely essential.

In conclusion, the Jay family is responding effectively to the management and treatment of Ellen's epilepsy. Ongoing community nursing involvement, if supportive and informative, is utilized by the Jays.

NURSING PROCESS

Assessment

The health problem: Epilepsy
Incidence and etiology. An estimated 2 million Americans—1% of the population—have epilepsy. Of the 100,000 new cases reported annually, the Epilepsy Foundation of America (1982) predicts that 75,000 will be young children or adolescents; the disease seems to affect both sexes and all cultural groups indiscriminately.

At least half of all seizure disorder cases have no identifiable cause or associated factor; this type of epilepsy is termed idiopathic. Patients whose seizures *can* be traced to a specific factor are said to have an "acquired" or "symptomatic" disorder. In infancy, recurrent seizures develop secondary either to perinatal anoxia and infections, or to metabolic or degenerative syndromes. Head trauma and ingestion of toxic substances, such as drugs or lead-contaminated substances, are additional factors in childhood seizure disorders (Chabria and Shope, 1982). Fortunately, the onset of seizure disorder in a young child rarely indicates a brain tumor; tumors in this age-group usually arise at the "base of the brain or the cerebellum, areas that, when involved, do not cause seizures" (Lechtenberg, 1984, p. 101). In the sense that head injuries, particularly from car accidents, falls, and poisonings, can be prevented, posttraumatic epilepsy can be considered avoidable; no primary preventive intervention has been identified for the idiopathic form, however.

Developed epilepsies are quite responsive to medication. Some 60% of affected children, regardless of seizure type, can maintain complete control; another 15% to 25% achieve partial control (Waechter, et al., 1985). Children with poor seizure control often have other neurologic problems.

Definitions and classification. A seizure is a sudden burst of electrical discharges resulting from an abnormality in the function of excitable neuronal membranes. These discharges interfere with behavior, perception, movement, consciousness, and other brain functions (Lechtenberg, 1984; McIntyre, 1982). Seizures tend to be very short in duration.

The term epilepsy refers to recurrent and more or less unpredictable seizures (McIntyre, 1982). Not all seizures indicate epilepsy. Febrile seizures in young children, which develop as body temperature rises, are examples of nonepileptic seizures. Even if another febrile seizure occurs at another time, the diagnosis of epilepsy does not necessarily apply. Febrile seizures occur in 50% of young children. However, epileptic children may be more prone to seizures when ill. Another condition in young children that mimics a seizure disorder occurs as a result of breath holding; in those cases, the child has usually been fussy and crying, and will have a prolonged expiration, turn limp and pale, and, in some instances, actually experience tremors.

To standardize terminology among clinicians and to facilitate communication, the International League Against Epilepsy has proposed a classification system, which is now in its second revision (Dreifuss, 1981). It categorizes seizures into two major classes: generalized (either of a convulsive or nonconvulsive form) and partial (focal or local). In the generalized form, the disruptive brain activity originates in both hemispheres simultaneously. The tonic-clonic (grand mal) event that most people associate with the word seizure is generalized, but so is the absence (petit mal) seizure. Such events are nonconvulsive and hence may be overlooked by those near the affected individual. Children having absence seizures often appear to be daydreaming or inattentive; all activities seem to go "on hold" for a few seconds. No convulsion occurs because the seizure activity does not spread to the appropriate areas of the brain. Other forms of generalized seizures include tonic, clonic, myoclonic, atonic, and infantile spasms.

Partial seizures, on the other hand, originate in one specific part of one cerebral hemisphere; that is, they are focal or local in nature. When presenting without a loss of consciousness, such seizures are called simple partial; one commonly recognized example is the Jacksonian seizure. Other seizures presenting with a loss of consciousness are called complex partial; the psychomotor or temporal lobe types fall into this group. Either type may progress into a generalized motor state, and the simple form can proceed to complex and then to generalized.

Lay people often fear that the child will die during a convulsive state, but the actual epilepsy mortality rate is quite low (1.3 per 100,000 population): it is, in fact, lower than the death rate from appendicitis (McIntyre, 1982). Not that seizure disorders are always innocuous. One major life-threatening event associated with seizure disorders is status epilepticus, which is a prolonged or continuous series of seizures without intervening recovery time. If the seizures are generalized tonic-clonic and compromise respiratory and cardiovascular status, they can be most problematic. Such cases constitute a medical emergency requiring aggressive intervention (Garvin, 1982; McIntyre, 1982). In contrast, petit mal status may present with mere staring, blinking, and unresponsiveness or prolonged periods of confusion, disorientation, and general slowness. The literature agrees that the most common cause of status epilepticus is abrupt cessation of anticonvulsant drugs.

Beyond any physiologic sequelae, epilepsy carries a host of psychological and social ramifications. It is considered a chronic disease even though the child looks, acts, and feels well most of the time. The acute phase, when the disease is most evident, occurs unpredictably and abruptly. The feeling of helplessness in the face of the seizure and a chronic fear that the child may die both undermine and discourage families of epileptic children.

Family developmental assessment. Two developmental frameworks applicable to life with a chronically ill child are those of Duvall (1977) and Carter and McGoldrick (1980). Duvall identifies the critical developmental tasks of the family with preschoolers: stimulating the child in growth-promoting ways and coping with energy depletion and lack of privacy as parents. The developmental tasks involved with the rearing of children include having an adequate financial base for expected and unexpected occurrences and making environmental allowances for the child. Additionally, the family should maintain an intimate level of communication within the home and motivate individual members to interact in the world outside the home, that is, with relatives and other community resources. This viewpoint matches the stages of the family life cycle as discussed by Carter and McGoldrick (1980). A key principle at this stage is acceptance of new members into the system. For the family to proceed developmentally, the marital system must make room for the children: parenting roles must be assumed and relationships with the extended family must be realigned to include the new parenting and grandparenting roles. Understandably, the demands and role adjustments required when any family member falls chronically ill can disrupt the flow and balance of family progress during any developmental stage.

In families with developmentally disabled children, systemic boundaries open more readily to the outside world and professionals tend to become attached to the family. This long-term connection to health and welfare professionals has been cited as one major difference between family life with a normal and a handicapped child (O'Hara, et al., 1980). The parents of an epileptic child must deal with many of the factors that characterize care in any childhood illness: multiple assessments over long periods of time, unknown or uncertain disease causes and prognosis, and the fact that care is provided by a team of specialists as opposed to a single physician, in any of several settings. Developmental tasks, particularly those involving intra- and extra-family communication, financial affairs, child care, and energy availability can potentially be overburdening when a child is chronically ill.

Many of the above points were illustrated by the Jays' case. Before Ellen was returned to her mother at age 3, Mrs. Jay had dealt only with routine child health matters, such as checkups and immunizations, in raising her five children. Now she is obligated to take Ellen from one specialized facility to another; to the local public health clinic, which is about 35 miles from home; to the hospital for outpatient physical therapy; and to the local health clinic for general care. She finds herself talking about Ellen and her family situation to a number of people, including nurses, physicians, and social workers. Even though she asked pointed questions of Ellen's kindergarten teacher regarding the child's academic status, she states she still doesn't understand what the teacher told her.

Impact of epilepsy on the family. The diagnosis of epilepsy unleashes a host of concerns and misconceptions. Ziegler (1982, p. 438) identified four questions raised implicitly or explicitly at the time of diagnosis: "Why did it happen to us/to our child?," "How can we manage normally in this abnormal situation?," "What activities are possible for us and our child?," and "What dangers adhere to each?" While still trying to comprehend the diagnosis, the family is suddenly forced to establish a medication schedule, learn the correct observational and interventional responses to an unexpected seizure, and plan future procedures and follow-up. Heisler and Friedman (1981) advise professionals to remember that clients come with varying degrees of knowledge, experience with the disease, and misinformation. Shock, denial, and anger may influence the family's ability to comprehend the implications of the diagnosis.

Ziegler (1982) also contends that seizure disorders affect both the individual's and the family's sense of control—that is, their autonomy—and the individual's sense of mastery, *i.e.*, competence in the environment. Lechtenberg (1984) suggests that the sense of helplessness that surrounds the epileptic condition leads some parents to exert control in the nonhealth-related areas of their child's life longer than is reasonable or appropriate. Conversely, the child may learn to control the family by capitalizing on parental guilt.

The literature is peppered with references to parental overprotection of the epileptic child and its deleterious effects on future development. Certainly there is some justification for this family response. A seizure can occur in the bathtub or on the swings at the playground, and therefore places the child in jeopardy. On the other hand, the epileptic child needs opportunities to develop social and motor skills. The fine art of achieving a balance on the protectiveness–permissiveness scale is not easily mastered.

Kerns and Curley (1985, p. 147), in discussing neurologic impairments and their effect on the family, state that the potential impact of such problems "may be measured in terms of restrictive social and vocational roles as they relate to the increased time spent caring for impaired family members, negative emotional reactions, financial burden, social stigma and the need to attend to a variety of important decisions." Using epilepsy as a prototype, Beniak and Beniak (1983, pp. 268-269) address the nursing diagnosis of social isolation. They state that social isolation "inevitably concerns setting the individual apart from whatever societal whole with which he or she could be expected to interact and affiliate." Social withdrawal evolves gradually, becoming progressively entrenched. By keeping this in mind, a nurse can often prevent this isolation with given interventions.

In families with an epileptic child, Long and Moore (1979) found that parents who were pessimistic about their child's development were more restrictive of the child. In comparing the influence of an epileptic child on family functioning relative to families in which a child had juvenile diabetes and families with healthy children, Ferrari, Matthews, and Barabas (1983) found problems in the child's self-concept and in the family's communication skills and cohesiveness. These children were of school age, however. Most research on children with epilepsy involves those who are in this developmental period.

Planning

In community settings, the nurse frequently encounters families who are poor and have the problems associated with poverty. Colon (1980) discusses differences in the family life cycles of multi-problem poor and middle-class families. Tracking these families across three generations, it appears that the poor transverse the developmental stages at a faster rate. "The multi-problem poor person leaves home, marries, has children, gets divorced, becomes a grandparent, gets old, and dies earlier than the middle-class counterpart. Poor families are subject to more abrupt loss of membership through cutoffs, deaths, imprisonment, and drug addiction" (p. 355). Their remaining members are expected to assume new roles and responsibilities before they are developmentally ready. Additionally, more children are born, prolonging the child rearing stage. This composite description outlines some of the structural and functional issues within this group of clients and has implications for the nurse in planning care. While the nurse's priority may be the family's response to the disease, family members may have more pressing concerns competing for their energies. The added dimensions of providing care for multi-problem poor families require the nurse to consider family values, experiences, and orientations when establishing treatment.

The aspects of seizure management to be incorporated in the care plan include comprehensive description of the seizure, management of the seizure at home, medication management, preparation for outpatient tests, financial planning, childhood activities of daily living, education, information and support issues, and family or community responses to the diagnosis. While these factors are classified as nursing interventions, the activity is actually managed by family members.

Intervention

Description of the seizure(s). Effective seizure control depends on choosing the medication most suitable for the particular seizure type. Therefore, seizure identification becomes a critical determinant of treatment. Because it is unlikely that the nurse in the community or even in hospital settings will have witnessed the child's seizure, asking the right questions becomes imperative.

Dividing seizures into four phases—interictal, aura, ictal, and postictal—can help systematize data collection. The interictal phase is the seizure-free period; the aura is the warning or alert phase; the ictal phase is characterized by manifestations of the seizure; and in the postictal phase the child/patient recovers.

Interictal phase. The interictal phase holds valuable clues to seizure causation, predisposing factors, and differential diagnosis.

Questions to ask the family:
• Was the child well, or were there symptoms of a cold, earache, sore throat, or other infection?
• What time of day or night did the seizure occur? (Epilepsy often manifests itself relative to sleep, just falling asleep or near waking.)
• What activities was he engaged in? Was he anticipating some event?
• What was his behavior like? Happy, sad, irritable, hyperactive, cooperative?
• Had the child recently engaged in activities that may have facilitated access to drugs, alcohol, or other toxic chemicals in the house or elsewhere?
• Any indication of injury? When?

Aura phase. The aura sometimes appears in generalized tonic-clonic seizure disorders, but it is more pronounced in focal seizures. Many auras occur in the sensory or motor mode (Chabria and Shope, 1982); the person may hear buzzing or strange sounds, or see spots. Most often the aura is described as a sensation rapidly ascending from the stomach to the head (Sugarman, 1984), but the child experiencing it cannot always describe it precisely. Some children will run toward a caretaker before a seizure, as if for protection, indicating that perhaps an aura was occurring.

Question to ask the family:
• Was there anything different or odd in the child's expression or posture just before the seizure?

Ictal phase. During the ictal phase, consider what drew attention to the child: was it a cry, an odd facial expression, or noise? The observer must think in terms of time and of changing manifestations, which is not an easy task, considering the fright many people experience when witnessing a seizure. Pay close attention to position, appearance, and activity, starting with the eyes, the mouth, and facial expression, then the individual extremities (upper and lower), and finally the body.

Questions to ask the family:
• Did the head deviate to either side?
• Were the eyes open, closed, deviating right or left, blinking, diverging, or converging? Did the child seem to grimace, drool, or be extremely rigid in the jaw?
• Did any movement of the extremities start in one specific area? If so, where? What were the positions of the right hand, left hand, arms, legs? Were there extremities that weren't moving?
• Was the body twitching, flaccid, or hyperextended? Was there any turning to the right? The left?
• Did the patient fall or was he or she walking? Any verbal responses? Incontinence of urine or feces? (Johnson, 1982)

Postictal phase. When evaluating the postictal phase, focus on the child's behavior and degree of alertness.

Questions to ask the family:
• Did the child seem groggy or confused?
• Did the child sleep? For how long?
• Did the child have trouble moving any extremity? If so, which one(s)? For how long?

It is probably easier for parents and others who are expected to provide data to record these observations in a simple checklist so that the information is standardized and can be easily compiled and retrieved.

Management of seizures. Appropriate care during a seizure varies according to seizure type. Absence seizures generally require no direct intervention other than to repeat what the child may have missed while in seizure.

Physical protection of the child is an overriding consideration during both tonic-clonic and complex partial seizures. The child who experiences an aura may learn to get himself to a safe or neutral place, such as the middle of a floor.

In tonic-clonic seizure disorders, the first symptom is often a cry resulting from air being forced out of the lungs by the contraction; it is *not* a pain response. If the child is in a wheelchair or on a sofa or other piece of furniture, he should be lowered to the floor. Sharp or otherwise dangerous objects should be kept at a distance. Tight clothing, belts, or high-buttoned shirts should be loosened. Turning the child to the side will facilitate airway maintenance and secretion drainage. (Never force objects into the child's tightened mouth. This well-meaning act can result in damage to jaw, teeth, and surrounding structures; the feared tongue-swallowing it is to prevent is impossible.) Because suffocation is a remote possibility, soft pillows should not be placed under the head. Finally, some well-intentioned people will try to restrain the convulsing child; this will not help terminate the seizure but may result in injury to child or helper (Beniak and Beniak, 1983).

During a complex partial seizure, the child may respond inappropriately or not at all; he may fidget with clothing, stand or walk about aimlessly, and make chewing or lip-smacking noises. If possible, the patient should not be restrained. Instead, one should attempt to remove harmful objects from the immediate environment or gently coax the child away from the harmful object. The child should be supervised until fully alert (Beniak and Beniak, 1983).

During the postictal phase of both these seizure types, the child may be confused or disoriented and want to sleep; supervision should be maintained until the child is fully alert. If another seizure begins, or if a single seizure lasts 5 to 10 minutes (depending on distance and available transportation to a hospital), emergency help is indicated.

Care of the child with status epilepticus is three-pronged: providing life support (maintaining airway patency), stopping the seizures (generally by administering anticonvulsants, often intravenously), and identifying the cause of the episode (which in epileptic children is often related to noncompliance with the treatment regimen) (McGrath, 1981).

Providing written material or booklets on seizure care to the family and day-care providers can be useful. Additionally, a list of health care providers, emergency room, and ambulance numbers should be compiled and made accessible to family members.

Medication administration. A constant reminder of the epileptic's condition is his need for daily—or even more frequent—administration of anticonvulsant drugs; this is a task for which the parents of the young child are responsible. Parents must learn many new behaviors: how to obtain and ensure an uninterrupted medication supply, how to measure and administer the drug, how to fit the child's regimen into the family schedule, and how to identify and report adverse effects. Flexibility is necessary since drugs or dosages are often adjusted or changed. The medication aspect of seizure management is a major nursing and family activity.

Anticonvulsant drugs must be tailored to the type of seizure as well as to the child's age and weight. A major breakthrough in seizure control has been the development of serum laboratory tests to measure drug concentration. While doses may vary, there is now a measurable safe serum range that is used as the basis for treatment. Depending on the drug, several weeks may pass until a steady state is achieved and the drug becomes maximally effective. If during that time the child has a seizure, it does not necessarily mean that the drug is not working.

In addition to drug efficacy, a major family and professional concern in childhood epilepsy is the possibility of adverse reactions. Adverse reactions to anticonvulsants can be categorized as either dose-dependent, nondose-dependent, or as drug interactions (Spunt and Black, 1982). Dose-dependent reactions may be acute, secondary to overdose, or cumulative over time. The central nervous system is often affected, with symptoms including drowsiness, irritability, ataxia, restlessness, dizziness, and diplopia. Nondose-dependent reactions include drug allergies and idiosyncratic reactions; they usually occur within a few hours to a few weeks of treatment onset. Problems may range from minor skin rashes to fatal toxicity; therefore, idiosyncratic reactions should be reported immediately. Drug interactions result when two or more drugs are administered; for example, when valproate is added to a phenobarbital schedule, the phenobarbital level substantially increases (possibly because the valproate inhibits phenobarbital metabolism) (McIntyre, 1982).

Childhood activities of daily living. The presence of epilepsy may require modifications in a child's care and activities. For instance, bathing, toileting, and dental hygiene skills are refined during the preschool period, but an over-full bathtub can be fatal to a child in seizure. When bathing, use as little water as possible. Showers or showering on a stool may be indicated if the seizures are not well controlled. During this activity or while toileting, the door should be neither locked nor completely shut; this may, however, be an affront to the preschooler's sense of independence and modesty.

Dental hygiene assumes greater than average importance if the child is on long-term hydantoin therapy. Approximately 25% to 50% of such patients develop varying degrees of gingival hyperplasia. In extreme cases, the entire tooth may be covered with gum overgrowth. This may create problems with eating and oral hygiene (Punwani and Anderson, 1982), particularly in the pediatric age-group. McIntyre (1982) suggests an aggressive preventive approach including careful brushing three times a day with a soft-bristled brush, massaging the gums with a finger dipped in baking soda or with a commercial dental massager, daily use of dental floss, and cleaning and scaling every 3 months by dental professionals.

Sleeping arrangements. Sleep-related seizures are common, particularly when the child is just falling asleep or near wakening. Ideally, the child patient's room should be near the parents'; the mattress and pillow should be firm, and the child should not occupy the upper platform of a bunk bed (Jan, et al., 1983). The child should not sleep in the parents' bed or room; if the parents feel a need for closer nighttime supervision, a wireless, plug-in intercom may be installed.

Play activities. Activities that involve running (such as softball) are suitable for all epileptic preschoolers. If the child has good seizure control and an informed supervisor is present, then some swimming or water activities, excluding underwater swimming and diving, are allowable (Jan, et al., 1983; Norman and Browne, 1983). When seizure control is uncertain, activities that involve heights, such as rope climbing, should be avoided.

Limit-setting. Another parental response to the child's problem is overpermissiveness, which can lead to a situation where the child rules the home in an almost tyrannical way (Lechtenberg, 1984). Being alert to this phenomenon in its early stage can avert sibling hostilities and create a greater sense of psychic comfort in the epileptic child.

Educating the preschool child about epilepsy. When working with the preschooler, certain developmental characteristics bear watching. Preschoolers' verbal skills are well practiced; they love to talk, to question, and can do so fairly correctly. Their fantasy lives are quite active, and contain a great deal of role playing and storytelling about monsters and other creatures. Perrin and Gerrity (1984) have elucidated selected developmental points with reference to preschoolers and illness. Children in this age-group have an oversimplified, magical view of how their bodies work. When asked about the components of their bodies, they usually mention that the body contains blood and skin, but they have no idea how these structures function. To them, the body is a big plastic bag filled with red liquid. The brain is seen as static and unidirectional—it makes one think. Without a brain a person would be stupid or couldn't think. A preschooler's idea of illness and causation is concrete, specific, and superficial. A specific event leads to a specific outcome, and interrelationships are not considered. The child's natural egocentricity—he may say to himself, "If I only did (or did not do) something, the illness would not have happened"—may lead to the belief that the epilepsy is a punishment for some thought or deed.

Much to the caretakers' relief, the preschooler soon develops into a more socialized being who can be a part of a play group, follow instructions, and wait for a turn. The preschooler also complies more during medical visits. However, if such painful procedures as blood tests are a usual part of the visit, anticipatory fear may develop. Preschoolers have the cognitive skill to cooperate in preparation for blood tests (which hurt but only for a minute or two) and EEGs (which cause wires to be stuck to your head, but don't give you a shock or hurt at all). The epileptic child may have little or no exposure to hospitalization because of his condition per se, since many such children are diagnosed and managed in community settings. When admitted to a hospital for the first time, the child may be in a crisis state, which precludes preparation.

Educational information and general supportive activities. The specialized educational information about epilepsy that the affected family will need ranges from a definition of the disorder to in-depth facts about etiology, drug effects, and the physiologic, educational, and social impact of the illness on the patient's future. On one level, there is a need for concrete data. On another level, each person must come to terms with that data. Not only parents require educational support; others who will need information include siblings, grandparents, babysitters, and day-care and preschool providers. Moreover, this information must be explained and interpreted. For many, the illness experience may be too new, the terminology too foreign, and/or the anxiety too high to allow immediate understanding of the situation. And if the family has multiple problems to cope with, epilepsy may just be one more pull on family energies.

On the positive side, a fair amount of literature on epilepsy and its management is available to both the public and the health professional. One prominent provider of these resources is the Epilepsy Foundation of America (EFA), located at 4351 Garden City, Landover, MD 20075. Nationwide, there are 134 organizations, some of them associated with EFA, that serve the needs of people with seizure disorders and their families (Shaw, 1983). Support advocacy, self-awareness, and community education groups all provide valuable assistance. There are also excellent current books for the lay public that explain the various aspects of living with epilepsy; the public library is also a good resource.

To reduce the burden of care, some states have instituted medication programs that supply anticonvulsants at greatly reduced or no cost. Also, most states provide highly specialized seizure or neurology clinics.

Entry into first grade and the beginning of formal education is a major transition for both preschooler and family. Should there be a question regarding the child's ability to complete this transition successfully, Public Law 94-142 provides for a diagnosis and evaluation to identify any special needs.

Nursing interventions must be based on sensitivity to potential or actual problems within specific epileptic families, as well as knowledge of the behavioral indices of these events. Depending on a number of factors, including the nurse's expertise, counseling may best be done by the nurse or by other members of the interdisciplinary team or outside resources. The goal is to help the family acquire a sense of mastery in the care of the child. In the event of backsliding or problems in the child's care, the nurse can help the family achieve a sense of competence by delineating and reinforcing positive behaviors as appropriate. Nurses must avoid giving mixed messages, *e.g.*, cautioning the parents not to make the child the focus of their lives, while demanding information or interventions that imply greater concentration on the epileptic child.

Evaluation

Seizure care. The goal of seizure management is to minimize seizure occurrence while encouraging normal life activities. But it is misleading for the nurse to use the number of seizures as a success criterion for her interventions, simply because the responsibility for identifying seizure type and prescribing the most appropriate medication resides with the physician. However, for those areas identified as nursing functions in the case of a preschooler with seizures, the following criteria are suggested:

Medication administration. In general, desirable outcomes related to epileptic drug therapy require correct and safe drug administration and storage, timely (1 week in advance of depletion) refill of prescriptions, and prompt family reporting of physical or behavioral indications of drug effectiveness and/or adverse drug reactions.

Seizure observations. Ideally, the family should be able to recall the details of the child's seizure(s), collect the data in report form, and maintain a seizure diary.

Seizure management. The following outcomes are desired:
• Family members will be able to describe appropriate management of the preschooler during the actual seizure.
• Parents will be able to describe acceptable practice regarding postseizure care.
• The family will communicate to significant others in the child's environment the need for seizure care for their child and enlist assistance, if needed, in making these suggestions.
• Over time, the parents will communicate a greater degree of comfort with their child's disorder or perhaps indicate that seizures disrupt family activities less.
• The preschooler will report memories and perceptions of the seizure event.

In the areas of medication, seizure observation and management, family members will at first seek validation of their observations and actions, and this behavior will gradually decrease over time. The need for reassurance depends largely on the nature and strength of the nurse-family relationship; the nurse should communicate to the family that seeking this confirmation is acceptable.

Epilepsy education. While not an exhaustive listing, the following outcomes seem reasonable:
• The parents, the affected preschooler, and siblings will verbalize their views of epilepsy—what it is and what it is not.
• All family members will be able to define epilepsy in terms of neural paroxysmal hyperactivity with resultant change in behavior, motion, and so on.
• Significant others' needs for epilepsy education will be identified and an educational approach hypothesized and eventually implemented.
• Parents, siblings, and the epileptic preschooler will identify the purpose of EEGs and blood tests, including what they do and do not measure.
• Parents will avail themselves of other opportunities, such as books and other written material and/or epilepsy education groups, to increase their understanding of the disorder.
• Resources will be used to reduce the financial and other burdens acquired secondary to the diagnosis.

Family issues. In situations where the nurse can initiate and maintain a relationship with the family over time, the following outcomes may be appropriate:
• Each parent will describe immediate accommodations made relative to the diagnosis of epilepsy.
• Parents will state their reactions, both short- and long-term, neutral and negative, and internally and externally directed to the diagnosis.
• A family perspective will be maintained with evidence that all problems not be centered on the child.
• The epileptic preschooler's limits and privileges will be age appropriate and in line with those used for other siblings.
• The family will indicate how their interactions within their nuclear, extended (family), and social groups have been modified subsequent to the diagnosis.
• Support systems, both personal and professional, will be delineated and contingencies for their use proposed.
• Family members will prepare for the transition to the next developmental stage (in this case, school) and attendant role readjustments by all family members.
• Family functions, particularly at work and at home, will be maintained or minimally modified.

CONCLUSIONS

The care of the young child with epilepsy resides primarily with the parents. Usually, seizures can be controlled effectively through treatment. Once epilepsy is diagnosed, the family must respond with a number of new behaviors, such as learning how to respond to the uncertain occurrence and outcome of the child's next seizure, dealing with emotional reactions (why us or our child), and other related direct care and psychosocial issues. The case study of the Jay family illustrated some of the thought processes and the effective coping behaviors of parents who are novices to seizure disorders and who also have to deal with other significant life concerns.

REFERENCES

Beniak, J.A., and Beniak, T.E. "Social Isolation," in *A Guide to Neurological and Neurosurgical Nursing.* Edited by Synder, M. New York: John Wiley & Sons, 1983.

Carter, E.A., and McGoldrick, M. *The Family Life Cycle: A Framework for Family Therapy.* New York: Gardner Press, 1980.

Chabria, S., and Shope, J.T. "Medical Aspects of Epilepsy: An Overview," in *Nursing Management of Epilepsy.* Edited by Black, R.B., et al. Rockville, Md.: Aspen Systems Corp., 1982.

Colon, F. "The Family Life Cycle of the Multi-Problem Poor Family," in *The Family Life Cycle: A Framework for Family Therapy.* Edited by Carter, E.A., and McGoldrick, M. New York: Gardner Press, 1980.

Dreifuss, F.E. "Proposal for Revised Clinical and Electroencephalic Classification of Epileptic Seizures," *Epilepsia* 22(4):489–501, 1981.

Duvall, E.G. *Marriage and Family Development,* 5th ed. Philadelphia: J.B. Lippincott Co., 1977.

Epilepsy Foundation of America. *Questions and Answers About Epilepsy.* Landover, Md.: Epilepsy Foundation of America, 1982.

Ferrari, M., et al. "The Family and the Child with Epilepsy," *Family Process* 22:53–59, 1983.

Garvin, J.S. "Status Epilepticus," in *Nursing Management of Epilepsy.* Edited by Black, R.B., et al. Rockville, Md.: Aspen Systems Corp., 1982.

Heisler, A.B., and Friedman, S.B. "Social and Psychological Considerations in Chronic Disease: With Particular Reference to the Management of Seizure Disorders," *Journal of Pediatric Psychology* 6(3):239–50, 1981.

Jan, J.E., et al. *Does Your Child Have Epilepsy?* Baltimore: University Park Press, 1983.

Johnson, B.M. "Nursing Priorities in the Management of Epilepsy," in *Nursing Management of Epilepsy.* Edited by Black, R.B., et al. Rockville, Md.: Aspen Systems Corp., 1982.

Kerns, R.D., and Curley, A.D. "A Biopsychosocial Approach to Illness and the Family: Neurological Diseases Across the Life Span," in *Health, Illness and Families: A Life-Span Perspective.* Edited by Turk, D.C., and Kerns, R.D. New York: John Wiley & Sons, 1985.

Lechtenberg, R. *Epilepsy and the Family.* Cambridge, Mass.: Harvard University Press, 1984.

Long, C.G., and Moore, J.R. "Parental Expectations for Their Epileptic Children," *Journal of Child Psychology and Psychiatry and Allied Disciplines* 20(4):299–312, 1979.

McGrath, D.M. "Nursing Management of the Child in Status Epilepticus," *Issues in Comprehensive Pediatric Nursing* 5–6:273–77, 1981.

McIntyre, H.B. *The Primary Care of Seizure Disorders.* Boston: Butterworths, 1982.

Norman, E.E., and Browne, T.R. "Nursing Management and Patient Education," in *Epilepsy: Diagnosis and Management.* Edited by Browne, T.R., and Feldman, R.G. Boston: Little, Brown & Co., 1983.

O'Hara, D.M., et al. "A Family Life Cycle Plan for Delivering Services to the Developmentally Disabled," *Child Welfare* 59:80–90, 1980.

Perrin, E.C., and Gerrity, P.S. "Development of Children with Chronic Illness," *Pediatric Clinics of North America* 31(1):19–31, 1984.

Punwani, I.C., and Anderson, A.W. "Dental Aspects of Epilepsy," in *Nursing Management of Epilepsy.* Edited by Black, R.B., et al. Rockville, Md.: Aspen Systems Corp., 1982.

Shaw, E.B. "Resources Available to the Patient with Epilepsy," in *Epilepsy: Diagnosis and Management.* Edited by Browne, T.R., and Feldman, R.G. Boston: Little, Brown & Co., 1983.

Spunt, A.L., and Black, R.B. "Drug Treatment of Seizure Disorders," in *Nursing Management of Epilepsy.* Edited by Black, R.B., et al. Rockville, Md.: Aspen Systems Corp., 1982.

Sugarman, G.L. *Epilepsy Fact Book: A Guide to Understanding Seizure Disorders.* St. Louis: C.V. Mosby Co., 1984.

Waechter, E.H., et al. *Nursing Care of Children,* 10th ed. Philadelphia: J.B. Lippincott Co., 1985.

Wright, F.S. "Epilepsy in Childhood," *Pediatric Clinics of North America* 31(1):177–88, 1984.

Ziegler, R.G. "Epilepsy: Individual Illness, Human Predicament and Family Dilemma," *Family Relations* 1(1):435–41, 1982.

17 Intervening with families of school-aged children with hypertension

Linda L. Jarvis, RN, EdD
Assistant Professor
Division of Nursing Studies
Curry College
Milton, Massachusetts

OVERVIEW

This chapter provides an overview of the issues associated with nursing the school-aged child with diagnosed hypertension. The focus is on family care, since hypertension is considered a chronic disease requiring lifelong treatment. The assessment for diagnosis, including taking a history, evaluating risk factors, and identifying family structure and function will be discussed, and blood pressure guidelines and treatment options delineated. The nursing process incorporates these main areas of concern when working with a family whose child is diagnosed as hypertensive.

CASE STUDY

Identified Client

Matthew Baxter is 11 years old. At his annual school physical examination, the nurse practitioner recorded an elevated blood pressure reading (150/95). This reading was obtained at the end of the health visit; 10 minutes later, a repeat check of Matthew's blood pressure revealed no change. At return visits 2 and 4 weeks later, his blood pressure ranged from 145/95 to 155/95, with no other apparent symptoms. Because of his elevated blood pressure and a strong family history of hypertension, Matthew was referred to a pediatric hypertension clinic for a complete evaluation.

At the clinic, family and medical histories were obtained. The physical examination included blood pressure measurements—sitting, lying, and standing—in both arms and both legs; height and weight measurement; funduscopic and cardiovascular examinations; and examination for such secondary problems as abdominal masses, decreased peripheral pulses, cushingoid stigmata, and abdominal bruit. All recommended (Lieberman, 1980; U.S. Department of Health and Human Services, 1984) laboratory studies—including urinalysis, complete blood count, blood urea nitrogen (to check for telltale creatinine), electrocardiogram, echocardiogram, chest X-ray, and intravenous urogram—were performed.

Findings

Both Matthew's parents and grandparents had a positive history of hypertension. His own medical history was unremarkable. The only health problems noted were occasional colds. No allergies were reported. Results of the physical examination were within normal limits with no evidence of disease. Blood pressure measured 150/95 in both arms in the sitting, standing, and supine positions. Height was in the 50th percentile and weight in the 75th percentile for the boy's age. Funduscopic and cardiovascular examinations were normal—no abdominal bruits or peripheral pulses were felt. Both electrocardiogram and echocardiogram were normal with no evidence of left ventricular hypertrophy; the chest X-ray was normal with no evidence of cardiac enlargement; the urogram was normal as was the urinalysis; the complete blood count (CBC) and blood urea nitrogen (BUN) results were all within normal limits; and no evidence of secondary causes, for instance, abdominal masses or cushingoid characteristics, was noted.

Diagnosis

Matthew was diagnosed as having primary hypertension and placed on a diuretic and salt-free, low-cholesterol diet. Activities remained unrestricted. Since his diagnosis, he has been seen monthly by the community center's nurse practitioner and every 6 months by the pediatric hypertension clinic. (See genogram, Figure 17.1.)

Figure 17.1 Genogram—The Baxter Family

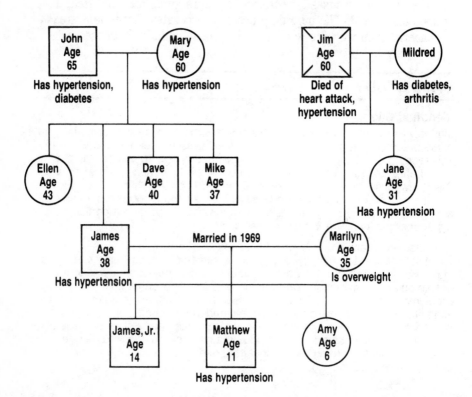

Family History
Matthew is the second child of Marilyn and James Baxter. He lives with his parents, a 14-year-old brother, and a 6-year-old sister in a three-bedroom home in a metropolitan suburb on the East coast.

Mother: Marilyn Baxter.
35 years old, high school graduate.
Homemaker and part-time waitress (Tuesdays, Wednesdays, and Thursdays from 10:00 a.m. to 2:30 p.m.) at a local restaurant. Has been working since Amy began school in September. Marilyn is also the leader of Matthew's Boy Scout troop and sings in the church choir.
25 pounds overweight. Still grieves over her father's death and expresses anger that he failed to comply with his health and medication regimen; worries about James's and Matthew's health compliance.

Father: James Baxter.
38 years old, two years of college.
Postal letter carrier, works Thursdays (day off from postal service) at a local gas station. Coaches James Jr. in competitive swimming; active in church (deacon and Sunday school teacher).
Primary hypertension first diagnosed at age 25. On diuretic and salt-free diet. Has complied with drug and diet regimen since Marilyn's father's death 1½ years ago from heart attack complicated by hypertension.

Children:
James Jr.
14 years old.
Freshman at Whitman High School, maintaining a B average academically. Active on junior varsity swim team and in local swim competitions during the rest of the year. Delivers newspapers before school; participates in church activities.
No identified health problems. Height in 80th percentile for age, weight in 35th percentile; blood pressure within normal limits.

Matthew.
11 years old.
Sixth grade student with a B− average. Plays Little League baseball and is a member of the Boy Scouts. Participates in church activities. See health history above.

Amy.
6 years old.
First grade, maintaining an A average. She participates in church activities and is taking swimming lessons. No identified health problems. In the 50th percentile for height and 40th percentile for weight. Blood pressure within normal limits for age.

All of the Baxters have yearly health evaluations at the community health center. Knowledge about hypertension varies among family members. Marilyn, for example, understands the need to reduce salt intake and does not place the salt shaker on the table; she does not enforce fat and cholesterol limitations as stringently, however. Since her father's death, she expresses increased fear of hypertension in herself and other family members. She and the other family members need additional nutrition counseling.

The Baxter children exercise daily, but James and Marilyn do not. Marilyn blames overweight on her inactivity; James walks daily on the job, but not at a pace that challenges his cardiovascular system.

Both James and Marilyn have smoked one pack of cigarettes per day since high school. Two years ago they changed to a low-tar, low-nicotine brand, and they have tried on several occasions to stop completely, though without success.

Family stress is moderate, resulting mainly from parental work schedules and family responsibilities for the children and the three remaining grandparents. Matthew's diagnosed hypertension has been met with concern and fear; both parents have expressed readiness to do whatever is necessary to control their son's high blood pressure and to prevent its development in other family members.

Culture and Family of Origin

The Baxters are a Black American family, middle-class socioeconomically with a family income of approximately $35,000 per year. They own both a house (in a suburban, racially mixed neighborhood) and a car. They are active Baptists, with extended family within 25 miles.

THE NURSING PROCESS

Assessment

The health problem: Hypertension. Hypertension is described either as primary—that is, caused by unknown factors—or as secondary— the result of identifiable factors such as renal disease, acute glomerulonephritis, cardiovascular disease, aortic coarctation, tumors, Cushing's disease, juvenile rheumatoid arthritis, hypercalcemia, and other endocrine disorders (Lieberman, 1980).

Most childhood hypertension is secondary, although the incidence of juvenile primary hypertension has been increasing over the past decade or so. The exact number of children and adolescents with primary hypertension is not known, but it is thought that between 0.5% and 1% of all prepubertal children and that 2% to 6% of all adolescents are affected (Loggie, 1977). The accuracy of these statistics should improve in the wake of increasing research into childhood hypertension.

The guidelines in Table 17.1 can help the nurse identify hypertension. The National Heart, Lung, and Blood Institute's Task Force on Blood Pressure Control in Children is currently revising its blood pressure guidelines. The new data should be available in the near future and can be obtained by writing the National High Blood Pressure Education Program, Task Force on Blood Pressure Control in Children, Bethesda, MD 20014.

Table 17.1   Guidelines for Identifying Childhood Hypertension

Age	Arterial Pressure (mm Hg) Systolic/Diastolic
Less than 6 years	+/− 110/75
6-10 years	+/− 120/80
10-14 years	+/− 125/85
14-18 years	+/− 135/90

Source: U.S. Department of Health and Human Services, 1984; Horan, 1985.

Diagnosis of hypertension, especially primary hypertension, is based on a series of elevated blood pressure readings over a given period of time. Because every reading must be accurate, the correct-size blood pressure cuff must be used and the measurement technique must be consistent. Once a pattern of hypertension has been identified, it is important, especially in children, to rule out secondary causes. Truly hypertensive children are often asymptomatic, while a healthy child's blood pressure may be quite labile. Therefore, a single elevated blood pressure reading does not necessarily indicate hypertension, a fact that must be communicated to parents.

There are two main categories of risk factors for childhood primary hypertension: nonmodifiable and modifiable. Nonmodifiable factors are those the individual cannot change, such as age, race, and family history. Modifiable risk factors include weight, smoking, salt and cholesterol intake, exercise, and stress level. Both family and individual nursing histories should identify both types of risks.

Families with school-aged children. Families with hypertensive children and/or adolescents must learn to cope with a chronic health problem that will probably have a marked impact on their life-style. The condition can have profound developmental implications, particularly in the adjustment of parent-child relationships, to help children move toward independence. In addition, many parents must deal simultaneously with the health problems and increased care demands of their own aging parents, as well as with the ongoing evaluation, negotiation, and change of their marital relationship.

Overprotectiveness, guilt, anger, blame-placing, and denial are typical parental reactions to a diagnosis of hypertension in their child. Nursing interventions are directed at helping the family come to terms with the child's diagnosis and treatment regimen, integrate needed life-style changes, and nurture the independence and maturation of each family member.

Family assessment becomes a major consideration in the formulation of nursing interventions. Family structure, function, developmental tasks, communication patterns, roles, and relationships take on primary importance. Therefore, the nurse's chosen family assessment model should be both familiar and easily utilized. Suggested options include the Calgary Family Assessment Model (CFAM) developed by Wright and Leahey (1984) or assessment models developed by Duvall (1977), Carter and McGoldrick (1980), Kantor and Lehr (1977), and/or Minuchin (1974).

Assessment of the Baxter family revealed that Marilyn and James married in 1969, and now have one adolescent child and two school-aged children. They also have parents who are entering old age and coping with two chronic disease conditions: hypertension and arthritis.

Developmentally, the family's tasks at this time are offering parental guidance while allowing their children to develop the independence appropriate to their chronologic and maturational ages; reviewing and possibly renegotiating marital responsibilities and reactions; and discussing, negotiating, and implementing responsibilities to and for parents.

The Baxter's marriage is solid. The parents share decision-making responsibilities; neither parents nor siblings feel that the children create difficulties beyond the bickering, tattling, stubbornness, daydreaming, and sloppiness considered normal for their ages. The children view their parents as strict but fair. The children's attachments are adaptive, with peer relationships encouraged but scrutinized by parents; childhood autonomy is based on age. All of the children are expected to contribute to home and family functioning through assigned chores and open communication.

The family is on fairly sound financial footing. Money has been set aside for the children's education, although additional financial assistance will be required. Mrs. Baxter's income is used for such luxuries as a VCR, vacation trips, and special clothing purchases.

The Baxters maintain open relationships with their parents/grandparents and the rest of their extended family. Although Marilyn's father died 1½ years ago from a heart attack complicated by hypertension, her mother cares for Amy and Matthew 3 days a week, between the end of school and Marilyn's return home from work at about 3:00 p.m.

Planning

Hypertensive children usually receive care in a community-based clinic or at home, although those with secondary hypertension may require hospitalization until the underlying condition is controlled. A team approach to hypertension treatment, involving the nurse, physician, nutritionist, psychologist, and others, has proven effective.

Nursing activities center around early diagnosis, prevention, teaching, and follow-up care all directed toward the following long-term goals:
• Maintain blood pressure within the normal range for age.
• Integrate needed life-style changes—such as salt restriction, fat/cholesterol restriction, weight loss, regular exercise, stress reduction, and smoking cessation—into the family routine.
• Prevent complications associated with hypertension.
• Maintain functional family unit.

Each family's care plan should be individual and based on continuing nursing assessment.

Care for childhood hypertension must be both individually and family focused. Ultimately, the child must learn to take responsibility for his condition. Individual and family life-style changes may be necessary. The family members and the nurse should recognize that such change may be slow and that backsliding often occurs. When this happens, attempts to determine the cause are in order so that plans can be developed to prevent recurrence.

Intervention

The hypertensive child. Close, *accurate* monitoring of the hypertensive child's blood pressure is crucial. Proper measurement requires carefully controlled equipment, technique, and environment. The sphygmomanometer, whether aneroid or mercury, should be checked every 3 to 6 months for accuracy and should fit the child being evaluated. The cuff should cover two thirds of the length of the upper arm between the olecranon and the acromion, without covering the antecubital fossa. The bladder should comfortably encircle the entire arm without gaps or overlaps (Lieberman, 1979). The stethoscope should be well maintained and fit comfortably in the ears; a Doppler head may be useful with neonates.

Seat the child with the right arm supported at heart level. If blood pressure is taken in the leg, the child should lie either prone or supine with one leg slightly flexed. Select an appropriately sized cuff and palpate the artery over the popliteal fossa. Record the first, fourth, and fifth phase of Korotkoff sounds, then inflate the cuff to 30 mm Hg above the palpable pressure (Lieberman, 1979). Maintain a quiet, comfortable environment throughout the evaluation, and always check blood pressure before any unpleasant procedures are performed.

The hypertensive child will require repeated blood pressure measurement on a timetable (usually weeks to months) varying with the amount of elevation noted and the practitioner's experience. In addition, a complete physical evaluation, including cardiac tests, height and weight recordings, urinalysis, BUN and/or creatinine test, as well as a chest X-ray and CBC will be necessary.

Even when the child with repeatedly high blood pressure readings is asymptomatic, encouragement to follow the prescribed regimen will probably be necessary. Encouraging normal activity and responsibility for the treatment program should therefore be a major nursing focus.

Since the etiology of a child's hypertension may have a profound impact on the nature of nursing intervention, it is worth noting that secondary hypertension is more common in prepubescent children (75% to 80% of all cases), while primary hypertension is more often diagnosed in the pubescent youngster (Lieberman, 1979).

The family. Through the family history, the nurse should look for hypertensive family members. Dietary history, obesity, smoking, exercise, and stress levels should also be assessed, particularly in diagnosed hypertensive family members (Table 17.2), and regular checks of all blood pressures should be done. Knowledge deficits related to hypertension also need to be addressed as in the case example (Table 17.3). Dietary supervision will be needed, especially in the area of salt and fat/cholesterol restriction. A nutritionist's assistance may be helpful. Regular supervised exercise that improves cardiovascular function should be encouraged. Finally, assess stress and guilt early on, and take steps to reduce their impact on the family unit.

Individually and collectively, the family is responsible for successful hypertension treatment. Life-style changes must be thoroughly discussed in terms of how they can be incorporated into family living patterns. As a unit, the family can reduce risk factors, modify hypertensive complications, and manage an effective treatment program with minimal health care support. Backsliding, which must be expected at times, should not be punished; instead, its etiology should be explored in order to prevent recurrence. Regular follow-up may be done in the clinic, home, or school with a check of blood pressure, reviews of diet, medication, exercise, and stress, and a question and answer session. See Table 17.4 for nursing interventions implemented in the Baxter case.

Evaluation

Evaluation of how well long- and short-term goals are met must begin with regular monitoring of blood pressure control. Modification of family risk factors is also important for long-term success, and opportunities for open questioning and clarification of the treatment regimen will be necessary during initial treatment and beyond.

Table 17.2   Evaluating the Hypertensive Members of the Baxter Family

Family Member	Assessment	Outcomes
James	• Discuss comprehension of diagnosis and medical instructions—diet, medication, exercise, smoking cessation, and stress reduction. • Determine compliance with medical instructions. • Check blood pressure. • Review medications—their purpose, dosage, frequency, and side effects. • Answer questions related to high blood pressure.	• Can discuss the meaning of the hypertensive diagnosis. • Describes, in accurate terms, dietary limitations. • States that fat and salt restrictions are the most difficult to adhere to, but that he has done so most of the time since Marilyn's father's death 1½ years ago. • Identifies the prescribed medication and takes it in the specified amounts. • Only exercise is walking (on the job). • Smokes one and a half packs of cigarettes (low-tar and low-nicotine type) per day. • States that his main life stressors relate to family members—Matthew's health, the deteriorating health of his parents, and the impact of hypertension on his family. Blood pressure is 125/80.
Matthew	• Discuss knowledge about hypertension. • Determine medication and diet compliance. • Discuss the impact of the hypertension regimen on his daily activities. • Check blood pressure. • Answer questions related to hypertension.	• Variable knowledge about hypertension. • Does not understand why medication and diet changes are necessary in absence of obvious symptoms. • Is reluctant to take a prescribed diuretic because increased voiding interferes with his play activities. • Unable to identify the actions and dosage of or schedule for his medications. Depends on mother's reminders to take them. • Eats high-salt foods with his friends without telling his parents. • Has not told his friends of his health problem because he is afraid they will abandon him. • Blood pressure is 125/75. • Does not seek information about his health problem.

Table 17.3   Evaluating Knowledge Deficits Related to Hypertension—The Baxter Family

Interventions	Outcomes
• Discuss knowledge about hypertension generally and in children. • Discuss relevant facts about diet, medications, exercise, smoking, and stress. • Provide reading materials from the American Heart Association. • Answer questions about high blood pressure. • Encourage the family to write down questions *when they arise,* for discussion with the nurse or physician. • Check and record individual blood pressures on a regular basis. • Encourage participation in hypertension support groups.	• Knowledge level about hypertension is adequate, but family still has difficulty integrating knowledge and life-style. • James is complying with his medications and diet regimens but finds it difficult at times, especially the salt and fat restrictions. • Marilyn is assuming responsibility for Matthew's diet and medication compliance. She expresses a great deal of guilt and considers herself responsible for her son's condition. She thinks Matthew is too young to take care of his health problem. • Both adults agree that they do not get enough exercise, although the children's activity level is adequate. They will consider starting a regular exercise program together beginning with a daily walking schedule. • Concerns and stressors about Matthew's illness and the impact it has on the family, as well as concerns about the grandparents, are greatest at this time. The Baxters agree that a hypertension support group might help them by showing how other families have coped with hypertension. • Blood pressure measurements are taken and recorded on individual family member forms; only Matthew shows a blood pressure elevation. An offer of reading material was enthusiastically accepted. Questions that arise will be written down to be discussed at next visit with the nurse. Matthew is reluctant to tell his friends about his hypertension.

Table 17.4   Family Interventions in Childhood Hypertension—The Baxter Family

Life-style factors	Interventions	Outcomes
Diet	• Discuss knowledge of dietary restrictions. • Discuss dietary compliance. • Provide dietary substitution information as needed. • Refer family to a nutritionist for dietary counseling.	• Marilyn, who is knowledgeable about the necessary dietary restrictions, prepares meals and shops for the family's food. Salt is seldom added to food while cooking, and no salt shaker is used at the table. • The children complain from time to time about the lack of salt; all report consumption of salty foods when away from home. • The family's fat consumption is high since the diet relies heavily on fried and high-fat foods. The nurse's suggestion that Marilyn use low-fat foods and bake or broil meat was acknowledged as important but difficult to adhere to. • An appointment was made for consultation with a nutritionist. • James complies with dietary restrictions most of the time, but Matthew has great difficulty doing so. James Jr. expresses interest in nutrition because of swimming. Amy eats what the rest of the family consumes; her primary complaints are about salt restriction.
Exercise	• Discuss family members' exercise levels. • Provide written material about exercise and cardiovascular health. • Assist with exercise program planning as needed. • Provide a list of exercise options and their cardiovascular benefits. • Explain the difference between aerobic and anaerobic exercises. • Answer questions about exercise. • Refer the family to a physical education consultant.	• The children participate in regular aerobic exercises at least three times per week, 20 minutes or more per session. • James continues to exercise only in the course of his work. • Marilyn does not exercise because she feels she is too heavy. • Both James and Marilyn express an interest in starting an aerobic exercise program and agree to a physical education consultation to plan and implement such a program.
Smoking	• Discuss family members' smoking behavior.	• Both James and Marilyn continue to smoke one pack of low-tar and low-nicotine cigarettes per day. Both have tried to stop smoking previously.

(continued)

Table 17.4 Family Interventions in Childhood Hypertension—The Baxter Family (continued)

Life-style factors	Interventions	Outcomes
Smoking (continued)	• Provide written material about the effects of smoking on cardiovascular health. • Assist with a smoking cessation program.	• Both parents acknowledge the health risks of smoking and express a readiness to cut down, but refuse to consider a formal smoking cessation program. They will begin smoking reduction by cutting down on the number of cigarettes smoked per day over a period of time. Week one: reduce by four cigarettes per day; week two: reduce by eight cigarettes per day; to be continued until they both cease smoking entirely.
Stress	• Discuss stress factors affecting the family unit. • Determine etiology of stress. • Explore ways to reduce stress. • Provide written information about reducing stress in daily living. • Answer questions related to stress and present family health concerns.	• Major assessed factors are Matthew's health status and the deteriorating health of James's and Marilyn's parents. • Marilyn expresses much anger and guilt about Matthew's hypertension and is not sure how to comply with necessary family behavioral changes. She also expresses anger about her father's failing to take better care of himself and dying. • James worries about Matthew's hypertension and fears it may develop in the other children. He expects himself to be a role model in hypertension control for Matthew. • Matthew views the hypertension treatment regimen as "stupid," since he feels fine. He is afraid it may keep him from playing baseball and admits to cheating on dietary restrictions. He takes his medications only when his mother reminds him and is unwilling to take responsibility for his treatment. • James Jr. has as little as possible to do with the hypertension issue, although he expresses some concern that he will eventually develop the condition. Swimming is his main interest.

(continued)

Life-style factors	Interventions	Outcomes
Stress *(continued)*		• Amy has started throwing temper tantrums since Matthew was diagnosed and has begun clinging to her mother. Her school performance has not been affected. She says that Matthew is sick and says she does not want to get sick and have to take pills all the time.
Fear and guilt about familial hypertension	• Discuss sources of fear and guilt concerning hypertension. • Provide written information about hypertension to children and adults. • Answer questions related to hypertension. • Help the family integrate new knowledge into its overall life-style. • Encourage open discussion about hypertension among family members. • Refer family for counseling if beyond nurse's competence and/or mandated in work setting.	• The nurse encourages family members to discuss their primary concerns about hypertension. • The family is encouraged to make a list of questions prior to each clinic visit. • The family is instructed to telephone the nurse if information needs clarification. • If family needs additional discussion or counseling, they are taught to use the health clinic's referral network. Both children and parents are encouraged to use this opportunity at each clinic visit. • James and Marilyn continue to express concern about their responsibility for Matthew's hypertension, suggesting that they should not have had children, since James had high blood pressure when they married. • Marilyn continues to express much anger at her father for not taking better care of himself. • The Baxters express relief when informed that medications can usually control high blood pressure symptoms; they need much more reassurance, however, that they can help control high blood pressure and that it need not prevent the family from normal activities. They are considering counseling to lessen their guilt.

(continued)

Table 17.4 Family Interventions in Childhood Hypertension—The Baxter Family (continued)

Life-style factors	Interventions	Outcomes
Fear and guilt about familial hypertension (continued)		• Reading materials have been devoured and have prompted many questions. • The Baxters have acknowledged their need for health and life-style changes, and have taken such positive steps as beginning smoking cessation, exercising, and seeking a nutritionist's assistance for dietary changes. • This is a very concerned family with a strong internal support system and good communication.

CONCLUSIONS

Childhood hypertension remains a relatively new area of research; the role of childhood hypertension in the development or presence of adult hypertension remains unknown. Hypertension in both children and adults can be understood only through conscientious tracking of blood pressure from childhood. Blood pressure measurement should be a part of every child's yearly health assessment, particularly after age 3 (National Heart, Lung, and Blood Institute's Task Force on Blood Pressure Control in Children, 1977).

Despite the fact that little is known about its origins, hypertension is an increasingly common phenomenon among school-aged children. Since victims are usually asymptomatic, treatment compliance may require creative approaches. Also, because all family members are at risk of developing this condition, efforts to improve cardiovascular health, reduce stress, and establish healthful dietary practices are in order.

Many parents express fear and guilt concerning their child's hypertensive diagnosis. These negative emotions can be allayed and the likelihood of treatment success improved through information and gradual revision of vital life-style patterns.

REFERENCES

Carter, E.A., and McGoldrick, M. *The Family Life Cycle: A Framework for Family Therapy.* New York: Gardner Press, 1980.

Duvall, E.M. *Marriage and Family Development,* 5th ed. Philadelphia: J.B. Lippincott Co., 1977.

Herz, F. "Family Crises and Emotional Disorders," in *Community Health Nursing: Keeping the Public Healthy.* Edited by Jarvis, L.L. Philadelphia: F.A. Davis Co., 1985.

Horan, M. Personal communication, 1985.

Kantor, D., and Lehr, W. *Inside the Family.* San Francisco: Jossey-Bass, 1977.

Lieberman, E. *Blood Pressure and Primary Hypertension in Childhood and Adolescence.* Chicago: Year Book Medical Pubs., 1980.

Lieberman, E. *Children Have Hypertension Too!* Los Angeles: American Heart Association, 1979.

Loggie, J. "Prevalence of Hypertension and Distribution of Causes," in *Juvenile Hypertension* (Kroc Foundation Series, Volume 8). Edited by New, M.I., and Levine, L.S. New York: Raven Press, 1977.

Minuchin, S. *Families and Family Therapy.* Cambridge, Mass.: Harvard University Press, 1974.

National Heart, Lung, and Blood Institute's Task Force on Blood Pressure Control in Children. "Report of the Task Force on Blood Pressure Control in Children," in *Pediatrics Supplement* (reprinted by U.S. Dept. of Health, Education & Welfare. Public Health Service, National Institutes of Health) 59(5):797–820, 1977.

The 1984 Report of the Joint National Committee on Detection, Evaluation, and Treatment of High Blood Pressure. Bethesda, Md.: U.S. Department of Health and Human Services, Public Health Service, National Institutes of Health, 1984.

Wright, L.M., and Leahey, M. *Nurses and Families: A Guide to Family Assessment and Intervention.* Philadelphia: F.A. Davis Co., 1984.

18 Intervening with families of adolescents with diabetes

Nancy C. Talley, RN, MN, ARNP
Division of Nursing
The University of Tampa
Tampa, Florida

OVERVIEW

There are two primary types of diabetes: insulin-dependent, which is also called Type I or juvenile onset diabetes, and non–insulin-dependent, which is also known as type II or adult onset diabetes. This chapter focuses on the more severe of the two, Type I, with specific attention to adolescent insulin-dependent diabetics and the family system response. Because adolescence is a time of accelerated developmental activity, additional attention will be paid to the needs and conflicts associated with this period. Both functional and dysfunctional family adaptation patterns will be discussed in order to identify those specific nursing interventions that enhance positive accommodation of chronic illness and promote family system growth.

CASE STUDY

Sandy Meyer was initially diagnosed as having juvenile diabetes at age 13. Typically, her premorbid history was that of a healthy preadolescent. Rapid weight loss and polyuria were the symptoms that first prompted her parents to seek consultation with their pediatrician. Dr. S's initial report was reassuring. She believed the symptoms indicated a urinary tract infection that would be easily managed with medication. Tests did not confirm this diagnosis, however, and further exploration revealed the problem to be juvenile diabetes. The family was suddenly confronted with the immediate need to accommodate an illness that demanded immediate attention, one that could be controlled, at best, but not cured.

Family Assessment

Mr. and Mrs. Meyer, Sandy's parents, have been married for 16 years. Mr. Meyer is a robust man who is self-employed as an auto mechanic. He is in excellent health. Mrs. Meyer is an attractive 35-year-old woman who has worked as a secretary in a physician's office since her marriage. She, too, enjoys excellent health.

Sandy is the oldest of three children; her siblings are Tom, age 11, and Joanne, age 9. Neither Tom nor Joanne has a history of health problems, although their social adjustment had deteriorated during the year prior to assessment.

Significantly, the family is very sports-minded. Each child has been active in a team sport; Mr. Meyer coached Tom's soccer team; Sandy played volleyball in junior high school.

Sandy's maternal grandmother, Mrs. Slive, was diagnosed as a Type II diabetic at age 52, 4 years prior to Sandy's diagnosis. Mrs. Slive's condition is controlled well with oral antidiabetic medication and a careful diet. There are no other diabetics in the family.

After emergency hospitalization for ketoacidosis resulting from noncompliance with her diabetic regimen, Sandy was referred to her pediatrician for counseling. Between the diabetes itself and Sandy's multiple hospitalizations, family system functioning was disrupted and each member was affected.

Mr. Meyer gave up coaching his son's soccer team and took a second job to meet the added expenses associated with Sandy's illness. Mrs. Meyer had, over a 3-month period, developed symptoms of reactive depression, including sleep and appetite disturbance as well as irritability. Tom had become angry and sullen, and Joanne, previously an honor roll student, was failing one subject at school. Sandy appeared angry and rebellious and had discontinued her participation in school sports. Obviously, because of the tremendous ripple effect of Sandy's diabetes, family-centered nursing intervention was essential.

Assessment began with an initial family interview, followed by individual sessions with each member. It was determined that each family member felt powerless in the face of Sandy's illness, and each was reacting destructively.

Family Intervention

The short-term nursing goal was to identify ways for each family member to regain enough internal control to prevent further deterioration. This was accomplished by reacquainting each member with areas of individual strength, identifying potentially supportive people and activities in the present environment, and examining exactly how the discovery of Sandy's diabetes had personally affected each of them. Initial stabilizing efforts were based on crisis intervention theory. Successful outcome was achieved in approximately 3 weeks through frequent (three per week) sessions.

Family nursing intervention in the Meyer case focused on diabetes education. There were many myths to dispel, most difficult of which was the notion that Sandy's diabetes could be equated with her grandmother's—that is, if Sandy controlled her diet, she would not require exogenous insulin. Myths such as this were confronted directly and replaced with accurate information about Type I diabetes.

Because Sandy was the family member most affected by the illness, it was also necessary to examine her (adolescent) developmental needs and tasks in light of how they could be addressed in the family context. Systems theory was employed.

Sandy needed encouragement to view herself holistically. Although she was a vital, multifaceted young woman, she had begun to see herself as only a diabetic. Sessions during this treatment phase were once weekly and consisted primarily of individual meetings with Sandy, meetings with her and her parents, as well as peer support group meetings for the three of them. The weekly education and counseling sessions were discontinued after 2 months, but support group participation continued.

Evaluation

All nursing goals—crisis stabilization, knowledge acquisition necessary for accommodation of and response to diabetes, and movement toward self-actualization in each family member—were met effectively after approximately 3 months. Sandy rejoined the volleyball team; her siblings made demonstrable social progress; Mr. Meyer could return to coaching; and Mrs. Meyer's depressive symptoms improved steadily. Sandy accepted, with few exceptions, responsibility for managing her illness and began using her parents as consultants rather than care providers.

NURSING PROCESS

Assessment

The health problem: Diabetes. Diabetes mellitus is the most common endocrine-related disturbance, affecting more than 10 million Americans and their families (Anderson and Kornblum, 1984). Although described as early as 1500 B.C. (in Ebers' Papyrus), diabetes etiology remains elusive. In fact, a glucose metabolism dysfunction may be the result of any of several genetic, physiologic, sociologic, and environmental factors. Additionally, predisposed individuals may develop the illness after viral infections of glandular tissue that stimulate a specific type of immune response. The disease probably results from the deterioration of insulin-producing islet cells in the pancreas, cells that produce insulin in response to environmental cues, genetic predisposition, diet, and lifestyle. Additionally, viruses are thought to have an etiologic role.

The islets of Langerhans, approximately 1,000,000 of which are found in the pancreas, are composed of several cell types. Beta cells secrete insulin, which reduces blood glucose levels, while alpha cells secrete its antagonist, glucagon. Delta cells, which are also found here, secrete gastrin (Tackett and Hunsberger, 1978).

Insulin functions as a catalyst, transferring glucose from the blood to fat and muscle cells and activating several other metabolic processes, including retention and synthesis of fat and protein (Patterson, et al., 1984). Insulin deficiency causes dysfunction in carbohydrate, fat, and protein metabolism by impeding glucose entry into cells. When glucose is not readily available, the body seeks alternative energy sources. Protein in skeletal muscles is catabolized (broken down), resulting in muscle deterioration, which in turn produces weakness and delays healing. Another emergency energy source is body fat. Tapping fat can produce dramatic weight loss, as well as accumulation of ketoacids and ketone bodies, which are by-products of fat metabolism, to potentially toxic levels. If corrective action is not taken, diabetic coma and ketoacidosis will occur.

Hyperglycemic symptoms indicating imminent coma include acetone or fruity breath odor, sluggishness, and deep, rapid breathing. The skin is warm and dry to the touch.

Type I diabetes typically appears suddenly in apparently healthy young people. There are no gradual signs or symptoms to facilitate adaptation. The clients typically present with complaints of sudden polyuria, polydipsia, fatigue, and weight loss. In 10% to 15% of diagnosed cases, ketoacidosis and coma occur prior to definite identification of the problem.

The use of exogenous insulin may produce episodic hypoglycemia—a potentially life-threatening complication—in juvenile diabetics. This condition results from either excessive insulin administration, a late or missed meal, or unusually strenuous exercise. The early symptoms include headache, sweating, and irritability, which, left untreated, can lead to confusion, rage, tremor, and seizure. When blood glucose levels fall below 50 mg/dl, immediate glucose administration is indicated.

Diabetic therapy is concerned with maintaining normal (70 to 130 mg/dl) blood glucose levels in order to prevent damage from hyperglycemia or hypoglycemia and to keep glucose available for normal functioning. This often becomes a formidable task, complicated by sensitive hormonal interplay, required alterations in diet and exercise, and difficulty in maintaining emotional stability in the face of stress.

Careful systemic assessment is particularly important in the nursing care of diabetics, since the results of dysfunctional glucose metabolism directly or indirectly affect all vital functions. Stress management capabilities, often treated lightly by assessing nurses, require close attention since stress accumulation greatly interferes with efficient insulin use. Conversely, reduced stress or increased exercise can markedly enhance insulin metabolism.

Families with adolescents. Diabetic adolescents and their families are thrust into a life-threatening crisis with absolutely no preparation. They have no choice but to comply with a strict treatment regimen that is especially restrictive for patients at this developmental stage. Such coping mechanisms as rebellion and denial, which are typically utilized by adolescents in response to overwhelming stress, serve only to escalate the family crisis and make the patient feel even more powerless. The entire family system is thrust into disequilibrium.

The nurse assessing an adolescent diabetic must consider the patient's developmental stage; otherwise, the illness can become a scapegoat for a vast array of insecurities and feelings of inadequacy, or a hindrance to the natural processes of youthful "breaking away" and parental "letting go." In short, the illness must be assessed as a component of one whole person residing within a family (Hanson and Henggeler, 1984).

The nurse providing family care to adolescent diabetics must assess several specific areas: family members' current stress levels and stressors; significant physical, psychological, and sociologic conflict or dysfunction; family recreational and nutritional patterns; members' existing knowledge and/or experience with diabetes; and interfamily support structures.

In sum, all aspects of individual and family life must be explored, since all might affect patient compliance (a change in family activity patterns during periods of stress, for instance, can change the patient's insulin demands). The nurse must communicate the significance of family life-style in diabetic management through holistic assessments. This will make the family more aware of how its actions affect the diabetic member, and help the client place the illness in an appropriate context.

Since insulin-dependent diabetes requires daily attention throughout the client's life, baseline information should be obtained on all aspects of the client's life pattern in order to determine possible areas for change. In all cases, modification will be directed toward the development of healthy living habits applicable to anyone—not just diabetics. In working with families of adolescents, this becomes a key issue; the nurse should not single out the "ill" family member but rather view the family as client. With the exception of insulin administration, most aspects of the therapeutic regimen can be adopted with benefit by each family member.

Adolescence is a time of paradoxes. The relationships between parents and their adolescent children may vacillate and polarize, making health care planning tricky at best. The basic task of adolescence, emancipation from parental dependence (Schuster and Ashburn, 1984), is viewed from both sides as threatening and overwhelming. Typically, both parents and adolescents emphasize the teenager's inadequacy in vain attempts to prolong the inevitable. This is not, however, done consciously. In fact, if questioned directly, both parents and adolescents will vehemently state that they "can't wait for the day of emancipation." Nurses must approach the subject cautiously and with a full understanding of the significance of all family members' behavior so that intervention will respond appropriately to the underlying conflict (Pasquali, et al., 1981).

As part of this pursuit of independence, adolescence is also a time for "trying on" adult roles, frequently through rebellious behavior. By its very nature, rebellion challenges someone else's—usually the designated authorities'—established behavior. Though it is on the one hand an attempt to gain power, rebellion is essentially a reactive statement; it produces no internally directed growth. The "noise" of rebellion may intimidate other family members, in which case they may allow fear rather than logic to dictate their response. When this occurs, as it does frequently among adolescent diabetics, parents often attempt to "take over" management of the diabetic regimen or to become more authoritarian. Such adolescents, however, need parental support to validate their ability to manage their illness. By "taking over," parents reinforce the adolescent's vulnerability, ultimately delaying positive adaptation. Though control is the message, chaos is often the result; the adolescent must own his illness in order to master it (Lidz, 1968; Group for the Advancement of Psychiatry, 1968).

Another phenomenon associated with adolescence, "peer clustering" (Schuster and Ashburn, 1984), is the tendency to bond with other adolescents in order to strengthen identity and defend against feelings of inadequacy. Within a group of adolescents, there may be multiple subgroups or clusters. In today's high schools, for example, there may be a cluster of athletes, a cluster of academic achievers, and a cluster of drug-involved persons. Largely because of this clustering, adolescents rarely establish an independent value system or thought pattern during this period. Clusters allow differentiation from parental values and thoughts without total dependence on self. The fears associated with emancipation are assuaged and hidden from consciousness by active group participation. Depending on the group norms, this can be ego-enhancing or devastating.

Once aligned, the adolescent becomes fiercely loyal to group values. When the new values conflict with those held by the family, many parents feel alienated, unloved, or even hated by their adolescent.

Cluster groups have tremendous influence, and the adolescent's need for peer acceptance must be considered in planning nursing interventions. If this is neglected, noncompliance will probably result.

Because of the intense developmental pressures, many adolescents become narcissistic in their thinking (Schuster and Ashburn, 1984). They may appear selfish and uncaring, but are actually self-absorbed. Most adolescents lack the psychic energy to keep their own physical, emotional, and sociologic demands in perspective and simultaneously to respond to others' needs. Because peers are essential to the adolescent's feelings of well-being, they come first; parents, being familiar and trusted, may be last on the adolescent's consideration list. Parents, having been left out of their child's mental arena, often find it difficult to accept that the very loving nature of their family relationship may be causing the adolescent's unresponsiveness (Erickson, 1968). Nurses can serve as behavioral interpreters during these times of miscommunication and promote linkage where connections are fragile or hostile.

Planning

To facilitate the healthy adaptation of the adolescent Type I diabetic, the nurse must plan interventions that respond not only to the demands of the illness but also to the developmental demands of the client. She must continually evaluate the rapidly changing internal and external stressors that will undoubtedly affect diabetic control. Rigid preparation and planning can defeat wellness promotion by preventing a spontaneous response to changes in the family climate.

As in most consultations, intervention timing is crucial. Crises require supportive and directive nursing responses, and nonessential teaching should be deferred until the physiologic or emotional storm has passed. This is especially important in today's health care delivery system, since most clients will be hospitalized only in times of crisis. Shorter stays may promote consumer responsibility but they also leave little time for the nurse to teach and plan. Too many nurses try to teach everything during hospitalization, when the client is often too frightened to retain information; indeed, it only serves to overwhelm him, and vital information is lost in the process. When the diabetic is a juvenile, counseling and education must follow hospitalization (Leahey et al., 1975); adequate patient understanding and adjustment requires time and a consultative relationship with a health care provider. With few exceptions, this is best accomplished in an outpatient setting.

Intervention

To be successful, nurses must develop and implement interventions based upon a thorough understanding of the dynamics of the adolescent patient and his family unit. Type I diabetes in particular requires life-style changes involving the total family and makes the family itself the client. The nurse must open up her professional "lens," accept the necessity of holistic family involvement, and structure her interventions accordingly (Tomm et al., 1977).

Discussion of nursing interventions should focus on specific behavioral hallmarks—rebellion, peer clustering, and self-absorption—in adolescent development. By combining principles from crisis management, teaching and learning theories, and communication skill education, the nurse can become an invaluable professional team member.

Initially, the nurse should respond to primary needs when they are expressed by each family member, even though the needs may not appear to be the appropriate priorities. What the nurse wants to teach must be compatible at all times with what the family wants to learn.

Intervening with rebelliousness. Rebellion is an awkward attempt to establish control. Therefore, initial interventions should identify "in-chargeness" and any other frustrations that may result from thwarted attempts to gain control. The first stage is to determine each family member's responsibilities in promoting positive adaptation. Reality dictates these individual responsibilities: the diabetic adolescent must control, for example, personal food consumption, exercise patterns, and academic performance; parents must control (by role model) dietary patterns, food availability (to a degree), granting of permissions, and other areas of support, guidance, and management. Adolescents instinctively "know" they are not capable of full life management, though they may boast of self-sufficiency.

After each family member has defined reality-based areas of control, nursing interventions must address validation and support when these boundaries are challenged from within the family. This is achieved by replacing "You made me" with "I choose to." The parents' most demanding task is to acknowledge the limits of their ability to protect their child. The nurse, sensitive to this vulnerability, must frame responses in supportive language, positively reinforcing the actual (and substantial) parental power to protect.

Intervening in peer alienation. Helping parents view peer clustering as positive and essential is another major component of nursing care of families with adolescents. At best, many parents personalize their child's peer focus if they have serious self-doubts or feelings of inadequacy. This tendency can prompt a major dysfunctional civil conflict within the family unit.

After diagnosis, many adolescent diabetics feel separate from and less accepted than their peers. The understanding nurse can be a catalyst in reestablishing peer linkages. Statements such as "Don't worry about other kids and what they think" do not help. The nurse must recognize the pivotal role of basic adolescent security and the importance of peer support in enhancing diabetic adaptation. Relating to other adolescent diabetics has proven to be extremely beneficial in combating feelings of peer group alienation. Most major cities have organizations such as the American Diabetes Association, which offer information regarding peer support groups for both adolescents and their parents.

The nurse can also help the adolescent diabetic communicate openly about his illness with "naturally occurring" peers so that they too can provide support. Peers usually accept the adolescent's illness and even encourage treatment compliance. Although he may not realize it, the adolescent diabetic retains all of his former talent, creativity, personality, and attractiveness. When this awareness is restored, the diabetic once again recognizes similarities to the peer group. On the other hand, adolescents who are allowed to "hide out" in their diabetes become firmly convinced of their difference. Depending on the adolescent's and his family's adjustment prior to the onset of diabetes, short-term counseling may be needed to establish stability, security, and positive identity.

Intervening with adolescent self-absorption. Self-absorption arises from the adolescent's need for periodic "time-outs" to organize and synthesize his rapid-fire developmental changes. The nurse must be aware of this, so that solitude is not mistaken for loneliness. Though long periods of isolation and withdrawal can be symptomatic of depression, episodic separation from others can also be a necessary step toward self-reliance—a pulling-in of energy and focus at a time of psychic overload. During these periods, parents and other family members should learn to accept the behavior as normal and not ascribe negative feelings to it.

Evaluation

In determining intervention effectiveness, the nurse must first examine all presenting symptoms of family dysfunction and patient noncompliance. Do family members communicate more directly? Do members display ownership of messages by relating in the first person? Have healthy adaptation patterns been reestablished? Does each member assume responsibility for defined control areas?

If these questions are answered affirmatively, the family is probably moving toward positive accommodation of Type I diabetes. Longitudinal reevaluation remains important (Caldwell and Pichert, 1985), however, as life and family stresses ceaselessly demand creative solutions.

The nurse provider collaborating with a client's physician must establish strategic consultation points. Once basic issues have been confronted and positively resolved, monthly contact (at least) is recommended for 1 year. After this, quarterly consultation sessions are usually sufficient to ensure continued compliance. Such contacts may, at times, be made by telephone.

If telephone consultation is utilized, the nurse must ask open-ended questions to promote a broader information exchange. For example, instead of asking "How is Sandy doing?," which would probably yield a "She's doing fine" response, say, "Could you describe the last couple of days in the life of the Meyer family?" Of course, effective phone consultation depends on the preestablishment of a solid, trusting therapeutic relationship. Without such a relationship, telephone consultation provides little reliable data and is contraindicated. Of course, hands-on contact is always preferable, since it provides opportunities to observe family processes and physical presentation, as well as to utilize multimodal communication channels.

CONCLUSIONS

Assisting the family of a diabetic adolescent is a most rewarding professional challenge for the nurse clinician. The nurse's holistic focus provides solid preparation for this multifaceted consulting role. Healthy adaptation is most effectively promoted when nursing interventions are grounded in a thorough understanding of the adolescent developmental demands, the existing family system, and the physiologic and emotional consequences of Type I diabetes.

REFERENCES

Anderson, B.J., and Kornblum, H. "The Family Environment of Children with a Diabetic Parent," *Family Systems Medicine* 2(1):17–27, 1984.

Caldwell, S.M., and Pichert, J.W. "Systems Theory Applied to Families with a Diabetic Child," *Family Systems Medicine* 3(1):34–44, 1985.

Erickson, E. *Identity: Youth and Crisis.* New York: W.W. Norton & Co., 1968.

Group for the Advancement of Psychiatry. *Normal Adolescence: Its Dynamics and Impact.* New York: Charles Scribner's Sons, 1968.

Hanson, C.L., and Henggeler, S.W. "Metabolic Control in Adolescents with Diabetes: An Examination of Systemic Variables," *Family Systems Medicine* 2(1):5–16, 1984.

Leahey, M., et al. "Pediatric Diabetes: A New Teaching Approach," *Canadian Nurse* 71:18–20, 1975.

Lidz, T. *The Person: His Development Throughout the Life Cycle.* New York: Basic Books, 1968.

Pasquali, E.A., et al. *Mental Health Nursing—A Bio-Psycho-Cultural Approach.* St. Louis: C.V. Mosby Co., 1981.

Patterson, H.R., et al. *Current Drug Handbook.* Philadelphia: W.B. Saunders Co., 1984.

Schuster, C.S., and Ashburn, S.S. *The Process of Human Development—A Holistic Life-Span Approach.* Boston: Little, Brown & Co., 1984.

Tackett, J.J.M., and Hunsberger, M. *Family-Centered Care of Adolescents.* Philadelphia: W.B. Saunders Co., 1978.

Tomm, K., et al. "Psychological Management of Children with Diabetes," *Clinical Pediatrics* 16(12):1151–55, 1977.

Williamson, P.R., and McCauley, E. "On Being a Diabetic Patient: A Simulated Experience," *Family Systems Medicine* 2(4):409–15, 1984.

19 Intervening with gay families and adolescent obesity

Frederick W. Bozett, RN, DNS
Professor, Graduate Program
College of Nursing
University of Oklahoma Health Sciences Center
Oklahoma City, Oklahoma

OVERVIEW

This chapter provides an overview of two major health problems, adolescent obesity and family dysfunctional communication within the context of the gay-father stepfamily. The case study approach is used, and the content is structured around it. The Calgary Family Assessment Model (Wright and Leahey, 1984) is used within the framework of the nursing process. Assessment of both adolescent obesity and communication in gay-father stepfamilies is addressed in order to arrive at family problems and strengths and family nursing diagnoses. The planning phase of the process is discussed, and specific interventions for adolescent obesity and dysfunctional communication in gay-father stepfamilies are highlighted. The need for nurses to examine their own feelings regarding sexuality, homosexuality, parenting, and family life-styles is stressed. The chapter concludes with a discussion of evaluation for the effectiveness of the interventions for the family's two identified health problems.

CASE STUDY

Family Structure
Bob Krasney, a 41-year-old city planner, and his 15-year-old son Josh live with Bob's lover, Mike Holmes, a 30-year-old interior designer. Although Bob's history of homosexual relationships dates from his late teens, he always enjoyed associations with women and thought of himself as bisexual. He developed a strong affection for his high school girlfriend, Eileen, whom he married after discharge from the Navy, when he was 22. Josh was born 2 years later. After 3 years of monogamous marriage, Bob began having occasional clandestine homosexual liaisons; as these social and sexual experiences became more frequent, it became increasingly clear to him that his sexual orientation was gay. Concurrently, Bob accepted the fact that he was not happy in his marriage.

Bob met Mike at a party, and they started seeing one another as often as possible. His affection for Mike provided the eventual impetus for Bob to disclose his homosexuality to Eileen. Although initially hurt and angry, she gradually became more understanding, although she continued to feel that she had been deceived throughout the course of their marriage.

The couple divorced when Josh was 13. Eileen was granted custody, and Bob was given unrestricted visiting rights, an arrangement that was satisfactory to both parents. Bob and Mike moved into a three-bedroom apartment while Eileen and Josh continued to live in the home they had lived in before the divorce. Two years later, Josh developed behavioral problems, primarily truancy from school. His weight problem—Josh had been 10% to 15% overweight for several years—also increased. Because Eileen could not control Josh's truancy, she and Bob decided that it would be best for him to live with Bob and Mike. Under Bob's firm, loving discipline, Josh began to attend school with only occasional unapproved absences; his weight, however, continued to increase. At the same time, Josh and Mike began arguing frequently. Josh resented Mike's taking on the disciplinary role of a second parent; similarly, Mike was bitter toward Josh because of the restrictions his presence in the household imposed on his and Bob's life-style. Mike also became jealous of Bob's attention to Josh and felt as though he had to compete for his lover's attention. All three family members became irritable with one another; tensions eventually led them to enter family counseling. On the advice of his pediatrician, Josh began attending an adolescent obesity outpatient clinic at a community hospital; Bob and Mike attended concurrent sessions for family members.

Presenting Problems: Obesity and Dysfunctional Family Communication

This family had two health problems: adolescent obesity in one member (treated as a family problem) and dysfunctional family communication as a result of structural change (Josh's arrival) that altered family role relationships and expectations. The family care contexts were the adolescent outpatient clinic at a community hospital and a community mental health center. Josh's obesity was assessed through such measures as triceps skin-fold measurements. He also underwent a complete physical examination with blood studies. A family history was obtained, revealing no pattern of obesity. Food intake, exercise, and routine self-concept were also determined. The initial family counseling interview (with all three members) consisted of a discussion of the members' relationships with each other, their perceptions of the problems, and hoped-for results of counseling. A nurse with graduate clinical nurse specialist (CNS) preparation in family counseling and psychiatric nursing determined that counseling was needed, and that the entire family would benefit from it.

Interventions for Obesity

The treatment plan for Josh's obesity was for him to attend 12 weekly sessions at the adolescent obesity clinic, while Bob and Mike participated in sessions for family members. Josh's goal was to come within 10% of his ideal weight in 6 months. The following interventions were utilized:
- Nutrition education
- Self-monitoring of food intake with emphasis on decreasing intake of high-calorie, low-nutrient foods
- Daily exercise

• Behavior modification techniques (e.g., eating only in specified places at designated times and eliminating other activities while eating)
• Bob and Mike's participation in a parents' group so they could obtain the knowledge and skills necessary to give Josh needed reinforcement and social support.

Interventions for Dysfunctional Family Communications

The counseling plan was based on weekly family interviews—probably no more than six to eight, since the systemic problems were not severe and all family members were eager to resolve them. The nurse also decided to work with all members together, at least for the first few sessions. Specific interventions were aimed toward achieving functional communication between all three family members, developing a time/attention framework at home so that each member spent adequate time with each other, and arranging times when all three members could be together. Having special time alone with each other helped all three work on vital role relationships. Much interview content centered on each member's feelings about his role in the household, its relationship to others' roles, and what he wanted/expected from other family members.

Another intervention called for the family to attend three consecutive sessions of the local gay fathers' group. This group met monthly to socialize, provide peer support, and discuss issues and concerns facing gay fathers and their lovers. Children met separately at the same time to discuss the issues and concerns, if any, that they faced living in a gay household.

Evaluation

Therapeutic goals were being achieved, although Josh's weight problem would require time to overcome. The family considered it a group problem, not Josh's alone; Bob and Mike altered their grocery shopping habits by purchasing fewer high-calorie, low-nutrient foods. All family members modified their eating habits, and Josh lost weight on schedule; as a result, his self-image improved. After 8 weeks of counseling, all family members were communicating more openly, and role relationships were much improved. Mike had a much better understanding of Josh's importance to Bob and was less intolerant of Bob's attention to his son. Mike also began to know Josh better; they have become friends. Also, Josh was more accepting of Mike's authority, and as a result of getting to know Josh better, Mike did not need to be as authoritative. Also, Josh accepted his father's need to have time alone with Mike.

NURSING PROCESS

Assessment

The health problem: Adolescent obesity. Obesity is a multidimensional phenomenon with racial, social, and cultural variables interacting in a complex and critical fashion (Brownell, 1984; Wells and Copeland, 1985). Defining obesity and approximating the number of overweight adolescents might appear to be easy, but it is not, since no means of accurately measuring the incidence of excessive fat within the population is available, nor are there accurate or consistent standards for determining when fat is excessive (Mahoney, et al., 1979). In the past, weight and weight loss were the basis for measurement, but the fact that children's vertical growth also increases their lean body mass was not considered. Now the relationship between weight and height in growing children is taken into consideration, as are the differences between boys and girls (Brownell, et al., 1983). However, any weight-based method of measuring childhood obesity may be unreliable simply because weight is not a direct measure of fat. Fatter children tend to be taller, have larger skeletal and muscular masses, and have greater mineral masses than nonobese children of the same sex and age. Thus, differences in lean body mass tend to make chronically obese children weigh more than lean children independent of body fat proportion. Moreover, children who, in the course of treatment, return to normal weight will weigh more than their lean counterparts due to the advanced development of lean body tissue.

Nurses should also remember that, in obesity treatment, only 70% to 90% of weight loss can be attributed to fat loss; the remainder comes from lost water and protein. The increased physical activity component of the treatment regimen further increases both lean body mass and weight. Thus, the use of weight as the sole treatment standard may be inaccurate (Mahoney, et al., 1979).

Because of the difficulties in using weight to evaluate obesity treatment, skin-fold measurements at the triceps and subscapular region combined with the Body Mass Index are the most practical method of indirectly assessing childhood body fat (Garn, et al., 1975; Womersley and Durnin, 1977).[1]

Even relatively standardized measurement techniques can be problematic in childhood obesity, primarily because there are no tables of desirable weight for children; the definition of childhood obesity is therefore somewhat arbitrary. For example, one study (Epstein, et al., 1980) defined children as obese if they were more than 20% above their "ideal" weight, without indicating how ideal weight was determined. Moreover, body composition varies considerably across race, ethnic, socioeconomic, and sex groups so that one standard of excessive fat is not likely to be appropriate for all adolescents.

Diagnosing adolescent obesity. Drabman and colleagues (1985) recommend combining three classification techniques to diagnose adolescent obesity. The first involves using height/weight/sex tables based on a stratified sample of black and white children in the United States. Although there is no cutoff point for defining obesity, the child's percentile ranking for children of comparable age can be determined. The child's

---

1. Body mass index is calculated by dividing nude weight (in kilograms) by the square of barefoot height (in meters). For example, an individual weighing 70 kg with a height of 180 cm would have a body mass index of 21.6 ($70 \div 1.8^2$). (Ackerman, 1983).

degree of overweight is then determined relative to the ideal figure listed on the chart; obesity is commonly defined at 120% or more of desirable weight. Drabman and colleagues (1985) also recommend comparing triceps skin-fold measures to percentile standards derived from normative data (Garn, et al., 1975). The 85th percentile is the standard used for defining childhood obesity. Drabman and colleagues (1985) also recommend using the "eyeball" technique in initial diagnosis; if two independent observers consider the person obese, a diagnosis of obesity is made. If the results of all three of these means are consistent, then the diagnosis of overweight or obesity seems warranted.

Although the stated prevalence of obesity in the population depends upon the means of measurement used; the operational definition employed (usually 110% to 120% of ideal weight); and the age, social class, and sex of the sample, it appears that 5% to 25% of children and adolescents in the United States are obese.

Determining the presence of obesity is only the first step; other factors also must be assessed. Foremost among these are patient and family eating patterns, including times of eating, location(s), activities accompanying eating, types of foods, and amounts ingested. The overweight adolescent's self-esteem and self-concept, both of which are often diminished, should also be assessed (Sallade, 1973). Obese adolescents often have difficulty fitting in with a peer group because of the stigma that accompanies being overweight. Physical activity must also be evaluated, since overweight adolescents seldom participate in sports or other group activities, favoring instead such sedentary leisure activities as watching television and eating (Langford, 1981).

Single-parent fathers. According to Hanson (1985), approximately 21% of all families with children in the United States are headed by single parents—a 111% increase since 1970. In other words, one in every five children lives with a single parent; 90% of the total live with their mothers and 10% with their fathers. The number of children residing with their fathers increased 101% between 1970 and 1982. Living arrangements are achieved through informal agreements between divorced parents, legal custody assignment, widowhood, and, less commonly, through child snatching and single-parent adoption.

Gay fathers. Accurate statistics on most aspects of homosexuality are virtually impossible to obtain, but rough estimates of the gay-father population are available. About 10% of the total U.S. population is gay and male (Churchill, 1971; Kingdon, 1979; Kinsey, et al., 1948), and about 20% of the gay male population marries heterosexually (Bell and Weinberg, 1978; Jay and Young, 1979; Spada, 1979). Twenty-five percent of married gay men become natural fathers (Bell and Weinberg, 1978; Miller, 1979). Thus, it is likely that at least 4 million gay men have been married, and 1 to 2 million of them are natural fathers. Finally, in light of the fact that some gay men marry more than once, and that some of them adopt children as single parents or when coupled with a wife or male lover, it is logical to assume that there are at least several million children of gay fathers. It is not possible to estimate how many of these men are primarily responsible for the care of their children.

Gay men marry for many reasons. Some may want children or permanent companionship; others may be in love, fear loneliness, desire stability, or succumb to parental pressures. Some gay men think that marriage will "cure" their homosexuality, while others may use marriage as a screen behind which their true orientation can be hidden (Bozett, 1982, 1984). It is likely that most married gay men remain married and have occasional homosexual liaisons, usually without their wives' knowledge. Many, however, do divorce and adopt a gay life-style, as did Bob.

Initially, most marriages of gay men to heterosexual women are satisfactory. Over time, however, the desire for sex with men intensifies, and the frequency of clandestine homosexual liaisons begins to increase. At the same time, sexual relations within the marriage commonly diminish in frequency, communication becomes dysfunctional, and the relationship deteriorates. This deterioration may involve sharp conflict or gradual distancing (Bozett, 1982). With exposure to the gay social scene and the possible development of a love relationship, cognitive dissonance (Festinger, 1957) intensifies as the man becomes torn between his dichotomous worlds. Eventually, when spousal incompatibility becomes unbearable, such men often disclose their homosexuality to their wives. Attempts to salvage the marriage through individual or marital therapy may be made, but are rarely effective. Separation and divorce usually ensue (Miller, 1978).

By entering the gay world, the man's marginality and resultant cognitive dissonance are reduced, but the gay father discovers what Fadiman (1983) calls the "double closet" phenomenon. After the man exits his closet in the heterosexual world by disclosing his homosexuality, he finds he must exit a second closet by revealing his fatherhood, which carries the potential for rejection within the new social group. Generally, however, the "second closet" is less confining than the first, since most gay fathers are deeply attached to their children (Bozett, 1980a; Miller, 1979). They usually do not develop close relationships with gays who reject their fatherhood or their children (Bozett, 1985a).

Because nonparents often have a low tolerance for children (Veevers, 1975), gay fathers, especially those with custody, may have difficulty establishing and maintaining long-lasting relationships with other men. Moreover, parental obligations often conflict with the single gay life-style. For example, most gay men do not have a long-term commitment to another person, have unrestricted use of time and money, and higher-than-average mobility. In spite of these differences, however, many gay fathers form couples with other men (Bozett, 1984).

Although there is considerable literature on the stepfamily (Bohannan, 1983; Fast and Cain, 1966; Pasley, 1985; Pasley and Ihinger-Tallman, 1984; Visher and Visher, 1979), writings on gay stepfamilies are con-spicuously absent. Hence, there are no theories or models specific to the assessment of these families. The model used in this chapter is the Calgary Family Assessment Model (Wright and Leahey, 1984), which is sufficiently general and inclusive to provide the nurse with a guide for a comprehensive assessment of these families.

The problems experienced by the Krasney-Holmes family are typical. One of the major problems in gay-father stepfamilies stems from the father's partner's unrealistic expectation that he will receive a majority of the father's time and attention. Because gay fathers have lived in a committed relationship, they have learned how to juggle their attention; they have also developed some notion of how to manage interpersonal difficulties. Their gay partners, most of whom lack similar experience, may find it difficult to vie with children for the father's affection.

Another common concern is the relationship between the child and the father's lover. The two may regard each other as rivals and react with mutual hostility, competition, and jealousy due to their feelings of insecurity and role confusion. Focal issues in such cases often include the child's refusal to accept the lover as an authority figure, the lover's unrealistic expectations of the child, and the child's resentment of the father's attention to the lover.

In sum, most of the problems faced by gay-parent stepfamilies arise from unclear role relationships and expectations.[2]

Structural assessment: The Krasney-Holmes family

Internal. This gay-father stepfamily consists of Bob, age 41; Bob's lover Mike, age 30; and Bob's son Josh, who is 15. Josh spends at least one weekend each month with his mother. However, since Bob and Eileen's relationship is amicable, exact visit frequency and length is negotiable depending upon Josh's desires or the special needs of Bob and Mike or Eileen.

---

2. There are multiple variations on the form and structure of gay-father families. Some of these men have custody while others do not; some are in love relationships with and without custody, while others are single; some gay fathers disclose their homosexuality to their wives and children, while others may remain married and never disclose to anyone. What is described here is one of the more common scenarios. Although lesbian mothers' issues and concerns are not identical, they are in some ways similar. However, the author cautions the reader to read the literature on lesbian mothers and not to rely on extrapolation from this chapter.

External. Bob's ancestors are Yugoslavian; he is a third-generation American. Bob's parents live 100 miles away, and he is an only child. Bob disclosed his homosexuality to his parents at the time of his separation from Eileen more than 2 years ago; they have gradually begun to accept that he is gay, although they say they don't understand it. This is not an uncommon reaction (Fairchild and Hayward, 1979). The elder Krasneys seem to like Mike. They visit Bob about every other month and Bob, Mike, and Josh spend occasional holidays with them. Bob's ex-wife Eileen resides in a nearby town, in the home she and Bob shared during their marriage.

Mike's parents were first-generation Americans. They were killed in an auto accident when he was 3, and he was raised by his paternal grandparents, who are now also deceased. Both his maternal and paternal grandparents emigrated from England after the Second World War. Mike has one brother and two sisters, all of whom are older, married, and living in divergent areas of the United States. Contact between any of them is rare. Mike feels that Bob is his only "real" family.

Bob and Mike both come from families that value hard work. However, both enjoy leisure activities and occasionally eat out, attend movies, socialize in gay bars, and have gay and nongay male and female friends in for dinner. Both men were reared as Catholics, but neither now attends church, nor are they members of *Dignity,* the affiliated fellowship for gay Catholics. Occasionally they attend Metropolitan Community Church (MCC), a nationwide interdenominational Christian church with a predominantly gay congregation. Religion and church attendance have not been a part of Josh's upbringing.

Developmental assessment. The Krasney-Holmes family is in the "Families with Teenagers" stage of the family life cycle, as it is defined by Duvall (1977). This stage begins when the first child becomes 13 and ends when that child leaves home. Duvall lists eight developmental tasks for this stage, such as "sharing responsibilities of family living" and "bridging the communication gap." However, this framework refers to the intact heterosexual family; some of the eight tasks—such as putting the marital relationship in focus—do not apply to gay families.

Certain social events and institutions, such as marriage and the children's departures from home, clearly delineate the stages of the heterosexual family life cycle. There are not comparable milestones for gay family units. Carter and McGoldrick's (1980) outline of developmental issues in remarried families, including "plan[ning] for maintenance of cooperative coparental relationships with ex-spouse" and "restructuring family boundaries to allow for inclusion of new spouse/ stepparent," although developed from the heterosexual family model, appear applicable to gay-father stepfamilies. The extent or degree of this applicability is uncertain.

Tasks. As an adolescent, one of Josh's primary developmental tasks is to increase his personal autonomy. Although problems in the Krasney-Holmes household are undoubtedly related to role conflict, the root of the problem might be a clash between Josh's pursuit of independence at a time when Bob, at age 41, is struggling with the difficult questions of mid-life. Because Bob made his transition to a homosexual life-style during the mid-life period, he, like Josh, might need affirmation of his identity and of the decisions he has made. Hence, another source of conflict may be father's and son's simultaneous encounters with the difficulties inherent in solidifying emergent identities (Bozett, 1985b). Around age 30, many men also experience a period of stress that culminates in a period of settling down (Levinson, 1978). Mike has already passed this crisis period; his task now is to concentrate on building his career, solidifying his relationship with Bob, and establishing a functional relationship with Josh.

Attachment. As noted in Figure 19.1, the Krasney-Holmes family displays elements of adaptive and maladaptive attachments. Although Josh's relationship with his father is strong and primarily adaptive, there is an element of maladaptation in the multiple developmental conflicts and in Josh's resentment of Bob's attention to Mike. Likewise, the interaction between Mike and Bob, while basically adaptive, has maladaptive elements in Mike's resentment of Bob's attention to Josh. The most maladaptive attachment is that between Josh and Mike. Competition for Bob's time and attention and an absence of clearly defined role relationships and expectations make their relationship a negative one.

The literature on heterosexual families after divorce indicates that remarriage may jeopardize connections between parent and child, and that the child may feel lost and abandoned (Grief, 1982). Josh may feel both loss and abandonment, as a result of Bob's attention to Mike and the absence of his mother's daily attention. Likewise, Mike, even though an adult, might harbor similar feelings because of Bob's attention to Josh. Josh's mood swings, characteristic of his developmental stage, also contribute to the maladaptation.

Figure 19.1   Attachments Among Bob, Mike, and Josh

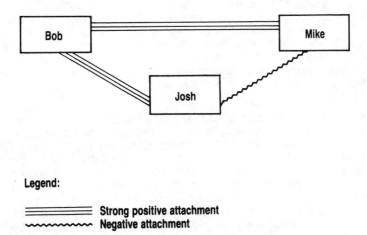

Legend:

═══════ **Strong positive attachment**
〜〜〜〜〜 **Negative attachment**

Functional assessment

Instrumental. Instrumental assessment involves evaluating such routine activities of daily living as preparing meals, house cleaning, and doing laundry. Before Josh moved in, Bob and Mike shared tasks they both enjoyed, and alternated doing the chores that neither of them liked. For example, both had a talent for cooking, so they often planned and prepared meals together. Neither enjoyed house cleaning, so they alternated doing it on a weekly basis. When Josh entered the household, his tasks were determined by mutual agreement. He agreed to put the trash out nightly, do the dishes every other week, and keep his own room clean. Like most boys his age, he occasionally complained about one or more of his chores, but Josh's fulfillment of household responsibilities rarely constituted a major problem.

Expressive. "Expressive functioning" refers to the emotional aspects of family life and includes such elements as communication, problem-solving, roles, control, beliefs, and alliances/coalitions (Wright and Leahey, 1984). All three members of the Krasney-Holmes household can express a range of emotions and feelings toward one another. Bob and Mike express their affection for one another by hugging or by a kiss, and do so in front of Josh; more demonstrative affection is expressed in private. No affection is demonstrated if Josh's friends are visiting. Bob and Mike have also agreed to discuss their differences at the time they arise rather than to harbor them; therefore, they rarely become angry with one another. Josh has little difficulty being expressive. He lets Bob know when he is sad or angry, although he can be moody and uncommunicative on occasion. At such times, he usually stays in his room and watches television. Bob and Mike leave him alone, knowing that within a day he will probably be back to normal. Bob attributes these periods of moody silence to normal adolescence. Josh also readily expresses his jealous anger at both Bob and Mike.

Periodically, Bob and Josh have "man-to-man" talks, one of which concerned sexuality, homosexuality, and Bob's relationship with Mike. Although Bob and Josh discussed Bob's homosexuality in a general way at the time of the separation and divorce, Bob thought that, at 15, Josh deserved a more complete explanation. Josh admitted that he was embarrassed by his father's homosexuality and kept it secret from everyone except his best friend. He also told Bob that, although he didn't care that his father was homosexual, he was afraid that his peers would accuse him of being gay, and he did not want to be similarly stigmatized. These reactions are common in children of gay fathers (Bozett, 1986).

This family's primary problem centers around a lack of role clarification and communication difficulties resulting in coalition problems. Mike attempts to set limits with Josh; Josh resents Mike's rule-making and becomes upset with his father when Bob supports Mike. On the other hand, Bob's attempts to support both Mike and Josh are inconsistent and increase stress among all family members. Rivalry and competition between Mike and Josh for Bob's time and attention further compound the family's problems; indeed, the most serious form of jealousy that any custodial gay father will encounter is that of other gay men who resent the father's attention to his children (Bozett, 1980b).

The overall results of the nursing assessment of Bob, Josh, and Mike appear in Table 19.1.

Planning

It is not possible to generalize goals for families with the types of problems displayed by Bob, Josh, and Mike. Each unit must be assessed individually to determine strengths and problem areas, and to establish mutual goals between family and nurse. In areas that are heavily laden with negative connotations, such as obesity and homosexuality, nurses must be aware of their own feelings in order to avoid devising inappropriate plans based upon stereotypic value judgments.

In the Krasney-Holmes case, the CNS (with input from the family) established realistic goals and collected evidence of their achievement through outcome criteria (Table 19.2). The family acknowledged that the goals were reasonable, and that all could be achieved within the mutually determined time frame. All members agreed to work toward attaining their goals.

Table 19.1 Assessment Results—The Krasney-Holmes Family

Family Problems	Major Family Strengths	Nursing Diagnoses
• Adolescent obesity • Diminished self-esteem (obese family member) • Dysfunctional intrafamily communication • Lack of clearly defined role relationships and expectations	• Motivation to adhere to weight reduction/treatment plan • Adults' love for one another • Father's love and concern for son/ patient • Father's desire to be a "good" father • Stepparent's willingness to negotiate a functional role relationship with son • Son's acceptance of the parent's homosexual relationship • Noncustodial parent's acceptance of homosexual relationship as a healthy home environment for son	• Adolescent obesity, chronic, related to difficulty adjusting to rapid and multiple complex alterations in family structure • Dysfunctional family communication, acute, related to role confusion and lack of role clarity

Interventions

Adolescent obesity
Diet. Although caloric restriction and weight loss must be emphasized in the treatment of adolescent obesity, modifying food selection behaviors is even more important (Epstein, et al., 1978, 1981).

Table 19.2   Care Plan—The Krasney-Holmes Family

Goals	Outcome Criteria

• All family members will participate in the family regimen prescribed for Josh's weight problem.
 • All family members will demonstrate decreased role confusion and increased role clarity, thus facilitating functional communication.
	• Within 6 months Josh will be within 10% of the normal weight for his sex, age, height, and body mass.
	 • Within 3 months:
	  a. Mike will be less envious of the time that Bob and Josh spend together.
	  b. Josh will be less envious of the time that Bob and Mike spend together.
	 • Within 2 weeks of beginning therapy, Josh and Mike will participate in activities together (*i.e.*, bicycle riding and working on Josh's homework).
	 • Within 1 month, Josh will begin to accept Mike as a friend.
	 • Within 2 months Josh will accept Mike's legitimate authority in the household.
	 • Within 1 month of beginning therapy, all family members will participate in leisure activities together.

A color-coded system (devised by Epstein and colleagues, 1978) of categorizing food was incorporated into Josh's plan; "red" foods were high in calories but low in nutritional value; "yellow" foods were high in both calories and nutritional value; "green" foods were highly nutritious and low in calories. Reduced consumption of red foods has been found to increase the consumption of green and yellow foods (Epstein, et al., 1981); attention to appropriate food selection in the treatment of childhood and adolescent obesity is therefore essential. Obese teenagers often skip breakfast and lunch and eat high-calorie "junk" foods after school; most consume few fresh fruits and vegetables. This behavior was characteristic of Josh, who also consumed numerous high-calorie soft drinks. These were forbidden on his diet. A reinforcement system was used whereby Josh's allowance was increased if he consumed fewer than four red foods per week. Other reinforcement came in the form of praise from both Bob and Mike for success in carrying out the therapeutic program and in losing weight.

In sum, a nurse must monitor and reinforce proper food selection and consumption during any weight loss program. It is not sufficient merely to count calories or monitor weight loss, especially among children and adolescents for whom inadequate nutrition could attenuate growth processes (Wells and Copeland, 1985).

In Josh's case, the nutritionist in the outpatient clinic instituted a self-monitoring program that involved keeping daily records of caloric intake, exercise, and weight. Each night before bed, Josh recorded each of these items in a special notebook. When he was uncertain of caloric values, either Bob or Mike would assist him, using a book provided by the nutritionist on the caloric content of food portions.

Altering food intake was only one of the behavioral modifications instituted with Josh. In light of evidence that obese children eat faster with fewer chews per bite than their normal weight counterparts (Drabman, et al., 1979; Keane, et al., 1981), the nutritionist suggested that Josh chew each bite thoroughly and replace his utensils on the table after each bite to slow the act of eating (Epstein, et al., 1976; Weiss, 1977).

Eating behavior in obese individuals is, to a great extent, regulated by external (environmental), rather than internal (hunger and satiety) cues. While there is some debate over this "externality hypothesis" (Rodin, 1981), techniques to reduce external stimuli to eating are commonly employed in behavioral treatment.

The following stimulus control techniques were used with Josh:
• The only *designated place for eating* at home was the dining room; at school, it was the cafeteria.
• The *designated times for eating* at home were the times when the family gathered for meals; at school, it was the designated lunch periods.
• *Other activities during meals,* such as watching television, were eliminated.
• Bob bought *opaque containers* to keep such high-calorie foods as cookies out of sight.
• Bob and Mike also altered their food selection patterns so that few of these foods were in the household at all.
• All family meals were served on *smaller plates and bowls.*
• At home, food was served *cafeteria style,* rather than family style (Aragona, et al., 1975; Coates and Thoresen, 1981; Weiss, 1977; Wheeler and Hess, 1976).
• Bob planned the meals so that all three family members ate the same food; by implementing this strategy, he made it more likely that Josh would adhere to his prescribed diet (Hagenbuch, 1982).
• Bob took Josh with him on the weekly grocery shopping trips, so that Josh could learn to plan nutritious low-calorie meals.

Exercise. The aforementioned treatment techniques focused on the intake side of the energy equation. However, obesity results from an imbalance between energy intake and energy expenditure; that is, it occurs when the amount of food consumed exceeds the amount needed for growth, maintenance, and activity. It appears that the primary cause of adolescent obesity is inactivity (Gutierrez, 1979). Therefore, a nurse must incorporate regular exercise into the treatment regimen. Exercise contributes to a negative energy balance, thus allowing the body to use energy stored in adipose tissue. Two types of exercise programs have been employed. One is "life-style" exercise in which the individual participates in common daily games and activities; the second is "programmed" activity such as daily aerobics. Research indicates that "life-style" exercise programs are more effective in long-term weight loss and maintenance (Epstein, et al., 1980).

Most obese teenagers seldom participate in sports, especially competitive sports (Langford, 1981), and this was true of Josh. Therefore, his planned exercise program was to ride his bicycle, which he enjoyed, at least 1 hour each day after school and on weekends. Mike, too, was a bicycle enthusiast, and often joined Josh on the weekends, when they would tour for more than an hour. Both Bob and Mike were athletic, and Josh's need for exercise stimulated them to renew the family's membership in the local YMCA.

Family involvement. From the foregoing, it is clear that both Bob and Mike were involved in Josh's treatment plan. For the nurse working from the family perspective, the patient is not overweight alone—the entire family is. Therefore, the whole family must be involved if treatment is to be effective. This is especially true in adolescent obesity, since the adults in the household usually do the menu planning, food shopping, and meal preparation. Thus, enlisting adult cooperation in modifying the intake of high-calorie foods and in other aspects of treatment is crucial; all family members must know what behaviors are targeted for change if the plan is to succeed.

In the case of the Krasney-Holmes family, the plan called for Bob and Mike to attend group meetings 1 night weekly for 12 weeks (the basic program) and then monthly (the maintenance program). The purpose of the meetings was to educate the family about adolescent obesity and its treatment; to teach basic nutrition, meal planning, and food preparation; to teach behavior modification techniques and exercise; and to discuss anxiety and other feelings that often accompany weight reduction. The definition of obesity as a family problem is stressed throughout the program. The adults in the household should be actively involved in learning the same information and skills that their overweight child learns, and they, too, might have the opportunity to vent their feelings. However, because adolescents have increased autonomy needs, they tend to do best when their parents meet in separate groups. The parents should learn how to provide reinforcement and support, but not to assume too much responsibility for daily treatment implementation (Brownell, et al., 1983; Wells and Copeland, 1985). When Bob and Mike attended the session for parents, one group member asked them why both of them were attending. Bob replied that Josh was his son, and that Josh lived with him and Mike. The answer seemed to satisfy the individual's curiosity.

Bob and Mike allowed Josh to monitor all aspects of his program, but Bob would periodically review Josh's daily diary and assist him with calculating calories as needed.

Through their weekend cycling trips, Josh gradually began to enjoy Mike's companionship. This activity helped them achieve one of the established outcome goals, that of developing a friendship.

It is important to note that both Bob and Mike attempted to model good nutrition behavior, although they found it difficult at times. On occasion they would both have high-calorie, low-nutrient snacks at night after Josh was asleep or when he was not at home.

In short, the best results in reducing childhood/adolescent obesity seem to come from programs that combine:
- A well-balanced, low-calorie diet
- Exercise, preferably with at least one other person
- Behavior modification
- Social support.

In addition, if there is evidence of psychological disturbance, as there was with Josh, counseling is helpful (Ackerman, 1983).

Dysfunctional family communication
Nurse's attitudes toward homosexuality. Several guidelines for nurses working with gay clients and/or stepfamilies should be discussed. First, nurses must examine their feelings about their own sexuality and about homosexuality in general. Nurses who lack knowledge about homosexuality and gay life-styles, who are uncomfortable with gays and with homosexuality as a sexual orientation, or who relate to gay families from the premise that the heterosexual life-style is superior, should refer gay client families to professionals who do not harbor such views (Baptiste, 1982; Bozett, 1984; DiBella, 1979). Moreover, nurses must examine their own values, attitudes, expectations, and standards regarding parenting and family life-style, since counseling cannot succeed if the family's and the nurse's views on these subjects differ too greatly (Bozett, 1984). Furthermore, the nurse should not be overly inquisitive or patronizing; assessment and interventions should center on the salient circumstances of the situation. Homosexuality should be the focus only if it is clearly relevant. This may seem obvious, but it is easy to overemphasize aspects of a family's situation that pique one's curiosity.

Research findings confirm that nonsexual psychological problems may be mistakenly attributed to persons of unconventional sexual orientation (Davidson and Griedman, 1981). Baptiste (1982) elaborates on this by remarking that "pseudo insight," which occurs when the counselor attributes family problems to the presence of homosexuality or another unusual circumstance, must be avoided. The family's own sense of need should guide therapy, not goals defined or redefined from the counselor's own value position (Baptiste, 1982).

Family interviews. The Krasney-Holmes family's treatment took place over a 2-month period, during which eight weekly counseling sessions were held. All family members attended seven of the sessions; Bob missed one because of a severe cold. Although the CNS was not gay, he had had considerable experience treating gay stepfamilies. From the outset he considered Bob, Mike, and Josh to be a two-parent family unit, and Josh's problem to be a family problem. The CNS knew that attempting to incorporate a child into an established gay relationship often creates strain and jealousy on the part of both child and lover since neither has the father's undivided love and attention (Woodman and Lenna, 1980). The CNS also realized the importance of openly discussing such matters as discipline, household responsibilities, child care, private time (separately and together), sleeping arrangements, adults' behavior in front of the child(ren), and other similar matters before the child(ren) moves in (Moses and Hawkins, 1982). Although Bob and Mike had briefly considered some of these issues, they had not dealt with them in depth. The CNS therefore used some sessions to discuss rules for managing the relationship and producing agreement, since lack of accord is often a major obstacle to lasting relationships among gays (Schrag, 1984).

Improving stepfather-adolescent relationship. Throughout the treatment period, all three members seemed motivated to succeed as a family unit. Interviews were focused on each family member's expectations for himself in relation to the others, and on each member's expectations of the others, in order to uncover inconsistent or potentially problematic expectations. Most importantly, Bob found out that Mike did not like to discipline Josh; Mike felt that he had been given the role of disciplinarian while Bob reserved for himself the role of being Josh's friend. This role conflict distanced Mike and Josh from one another and created mutual hostilities. The CNS explained that, in the early stages of the stepfamily life cycle, the biological parent should be the one responsible for setting and enforcing limits on the child(ren). If the stepparent needs to enforce established rules, he should use the phraseology "Your parent said you should...," so that the stepparent does not assume the disciplinarian role (Mills, 1984). The CNS also directed Mike to develop specific friendship affiliation behaviors with Josh. Stern (1982) has found that affiliating strategies improve the stepfather-stepchild relationship. The strategy most natural to Mike was to *spend time* with Josh through bicycle riding. As a result, both Josh and Mike got to know one another better and relate more as friends than as stepfather/stepchild. As a consequence of Mike's increased attention to Josh in a nonthreatening situation, Josh gradually became less resentful of Mike and of Bob's attention to him.

Improving the father-son relationship. Concurrently, the CNS recommended that Bob and Josh set time aside for each other each week. During those special times Bob would help Josh with his homework; occasionally they would eat out if Mike was working late. On weekends they would attend a movie, go bowling, or participate in some other activity. As a result of Mike's and Josh's increased knowledge of and liking for each other, Mike became less resentful of Bob's attention to his son.

Finally, the CNS assigned Bob and Mike to plan time together without Josh. They reserved weekend time at least twice a month, usually when Josh was visiting his mother, in order to be together without any parental obligations.

Dealing with stigmatization. Although adolescent children are often embarrassed by a gay parent, Josh accepted his father's homosexuality and his relationship with Mike. Although Josh did not bring the topic up, the CNS knew the subject was important enough to explore with Josh.

The boy discussed the issue with some reluctance. Baptiste (1982) emphasized that it is difficult for a child to be a member of a family that society labels deviant or pathological. The need to maintain secrecy may cause isolation, especially when adolescents avoid bringing friends home for fear of discovery. The children themselves may also fear visiting friends' homes lest they be asked probing questions. Although Josh occasionally brought his best friend home, he admitted that he had these concerns. The CNS explored potential interventions, such as having Josh refer to Mike as an "uncle." Also, since the apartment had three bedrooms, it could be made to appear that Mike and Bob slept separately. It was also important to Bob and Mike, however, that Josh understand that they believed that their relationship was natural, good, and moral, and that there were millions of other gay men and lesbians, as well as millions of nongays, who believed as they did. Josh understood this. Josh explained that his school chums had made derogatory remarks about him because of his obesity and that, because of this, he knew what it felt like to be stigmatized; he could thus identify with the differentness that his father must feel. He also remarked that neither his dad nor Mike displayed any of the effeminacy or other mannerisms stereotypically associated with gay men, and was therefore comfortable with them in public. This supports the research findings of Bozett (1986) who found that children of gay fathers who feel that they are different from their peers and whose father's homosexuality is not perceived by the children to be overt, are less likely to conceal the father's homosexuality.

Increasing family's social support. The CNS assigned the family to attend three consecutive monthly meetings of the local gay fathers' group, which was affiliated with The International Gay Fathers Coalition (P.O. Box 50360, Washington, DC 20004). The purpose of this intervention was for Bob and Mike to discuss their family situation and the relationship problems they had had since Josh moved in with men who had successfully navigated this stage of the gay stepfamily life cycle. Social support with peers in similar circumstances has been found to be an important element in promoting longevity in gay/lesbian relationships (Tanner, 1978; Mendola, 1980). Often the involved children meet separately, at the same time as their parents/stepparents. The absence of the fathers leads to less inhibited discussion of feelings and potential ways to manage the various awkward situations that may arise as a result of their fathers' homosexuality. Also, the children learn that they are not unique, that other children also have gay fathers. Although Josh was initially resistant, after attending two meetings he developed a new friendship, which motivated him to attend regularly. Within several months Josh was dating one of the girls in the group. She was also on a plan to lose weight, and they could provide mutual support and reinforcement.

In sum, because the Krasney-Holmes family was deemed compliant, direct interventions were employed. Some of these measures were applied at the cognitive and affective levels, but most were behavioral and involved assigned family tasks outside of the interview sessions. These behavioral interventions were targeted at facilitating intrafamily communication so that interactions and behaviors would be consistent with functional role relationships (Wright and Leahey, 1984).

Evaluation

Adolescent obesity. Evaluation is accomplished by determining the extent to which the goals and outcome criteria established during planning have been achieved. The goal of all family members participating in Josh's weight control program is currently being accomplished. The family has just completed the 3-month structured weight reduction program. No sessions were missed. They intend to return to the clinic for scheduled monthly follow-up sessions. Because of the family's demonstrated adherence to the treatment program and the members' obvious motivation, they will probably do so. Although Josh has not lost a great deal of weight, he is also getting taller, so that he appears thinner. He admits that he occasionally cheats on his diet by eating forbidden foods after school. Also, he and Kathy, his girlfriend from the gay fathers' children's group, sometimes indulge in candy and buttered popcorn at the movies. But, generally, Josh adheres to his dietary regimen and receives the promised increase in his allowance most weeks.

Recently, Josh was asked to try out for a school play. Bursting with pride, he could hardly wait until Bob and Mike arrived home that evening to tell them. When they came in, he explained that he probably would not have been offered the part if he had not lost weight. The possibility of performing in the school play seemed to boost his self-esteem, which had already been lifted by regular praise from Bob and Mike. This kind of reinforcement not only encourages Josh to continue positive nutritional and exercise behaviors, but also helps to raise his self-confidence. Also, Kathy is the first girl who has demonstrated consistent interest in Josh. Her liking for and support of him also fosters Josh's sense of self-worth. If Josh continues his treatment program, and he *is* motivated to do so, he will probably achieve the outcome criterion of being within 10% of his normal weight within the first 6 months.

Dysfunctional family communication. The nurse's therapeutic effectiveness with gay stepfamilies may be difficult to evaluate because of the lack of models, theory, and literature. The nurse cannot be certain that the heterosexual stepfamily model is capable of determining function in a gay stepfamily; nor is such a model necessarily useful for validating the effectiveness of nursing interventions. Thus, continuous feedback from the family is crucial. Moreover, evaluation of each family member's progress toward his goal is essential. Also, familiarity with functional gay-stepfather (or lesbian-stepmother) families would provide a useful baseline against which to make judgments. One suggested strategy for this would be to offer multiple-family therapy for gay-stepfather (or lesbian-stepmother) families. The families could provide each other with needed validation, thus helping the nurse evaluate progress (Bozett, 1984).

It is now 1 month since the family terminated its program with the CNS. The relationship between Josh and Mike has become closer; they bicycle regularly and on one occasion went on an all-day outing without Bob. Also, Josh sometimes seeks Mike's, rather than Bob's, assistance with his nutrition diary or homework. Josh is making a conscious effort to be a positive force within the household. He readily admits that his discussions with Kathy about having a gay father and living with Mike are very helpful. He is still moody on occasion, but Bob and Mike allow him to seclude himself in his room when he feels the need; his moods are not a family problem. Bob and Josh, and Bob and Mike are spending time together. Regular activity involving all three family members, however, has not yet been instituted, although they plan to take a water aerobics class together at the YMCA beginning next month. Envious feelings are almost absent. Mike still resents Bob's attention to Josh but not as severely as before counseling.

It is often difficult to adjust to living with an adolescent, especially when one has never before experienced parenting. Thus, more than several months are needed to resolve all problem areas. Mike did have one additional session with the CNS to discuss his feelings privately. Generally, the family is progressing well. Each outcome criterion has been, or is in the process of being, met.

CONCLUSIONS

Working with a family unit is rarely simple. Families are multicomplex systems, and often require nursing knowledge and sophisticated therapeutic strategems to achieve effective outcomes. Families of obese adolescents are especially challenging because of frequent difficulties with compliance. Although Josh occasionally ate forbidden foods, he was more compliant than most children his age. This was due in part to the effectiveness of the CNS's interventions and to Bob's and Mike's support of the weight reduction program. Their support was not surprising; it has been found that gay fathers often make special efforts to meet the highest parenting standards. Explanations given for this behavior are that gay fathers want to prove the inappropriateness of social sanctions against gays as parents, that they feel the need to protect custody or visitation rights (Bozett, in press; Turner, et al., 1985), or that they place greater emphasis on paternal nurturance than non-gay fathers (Scallen, 1981). These reasons may also explain Bob's and Mike's efforts to improve their own communication and clarify their role relationships. Stepfamily cohesion always takes time, and it is often an arduous process. Gay-father stepfamilies have similar difficulties compounded by the presence of homosexuality and the attendant problems imposed by a homophobic society.

Nurses who work with families in which a member is overweight or with families of gays need to be accepting, knowledgeable, receptive to learning, and willing to examine their own value systems. From such experiences and introspection, nurses mature in their professional capabilities, thus becoming of greater assistance to families in need. Also, immense satisfaction is derived from knowing that stigmatized populations have been well served.

REFERENCES

Ackerman, S. "The Management of Obesity," *Hospital Practice* 18:17–140, 1983.

Aragona, J., et al. "Treating Overweight Children Through Parental Training and Contingency Contracting," *Journal of Applied Behavioral Analysis* 8:269–78, 1975.

Baptiste, D.A. "Issues and Guidelines in the Treatment of Gay Stepfamilies," in *Questions and Answers in the Practice of Family Therapy,* vol. 2. Edited by Gurman, A.S. New York: Brunner-Mazel, 1982.

Bell, A.P., and Weinberg, M.S. *Homosexualities: A Study of Diversity Among Men and Women.* New York: Simon & Schuster, 1978.

Bohannan, P., ed. *Stepfamilies: A Partially Annotated Bibliography.* Palo Alto, Calif.: Stepfamily Association of America, 1983.

Bozett, F.W. "Gay Fatherhood," in *Fatherhood Today: Men's Changing Role in the Family.* Edited by Bronstein, P., and Cowan, C.P. New York: John Wiley & Sons, in press.

Bozett, F.W. "Gay Fathers: How and Why They Disclose Their Homosexuality to Their Children," *Family Relations* 29:173–79, 1980a.

Bozett, F.W. "Gay Men as Fathers," in *Dimensions of Fatherhood.* Edited by Hanson, S.M.H., and Bozett, F.W. Beverly Hills, Calif.: Sage Publications, 1985a.

Bozett, F.W. "Heterogenous Couples in Heterosexual Marriages: Gay Men and Straight Women," *Journal of Marital and Family Therapy* 8:81–89, 1982.

Bozett, F.W. "Identity Management: Social Control of Identity by Children of Gay Fathers When They Know Their Father Is a Homosexual," Paper presented at the Seventh Biennial Eastern Nursing Research Conference. New Haven, Conn., April 1986.

Bozett, F.W. "Jealousy in Gay Father Relationships," Paper presented at the annual meeting of the National Council on Family Relations. Portland, Ore., October 1980b.

Bozett, F.W. "Male Development and Fathering Throughout the Life Cycle," *American Behavioral Scientist* 29(1):41–54, 1985b.

Bozett, F.W. "Parenting Concerns of Gay Fathers," *Topics in Clinical Nursing* 6:60–71, 1984.

Brownell, K.D. "New Developments in the Treatment of Obese Children and Adolescents," in *Eating and Its Disorders.* Edited by Stunkard, A.J., and Stellar, E. New York: Raven Press, 1984.

Brownell, K.D., et al. "Treatment of Obese Children with and without Their Mothers: Changes in Weight and Blood Pressure," *Pediatrics* 71:515–23, 1983.

Carter, E., and McGoldrick, M., eds. *The Family Life Cycle: A Framework for Family Therapy.* New York: Gardner Press, 1980.

Churchill, W. *Homosexual Behavior Among Males: A Cross-Cultural and Cross-Species Investigation.* Englewood Cliffs, N.J.: Prentice-Hall, 1971.

Coates, T.J., and Thoresen, C.E. "Obesity Among Children and Adolescents: The Problem Belongs to Everyone," in *Advances in Clinical Psychology.* Edited by Lahey, B., and Kazdin, A. New York: Academic Press, 1981.

Davidson, G., and Griedman, S. "Sexual Orientation Stereotypy in the Distortion of Clinical Judgement," *Journal of Homosexuality* 6:37–44, 1981.

DiBella, G.A.W. "Family Psychotherapy with the Homosexual Family: A Community Psychiatry Approach to Homosexuality," *Community Mental Health Journal* 15(1):41–46, 1979.

Drabman, R.S., et al. "Childhood Obesity: Assessment, Etiology, Risks, and Treatment," in *Assessment and Treatment of Developmental Disorders*. Edited by Doleys, D.M., et al. New York: Spectrum, 1985.

Drabman, R.S., et al. "Developmental Trends in Eating Rates of Normal and Overweight Preschool Children," *Child Development* 50:211–16, 1979.

Duvall, E. *Marriage and Family Development*. Philadelphia: J.B. Lippincott Co., 1977.

Epstein, L.H., et al. "Child and Parent Weight Loss in Family-Based Behavior Modification Programs," *Journal of Consulting and Clinical Psychology* 49:474–85, 1981.

Epstein, L.H., et al. "Comparison of Family-Based Behavior Modification and Nutrition Education for Childhood Obesity," *Journal of Pediatric Psychology* 5:25–36, 1980.

Epstein, L.H., et al. "Descriptive Analysis of Eating Regulation in Obese and Nonobese Children," *Journal of Applied Behavioral Analysis* 9:407–15, 1976.

Epstein, L.H., et al. "A Nutritionally Based School Program for Control of Eating in Obese Children," *Behavior Therapy* 9:766–78, 1978.

Fadiman, A. "The Double Closet," *Life* 76–78, 80, 82–84, 86, 92, 100, 1983.

Fairchild, B., and Hayward, N. *Now That You Know: What Every Parent Should Know About Homosexuality*. New York: Harcourt Brace Jovanovich, 1979.

Fast, I., and Cain, A.C. "The Stepparent Role: Potential for Disturbances in Family Functioning," *American Journal of Orthopsychiatry* 36(3):485–91, 1966.

Festinger, L. *A Theory of Cognitive Dissonance*. Stanford, Calif.: Stanford University Press, 1957.

Garn, S.M., et al. "Growth, Body Composition, and Development of Obese and Lean Children," in *Childhood Obesity*. Edited by Winick, M. New York: John Wiley & Sons, 1975.

Grief, J.B. "The Father-Child Relationship Subsequent to Divorce," in *Family Therapy Collections: Collection II*. Edited by Messinger, L. Rockville, Md.: Aspen Systems Corp., 1982.

Gutierrez, Y. "Nutrition and the Adolescent," in *Perspectives on Adolescent Health Care*. Edited by Mercer, R.T. New York: J.B. Lippincott Co., 1979.

Hagenbuch, V.E.G. "Obesity and the School-Aged Child," *Nursing Clinics of North America* 17:207–16, 1982.

Hall, M. "Lesbian Families: Cultural and Clinical Issues," *Social Work* 23:380–85, 1978.

Hanson, S.M.H. "Single Fathers with Custody: A Synthesis of the Literature," in *The One-Parent Family in the 1980's*. Edited by Schlesinger, B. Toronto: University of Toronto Press, 1985.

Jay, K., and Young, A. *The Gay Report*. New York: Summit, 1979.

Keane, T.M., et al. "A Parametric Investigation of Eating Styles in Obese and Nonobese Children," *Behavior Therapy* 12:280–86, 1981.

Kingdon, M.A. "Lesbians," *The Counseling Psychologist* 8:44–45, 1979.

Kinsey, A.C., et al. *Sexual Behavior in the Human Male*. Philadelphia: W.B. Saunders Co., 1948.

Kirkpatrick, M., et al. "Lesbian Mothers and Their Children: A Comparative Survey," *American Journal of Orthopsychiatry* 51:545–51, 1981.

Langford, R.W. "Teenagers and Obesity," *American Journal of Nursing* 81:556–59, 1981.

Levinson, D.J. *The Seasons of a Man's Life.* New York: Alfred A. Knopf, 1978.

Lewin, E. "Lesbianism and Motherhood: Implications for Child Custody," *Human Organization* 40:6–14, 1981.

Lewin, E., and Lyons, T. "Everything in Its Place: The Coexistence of Lesbianism and Motherhood," in *Homosexuality: Social, Psychological, and Biological Issues.* Edited by Paul, W., et al. Beverly Hills, Calif.: Sage Publications, 1982.

Mahoney, M.J., et al. "Assessment of Human Obesity: The Measurement of Body Composition," *Journal of Behavioral Assessment* 1:327–49, 1979.

Mendola, M. *The Mendola Report: A New Look at Gay Couples.* New York: Crown, 1980.

Miller, B. "Adult Sexual Resocialization: Adjustments Toward a Stigmatized Identity," *Alternative Lifestyles* 1(2):207–34, 1978.

Miller, B. "Gay Fathers and Their Children," *The Family Coordinator* 28:544–52, 1979.

Mills, D.M. "A Model for Stepfamily Development," *Family Relations* 33:365–72, 1984.

Moses, A.E., and Hawkins, R.O. *Counseling Lesbian Women and Gay Men: A Life-Issues Approach.* St. Louis: C.V. Mosby Co., 1982.

Pasley, K. "Stepfathers," in *Dimensions of Fatherhood.* Edited by Hanson, S.M.H., and Bozett, F.W. Beverly Hills, Calif.: Sage Publications, 1985.

Pasley, K., and Ihinger-Tallman, M., eds. *Family Relations* (Special issue on remarriage and stepparenting) 33(3), 1984.

Rodin, J. "Current Status of the Internal-External Hypothesis for Obesity: What Went Wrong?" *American Psychologist* 36:361–72, 1981.

Sallade, J. "A Comparison of the Psychological Adjustment of Obese vs. Non-Obese Children," *Journal of Psychosomatic Research* 17:89–96, 1973.

Scallen, R.M. "An Investigation of Paternal Attitudes and Behaviors in Homosexual and Heterosexual Fathers," *Dissertation Abstracts International* 42(9):3809–B, 1981.

Schrag, K.G. "Relationship Therapy with Same-Gender Couples," *Family Relations* 33:283–91, 1984.

Spada, J. *The Spada Report.* New York: New American Library, 1979.

Stern, P.N. "Affiliating in Stepfather Families: Teachable Strategies Leading to Stepfather-Child Friendship," *Western Journal of Nursing Research* 4:75–89, 1982.

Tanner, D.M. *The Lesbian Couple.* Lexington, Mass.: D.C. Health, 1978.

Turner, P.H., et al. "Parenting in Gay and Lesbian Families," Paper presented at the meeting of the first Future of Parenting Symposium. Chicago, 1985.

U.S. Bureau of the Census. *Statistical Abstracts of the United States: 1984,* 104th ed. Washington, D.C.: U.S. Government Printing Office, 1983.

Veevers, J.E. "The Moral Careers of Voluntarily Childless Wives: Notes on the Defense of a Variant World View," *Family Coordinator* 24:473–87, 1975.

Visher, E.B., and Visher, J.S. *Stepfamilies: A Guide to Working with Stepparents and Stepchildren.* New York: Brunner-Mazel, 1979.

Weiss, A.R. "A Behavioral Approach to the Treatment of Adolescent Obesity," *Behavior Therapy* 8:720–26, 1977.

Wells, K.C., and Copeland, B. "Childhood and Adolescent Obesity: Progress in Behavioral Assessment and Treatment," *Progress in Behavior Modification* 19:145–76, 1985.

Wheeler, M.E., and Hess, K.W. "Treatment of Juvenile Obesity by Successive Approximation Control of Eating," *Journal of Behavior Therapy and Experimental Psychiatry* 7:235–41, 1976.

Womersley, J., and Durnin, J.V.G.A. "A Comparison of the Skinfold Method with Extent of Overweight and Various Weight-Height Relationships in the Assessment of Obesity," *British Journal of Nutrition* 38:271–84, 1977.

Woodman, M.J., and Lenna, H.R. *Counseling with Gay Men and Women.* San Francisco: Jossey-Bass, 1980.

Wright, L.M., and Leahey, M. *Nurses and Families: A Guide to Family Assessment and Intervention.* Philadelphia: F.A. Davis Co., 1984.

20 Intervening with families at the launching stage and premenstrual syndrome

Bonnie Zwack, RN, MN
Director of Medical and Mental Health Nursing
Rockyview General Hospital
Calgary, Alberta, Canada

OVERVIEW

This chapter discusses the impact of premenstrual syndrome (PMS) upon a family at the launching stage of its developmental cycle. PMS incidence and characteristics are surveyed with reference to current theories regarding etiology and pathophysiology.

An approach to family assessment, based upon both general systems theory and the Calgary Family Assessment Model (CFAM), is also presented. Direct interventions are outlined, each designed to help the clinical nurse specialist teach the family to alleviate the symptoms of moderate PMS.

Throughout, the need for clinical research to improve the quality of nursing care for PMS families is emphasized.

CASE STUDY

Janet Turner, age 42, a high school English teacher, and her husband John, age 43, live in a middle-class suburb with their three children: Paul, age 18, who is graduating from high school and will be attending university 1,000 miles from home; Karen, age 16; and Sarah, age 14, in grades 11 and 9, respectively. John is a petroleum land consultant; the family has two stable incomes and is financially secure.

During the past year, Janet has been "feeling stressed" at work, and it has affected her performance. For the first time in 20 years of teaching, she has been approached by the assistant principal because of complaints from students about her irritability, impatience, shouting, and increasing anger in the classroom. Her students claim that these outbursts are "almost cyclic" and that for a week of each month their teacher's mood is intolerable.

Janet admits that for about 10 days of each month, before menstruation, she becomes extremely fatigued, depressed both at home and at work, and at times unable even to "drag" herself to work. Her menstrual periods have been increasingly heavy for the past year, and before each menstruation she has experienced severe headache, abdominal bloating, and a feeling of general heaviness. She cries a great deal at home and gets "so tense."

Janet told her gynecologist that, on the basis of a television documentary the family viewed 3 months ago and a subsequent reading of *Once a Month* by Dr. Katharina Dalton, she belives she has premenstrual syndrome. Her gynecologist recommended a dilatation and curretage (D&C) to help identify the cause of Janet's heavy menstruation. Janet and her physician agreed that, upon her hospital admission, she and her family would be assessed by the clinical nurse specialist (CNS) on the gynecology unit. She reported that she was almost "looking forward" to the operation.

In the hospital, a patient history was obtained by the primary nurse assigned to care for Janet. Specific information regarding previous admissions, health history, allergies, and use of medications or other therapy pertained to Janet alone, but the nurse also sought information about the family. With Janet and John's assistance, the primary nurse developed a genogram (Figure 20.1), providing structural (and some developmental) information about the family, as outlined in the CFAM (Wright and Leahey, 1984).

Routine physical assessment was also carried out by the resident physician; the primary diagnosis was menorrhagia, to be confirmed and treated by D&C. Upon the advice of Janet's gynecologist, who concurred that Janet's described cluster of biophysical, emotional, and behavioral symptoms seemed indicative of PMS, the resident also ordered a consultation with a CNS. Before seeing Janet, the CNS met with the primary nurse to review the data gathered to date and note the family's developmental stage.

Family Assessment

The CNS met Janet for a brief introductory interview prior to the surgery; a family interview was scheduled for the next evening at 7 p.m. *after* the D&C and *prior* to Janet's discharge. Further assessment data was gathered during this interview utilizing the CFAM.

The CNS observed that, while instrumental functioning was still achieved through participation of all family members, expressive functioning was becoming extremely difficult during Janet's premenstruum. The CNS used a circular communication diagram (Figure 20.2) (Tomm, 1980; Wright and Leahey, 1984) to demonstrate the reciprocal communication patterns that had developed between Janet and all the other members of her family to help them through the stresses of premenstruum (Watzlawick, et al., 1967); nods from the family confirmed its accuracy. The CNS also found it useful to "gossip in the presence of the other" (Weeks and L'Abate, 1982), using conversation with one family member to help assess communication patterns between two others. By involving all members in the interview and utilizing "difference questions" (Hoffman, 1981; Penn, 1982), the CNS was able to develop a mental picture of the family's expressive functioning and identify the members' common goals to (a) "help" mom feel better and (b) promote a happier home environment.

Janet realized from her reading of *Once a Month* that the *timing* of recurrent symptoms was extremely important. Therefore, she had charted her symptoms (according to Dalton's suggestion) to confirm that these manifestations did

Figure 20.1 Genogram—The Turner Family

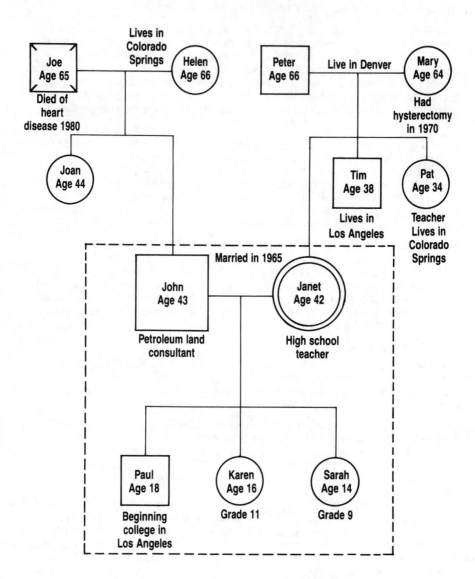

Figure 20.2   Circular Communication Pattern Diagram—The Turner Family

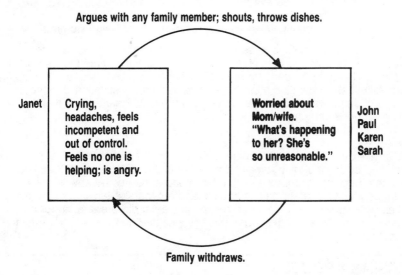

Argues with any family member; shouts, throws dishes.

Janet | Crying, headaches, feels incompetent and out of control. Feels no one is helping; is angry.

Worried about Mom/wife. "What's happening to her? She's so unreasonable." | John Paul Karen Sarah

Family withdraws.

in fact occur cyclically during the premenstruum. Among the phenomena she documented were shakiness and a craving for chocolate. In general, she could not cope with the stresses of her everyday life during the premenstrual period, citing the imminent departure of her son for college as a particular source of anxiety. The appearance of minor premenstrual symptoms in her daughters also caused her concern and was an additional reason for family participation in treatment. A strong marital bond between Janet and John and mutual family caring were evident. The CNS recognized the importance of emphasizing the family system's strengths as well as identifying its problems (Wright and Leahey, 1984).

Intervention

Following the assessment interview and a brief break, the CNS outlined a direct intervention program for the family. Her objectives were as follows:
- To commend the family for the strong, positive bond among its members
- To educate the family about hormonal changes/functions throughout the menstrual cycle and the imbalances that seem to precipitate PMS
- To facilitate life-style changes therapeutic for the whole family, which would result in both PMS symptom control and improved family interaction
- To work in consulation with the gynecologist, if necessary, to alleviate premenstrual symptoms within 3 to 4 months.

After "stroking" family members for their interactive strengths and common purpose, the CNS prescribed the following:
- Recording of menstrual symptoms by Janet and her daughters (to be continued indefinitely)
- Specific dietary/nutritional recommendations

- A daily exercise program, individually chosen by each member, to be continued throughout the cycle (30 minutes of pleasurable physical activity daily)
- Family discussion of expected stressful events at the beginning of Janet's cycle, followed by active planning to avoid or reschedule stressors
- Family commitment to an average of 8 hours sleep per night; relaxation exercises as taught by the CNS
- Use of a mild, nonconstipating analgesic for premenstrual discomfort

These direct interventions, prescribed for a cooperative family, were to be initiated immediately and continued for 2 months, at which time the CNS would see the family again. Depending upon the symptoms presenting at follow-up, pharmaceutical intervention might be considered (in consultation with the physician). Janet was encouraged to contact the CNS before the 2 months' interview if her symptoms worsened.

Evaluation

To a large extent, the prescribed therapeutic measures were effective. Headaches and abdominal pain remained a problem, though to a lesser degree. Janet noted particular improvement in her mood at home and at work; she became committed to her daily aerobics, and felt that the family was generally healthier. Her physician prescribed an antiprostaglandin preparation for her remaining symptoms; progesterone therapy was held in reserve and, in fact, was not required.

NURSING PROCESS

Assessment

The health problem: PMS. Premenstrual syndrome (PMS) is defined as the cyclic recurrence of clusters of symptoms during the premenstruum, with absence of postmenstrual manifestations. Such symptoms, which vary in presentation and severity, affect 40% of women (Dalton, 1984). The phenomenon tends to worsen with increasing age and parity, and occurs in all cultures and races (Dalton, 1984). Dalton refers to studies demonstrating the prevalence or absence of specific symptoms within specific cultures; abdominal pain, however, is reported to be virtually universal.

PMS demonstrates a familial tendency and, in fact, is often present simultaneously in several female members of a family unit. Similar cycles and synchronal menstruation of family members, a frequent occurrence, can precipitate additional stress and increase discord when accompanied by premenstrual discomfort (Dalton, 1984).

Characteristics of PMS. PMS symptoms generally appear 4 to 10 days prior to menstruation; some women are affected from ovulation to menses (the luteal phase). Although physiologic symptoms (Table 20.1) might be quite pronounced, many PMS sufferers cite such behavioral manifestations as lethargy/apathy, depression, and/or irritability as their primary complaints. "Emotionally, I'm completely out of control" is

Table 20.1 Physiologic Characteristics of PMS

Moderate	Severe
• nausea/vomiting • headache • fatigue • breast swelling/tenderness • peripheral swelling • abdominal pain/bloating • constipation • increased thirst/appetite • craving for sweet or salty foods (chocolate is common)	• epileptic seizures • asthma or other allergic reaction(s) • migraine • glaucoma

a classic lament. Affected women might display such extreme behaviors as uncontrollable crying, suicidal ideation, or even violence. Irrational behavior may be directed toward family members or society in general, through crime or other antisocial activity. The physical and psychological symptoms, so repetitive in nature, diminish the victim's confidence and self-esteem, which has definite implications for the larger systems and subsystems of which she is a part.

PMS and the launching stage family. Beginning with the actual departure of the first child from the home and continuing until the youngest child has left (Carter and McGoldrick, 1980; Duvall, 1977; Wright and Leahey, 1984), a family is said to be at the launching stage developmentally. Tasks to be accomplished during the launching stage are:
• Establishment of independent identities for parents and young adult(s)
• Renegotiation of the marital relationship.

The Turners' history and genogram indicated to the CNS that they were entering the launching stage. The family also tended to fit into the stage of families with teenagers; developmental tasks are similar. It is not unusual for families' developmental stages to overlap and for illnesses and problems to present as a family unit attempts to move smoothly from one stage to another (Wright and Leahey, 1984).

The March 1984 U.S. Survey of Current Household and Family Characteristics estimated the total number of families with children at home to be 36.9 million. Of these, 13%, or 4.79 million, contained at least one child between age 18 and 25 and at least one child 17 years or younger (U.S. Bureau of Census, 1985). Similarly, the 1981 Canadian census identified 657,150 (15.2%) Canadian families containing children in these age-groups (Government of Canada, 1985).

As Wright and Leahey (1984) state, families are in a constant state of flux. Therefore, when chronic illness strikes a family, particularly the "lynchpin" (i.e., the mother) (Dalton, 1984), and is manifested cyclically through both physical and emotional behaviors, *all* family members are affected (Wright and Leahey, 1984). This situation substantially complicates completion of developmental tasks.

For PMS families this constant flux becomes a struggle, an attempt to capitalize on the "good days" when mother is cheerful and efficient and to prepare for that crucial time each month when she is inefficient, depressed, physically ill, and perhaps irrational in her behavior toward her children and spouse. Husbands state that they are baffled by cyclically recurrent crying, depression, and/or wild, abusive behavior, any of which may be accompanied by inefficiency and forgetfulness concerning such normally nonthreatening responsibilities as cooking, running errands, or driving a car (Norris and Sullivan, 1983).

PMS' many and varied behavioral manifestations threaten family relationships and family unity; women who have experienced the syndrome for many years without assessment and intervention attribute family violence, divorce, and parent–child conflict to the cyclic physical and emotional dysfunction (Dalton, 1984; Lauersen and Stukane, 1983; Norris and Sullivan, 1983).

PMS does not occur only at the launching stage; it is well known that girls can display premenstrual symptoms soon after puberty and that these symptoms will probably worsen with age and parity. By adulthood, the affected woman may be involved in different subsystems, for instance marriage or career, thus expanding the impact of her PMS. Adaptation to, and enjoyment of, the motherhood role, as well as normal child development, will be influenced. As children reach the teen years and prepare for separation from the family, at a time when parental support, guidance, and understanding are most important, a mother's PMS may contribute to potential conflict that can pervade all family systems and subsystems. Even the marital dyad is vulnerable to tension regarding children's welfare and future.

The author believes that the launching stage family is particularly subject to PMS-related disruption. Family members, particularly the husband, frequently decide that they can no longer tolerate PMS manifestations and that separation is the only answer. At the same time, the psychological effects of PMS may well have become too much for the woman to endure alone, and the suicidal thoughts experienced by so many PMS victims may have become more prominent. On the positive side, the threat of losing one's spouse or other family members, plus the fact that physical and emotional symptoms may be at their peak, often provide the stimulus necessary for women with PMS to seek diagnosis and treatment. Nevertheless, Dalton (1984) cites numerous cases of women whose family relationships have been severed before the woman discovers PMS to be the reason for her chronic ill health.

Causal theories. Reid and Yen (1981) described premenstrual syndrome as a "multifactorial psychoneuroendocrine dysfunction" resulting from luteal phase sensitivity to the neuropeptides beta-endorphin and alpha-melanocyte-stimulating hormone. Other theories (Abraham, 1980; Nazzaro, et al., 1985) assign a nutritional base to PMS. Abraham, for instance, attributes etiology to nutritional deficiencies (magnesium and pyridoxine) and stress. Dalton (1984) and Budoff (1981) relate PMS pathophysiology to progesterone and prostaglandin imbalances respectively. Other hormonal imbalances are similarly cited as causative. Health professionals must study the convergence and interrelationship of these many factors to facilitate complete patient/family assessment.

Family assessment models. Health professionals have only recently become involved in PMS assessment and intervention; yet they now perform such duties in hospitals, community health and PMS clinics, and in the home. Knowledge of systems theory facilitates nursing assessment of family dynamics when one or more members present with complaints suggesting PMS. The nurse should recognize that the illness of one family member affects the others, and that rehabilitative change in the identified patient will precipitate changes in the whole family and in other systems—e.g., the workplace—of which the identified patient is a part (Wright and Leahey, 1984). Use of CFAM as a major assessment model and creative expansion of the model's structural, developmental, and functional components allow development of a *picture* of the family: its beliefs, attitudes, and interactional patterns, within both its own boundaries and larger systems.

Such structural tools as the genogram (Figure 20.1) and ecomap are extremely useful in illustrating the features, connections, possible trends (e.g., the menstrual cycle), and repetitive behaviors that make the client family unique. Interviewing the family also demonstrates, to a degree, the manner in which tasks of the identified developmental stage are being met, as well as existing interactional communication patterns.

Dr. Katharina Dalton has provided an extremely helpful menstrual chart for PMS assessment. Using it to record symptoms month after month will confirm whether they are indeed characteristic of the luteal phase or are occurring randomly throughout the cycle. Symptom *timing* is crucial in the diagnosis and subsequent treatment of PMS patients and families (Dalton, 1983, 1984). Other charts and menstrual diaries have been developed, but Dalton's is simple and clearly illustrates recurring symptoms.

Planning

Many families will have suffered PMS effects for many years with little or no relief. It may well be that the launching stage family, struggling with this chronic illness's severe impact, is seeking help for the first time. Nursing care must be planned individually for each client family. It is important to determine whether or not the patient/family has sought previous therapy for PMS symptoms. If so, which measures were effective? Which were not?

Goals and objectives must be set, the importance of change ascertained, and the degree of family commitment to correcting negative patterns explored. What particular changes does the family seek? What will happen to this family if identified problems persist? What aspect of the illness affects the family most? Why is *this* particular time crucial?

The nurse responsible for planning care must consider the family's life-style, work habits, educational level, general health, and commitment to change; determine whether the family will resist or attempt to perform assigned tasks; and recognize that life events may require changes in the plan. The plan itself should clarify mutual goals, educate the family regarding PMS, provide a program for symptom alleviation, and solicit physician participation in follow-up therapy and plan revision and modification.

Intervention

Family intervention for PMS is indicated when the woman experiences symptoms that directly or indirectly affect her family as a whole. Self-help family intervention is currently a popular approach, particularly in mild to moderate PMS. The large amount of self-help literature describing PMS and offering intervention guidelines that has become available since 1980 has both encouraged and complicated this approach. Such material often contains controversial explanations of PMS etiology and pathophysiology, but little good advice regarding changing life-styles to alleviate symptoms. Various pharmaceutical approaches are suggested, dependent upon the author's preferred pathophysiologic explanation.

Most pertinent scientific research to date has centered upon subject response to pharmaceutical preparations. Dalton (1979, 1984) also cited studies confirming PMS incidence, effects on work/school performance, and sociologic significance. Her recorded data assessing more than 35 years of PMS intervention has assisted and expanded the development of PMS clinics in North America.

Another growing self-help resource for PMS sufferers is the support group, although the therapeutic value of such an approach remains inconclusive. Inclusion of family members in assessment and intervention is another relatively new but essential idea; indeed, it may prove to be the crucial approach to primary prevention. Family therapy may be indicated if marital or family problems are present, when suicide is a threat, or when symptoms include crime and/or violence.

Assessment as intervention. As the case study illustrates, the assessment process itself can unite the family by clarifying the presenting problem and identifying and prioritizing goals for change.

Nutritional measures. While PMS etiology is unclear, theorists agree that nutritional measures facilitate alleviation of mild to moderate symptoms. A typical nutritional approach might include:

Avoiding caffeine. Caffeine, a xanthine derivative present in varying amounts of coffee, tea, cocoa/chocolate, and colas, is believed to increase breast tenderness, a common PMS complaint, through stimulation of prostaglandin production. Caffeine is also known to increase PMS-related irritability, hyperactivity, and headaches, possibly due to its effect upon neurotransmitters in the brain. Because irritating oils in coffee can precipitate nausea and vomiting in sufferers, even decaffeinated preparations might not resolve every coffee-related symptom (Budoff, 1981). (The client should be warned of this.)

Avoiding salt. It is suggested that salt use, both in cooking and at the table, be restricted for 10 days prior to menstruating. This should reduce fluid retention and related abdominal bloating, peripheral edema, increased intraocular pressure, and weight gain. Avoidance of such high-salt prepared foods as commercial salad dressings, gravies, snacks, canned or dried soups, ham, bacon, peanut butter, pickles, and many condiments will facilitate achievement of this goal; it may also reduce the need for diuretics, which carry the risk of potassium imbalance.

Vitamin and mineral supplementation. Researchers since the time of Biskin (1943) have studied the etiologic and therapeutic roles of vitamins in PMS. Biskin's theory that a lack of pyridoxine (vitamin B_6) would impair estrogen metabolism lost favor. Pyridoxine, however, *has* been found to act as a coenzyme in the conversion of tryptophan to dopamine and serotonin and thus may be an etiologic factor in PMS-associated depression; many women do find relief from psychological PMS manifestations through vitamin B_6 supplementation. A more recent study by Nazzaro and colleagues (1985) cites pyridoxine's diuretic effect in reducing premenstrual fluid retention. The other B vitamins, the "energy vitamins," may help to offset the fatigue and lethargy felt by the woman with PMS (Nazzaro, et al., 1985).

B-complex vitamin supplements can be purchased at every pharmacy; specific food sources follow:

- B_1 (thiamine) and B_2 (riboflavin): liver and organ meats, pork, brewer's yeast, lean meat, eggs, green leafy vegetables, whole grain breads and cereals, nuts, and legumes
- B_3 (niacin): liver and organ meats, fish, tuna, dried peas and beans, whole grains, nuts, eggs
- B_6 (pyridoxine): yeast, wheat, corn, liver, kidney, red meats
- B_{12} (cyanocobalamin): organ and muscle meats, milk, eggs, brewer's yeast, seafood (especially clams, oysters, and shrimp).

Zinc and magnesium levels are also known to be depleted during the premenstruum. Zinc is necessary for protein synthesis, cell growth, and connective tissue formation. It is also essential for proper metabolism of other minerals, including magnesium, which in turn is believed to be associated with the mood swings, nervous tension, bloating, and breast tenderness characteristic of PMS. Chocolate, one food source of magnesium, should be avoided for reasons previously discussed. Better sources include whole grains, green leafy vegetables, legumes, nuts, seeds, cereals, and shellfish (Norris and Sullivan, 1983).

Maintaining adequate blood glucose levels. Many women with PMS have flattened glucose tolerance curves (Norris and Sullivan, 1983; Reid and Yen, 1981), perhaps due to an increased insulin receptor concentration. Hunger, cravings, fatigue, nervousness, sweating, and gastrointestinal complaints may also be due to endorphin activity on glucose metabolism. A regimen of frequent feedings (three meals and three snacks per day) of low-carbohydrate, low-fat, high-protein foods should alleviate the symptoms; consumption of fresh fruits as a replacement for refined sugars should be encouraged.

High-fiber diet. Foods high in roughage, in conjunction with physical exercise, help reduce the constipation frequently associated with PMS. Avoidance of codeine-containing analgesics further diminishes the constipation problem.

Menstrual synchrony and the strong familial incidence of PMS should encourage at least female family members to adopt these usually effective nutritional measures. The nurse can provide lists of preferred foods and foods to be avoided, and can develop sample menus according to the family's likes and dislikes.

Stress avoidance. Families with one or more PMS sufferers should strive to work together to limit stressful events or responsibilities during the premenstruum. When caring for the PMS family, encourage discussion of stress and stress avoidance; valuable input from every member will help identify problems and promote cooperation in altering stress-producing life habits or pursuits. Stressful work or personal commitments, examinations, surgery, or other treatments are better postponed until non-PMS times.

The family should also plan leisure activities and some form of pleasurable daily exercise for each member. Thirty minutes of daily activity, such as walking, aerobics, swimming, or floor exercises, will provide both physiologic and emotional benefits, and should be continued through both premenstruum and paramenstruum, that is, through the whole cycle (Harrison, 1982; Norris and Sullivan, 1983). Along with appropriate nutritional measures, exercise might control moderate PMS.

The Turners' CNS demonstrated relaxation techniques advocated by Norris and Sullivan (1983). The family was given printed material to encourage this practice, particularly by Janet and her daughters, during the premenstruum.

Extra rest and sleep, with or without preparatory relaxation exercises, is a most important part of therapy, one to be undertaken by the whole family.

Drug therapy. A great deal of recent PMS research has centered upon the response of subjects to pharmaceutical intervention. PMS families frequently respond dramatically after just 1 or 2 months of nonpharmaceutical therapy, but in cases where symptom reduction is minimal, drug administration should be considered. That approach is best pursued through consultation with a physician who also considers the family to be the primary unit of care (Wright and Leahey, 1984).

Dalton (1984), who believes that a dramatic drop in the progesterone level during the late luteal phase is the main etiologic factor in PMS, recommends progesterone replacement. She reports significant success with such treatment for both patients and families coping with severe biophysical and emotional PMS. Other preparations used by physicians include diuretics, antiprostaglandins, and antiprolactins. Although every nonpharmaceutical option should be considered, the physician should be consulted if medication is indicated.

Indirect intervention. The interventions just described involve direct action to alleviate PMS. If certain difficult psychological symptoms predominate, or if the family resists the therapeutic regimen, indirect interventions may be indicated. These indirect interventions may take the form of a "reframe," paradoxical directive, or a ritual (Wright and Leahey, 1984; Weeks and L'Abate, 1982).

Evaluation

Nursing assessment of and intervention with PMS families is relatively new (Zwack, 1985), and as such has not been evaluated extensively. Assessment tools and intervention alternatives continue to be developed and promise to be targets for clinical research in the future. Nurses as professionals, as members of family systems, and as women must consider the personal impact of PMS upon their clients' self-concepts, goal achievement, and ultimate self-actualization.

CONCLUSIONS

Premenstrual syndrome is a phenomenon that continues to provoke controversy despite more than 50 years of research. Etiologic theories remain inconclusive, and presentation varies with developmental status. Intervention is frequently delayed and must continue indefinitely. Nurses, with their ever-expanding assessment skills and family-oriented intervention repertoire, and with their increasing availability in homes, communities, and active care centers, are the most appropriate health care consultants for families coping with PMS.

REFERENCES

Abraham, G.E. "The Premenstrual Tension Syndromes," in *Contemporary Obstetric and Gynecologic Nursing.* Edited by McNall, L. Toronto: C.V. Mosby Co., 1980.

Biskin, M.S. "Nutritional Deficiency in the Etiology of Menorrhagia, Metrorrhagia, Cystic Mastitis and Premenstrual Tension: Treatment with Vitamin B Complex," *Journal of Clinical Endocrinology and Metabolism* 3:227–34, 1943.

Budoff, P.W. *No More Menstrual Cramps and Other Good News.* New York: Putnam, 1981.

Carter, E., and McGoldrick, M. "The Family Life Cycle and Family Therapy: An Overview," in *The Family Life Cycle: A Framework for Family Therapy.* Edited by Carter, E., and McGoldrick, M. New York: Gardner Press, 1980.

Dalton, K. *The Premenstrual Syndrome and Progesterone Therapy.* New York: Oxford University Press, 1979.

Dalton, K. *Once a Month.* Claremont, Calif.: Hunter House, 1983.

Dalton, K. *The Premenstrual Syndrome and Progesterone Therapy,* 2nd ed. Southampton: Camelot Press Ltd., 1984.

Duvall, E. *Marriage and Family Development,* 5th ed. Philadelphia: J.B. Lippincott Co., 1977.

Government of Canada. *Statistics Canada.* Ottawa, 1985.

Harrison, M. *Self-Help for Premenstrual Syndrome.* Cambridge, Mass.: Matrix Press, 1982.

Hoffman, L. *Foundations of Family Therapy.* New York: Basic Books, 1981.

Lauersen, N.H. "Recognition and Treatment of Premenstrual Syndrome," *The Nurse Practitioner* 10(3):11–21, 1985.

Lauersen, N.H., and Stukane, E. *PMS: Premenstrual Syndrome and You.* New York: Pinnacle Books, 1983.

Nazzaro, A., et al. *The PMS Solution.* Montreal: Eden Press, 1985.

Norris, R.V., and Sullivan, C. *PMS: Premenstrual Syndrome.* New York: Berkley Publishing, 1983.

Penn, P. "Circular Questioning," *Family Process* 21(3):267–69, 1982.

Reid, R., and Yen, S. "Premenstrual Syndrome," *American Journal of Obstetrics and Gynecology* 85:85–104, 1981.

Tomm, K. "Toward a Cybernetic Systems Approach to Family Therapy at the University of Calgary," in *Perspectives on Family Therapy.* Edited by Freeman, D. Vancouver: Butterworth & Co., 1980.

U.S. Bureau of Census. *Household and Family Characteristics, March, 1984.* U.S. Bureau of Census Current Population Reports. Washington, D.C.: U.S. Government Printing Office, 1985.

Watzlawick, P., et al. *Pragmatics of Human Communication.* New York: W.W. Norton & Co., 1967.

Weeks, G.R., and L'Abate, L. *Paradoxical Psychotherapy: Theory and Practice with Individuals, Couples, and Families.* New York: Brunner-Mazel, 1982.

Wright, L.M., and Leahey, M. *Nurses and Families: A Guide to Family Assessment and Intervention.* Philadelphia: F.A. Davis Co., 1984.

Zwack, B. "Premenstrual Syndrome," *The Canadian Nurse* 81(1):51–53, 1985.

21 Intervening with middle-aged families and chronic pain

Mary Ann Norfleet, PhD
Director of Clinical Services
Mental Research Institute
Palo Alto, California

OVERVIEW

This chapter presents a learning and systems theory framework for assessing and intervening with middle–aged chronic pain families, in the context of a multidisciplinary comprehensive treatment program. A case study illustrates diagnosis and treatment. Developmental issues are discussed and characteristics of chronic pain families given, along with a summary of the functions chronic pain serves in the family and rationale for planning interventions. Treatment is described as a process that changes the family's response to pain and encourages adaptive patient functioning. The intervention program is described and suggestions made for program evaluation.

CASE STUDY

Mrs. Martinez, a 43-year–old married homemaker with three children, presented to an inpatient multidisciplinary comprehensive pain center complaining primarily of low back pains. The pain, described as sharp and stabbing, had begun while she was vacuuming her carpets 6 years before. She had had a ruptured lumbar disk (L4–5) repaired; 4 months later a radiopaque marker and other residual material were removed from the surgical site. Since then, she has experienced intermittent pain, spends progressively more time in bed, and has become addicted to pain medications. Conservative treatment—physical therapy, bed rest, and aspirin—failed, and the patient showed increasing psychological and physiologic signs of depression. The family waited on her and indulged her decreased activity. As she ceased attending social activities outside the home and became unable to participate in outings with her family, they began to leave her out of their plans. Sexual activity stopped, and her husband became absorbed in a new hobby. Concealed conflict manifested itself in tension between the patient and her husband, and was occasionally addressed indirectly through sarcastic references to finances and home chores.

NURSING PROCESS

Assessment

The health problem: Chronic pain. The term "chronic pain" is used to designate chronic benign discomfort. It is generally "considered to exist when pain persists longer than 6 months and does not respond to traditional medical and/or surgical treatment" (Norfleet, et al., 1982, p. 302). Crue (1985, p. 32) has recently given an alternative definition for what he terms the "Chronic Intractable Benign Pain Syndrome" (CIBPS): "chronic pain with poor patient coping: pain becomes central focus of the patient's existence (no known nociceptive peripheral input)."

Chronic pain patients usually display a constellation of problems in six different dimensions: family and social, occupational, pharmacologic, physical, psychological, and interpersonal. Effective treatment begins with assessing each dimension, then implementing an organized treatment approach addressing the total biopsychosocial context. Comprehensive treatment of chronic pain attends to each of the six dimensions concurrently.

This chapter discusses family-oriented treatment of chronic pain, but it cannot be overemphasized that effective treatment requires concurrent multidisciplinary treatment of all six affected dimensions. Family intervention must be implemented in accordance with an integrated treatment plan that addresses the problems identified by *complete* pretreatment evaluation.

Chronic pain patients readily seek medical assistance and can easily become overdependent on health care personnel. Their frequent disability leads to tremendous social, psychological, and financial costs. Bonica (1980) has stated that when lost wages, medical costs, workers' compensation, and related expenses are included, annual chronic pain expenditures are in the $60 billion range in the United States alone.

Chronic pain can occur at any stage of the life cycle. It usually begins with a physical problem, often associated with an accident or injury that produces strains, sprains, lacerations, or fractures. The back is the most common site of chronic pain; it often results from lumbar or cervical disk degeneration. Other common locations of chronic pain are the neck, abdomen, and the extremities. (Headaches are considered to be acute *intermittent* pain.) Chronic pain also occurs frequently with such conditions as endometriosis and fibrositis.

Iatrogenic problems may arise when such traditional medical treatments as medication and/or surgery are unsuccessful. When patients receiving all medically indicated treatments continue to feel "sick," they often seek additional medical or allied health treatment from one caregiver after another. This situation is generally complicated by the fact that the patient might have other health problems requiring medical treatment, such as hypertension or ulcers. In addition, such patients are usually out of condition and overweight.

Depression is almost always seen in the chronic pain patient. Lukensmeyer (1979, p. 335) has pointed out that "Pain may be a physiological manifestation of depression and may occur with other physiological symptoms of depression including psychomotor retardation, sleep disturbance, and alteration of diurnal rhythms." Other signs associated with depression in chronic pain patients are poor concentration, irritability, low energy, and weight loss or gain.

Middle-aged families. Estimates of the percentage of chronic pain families run as high as 10% of the total family population. Although chronic pain occurs in patients from childhood to old age, a large part of the affected population is middle–aged, from 40 to 60 years old.

Middle–aged families are occupied with the developmental issues associated with sending grown children into the world. In addition to coping with the adjustments required when children leave home, many chronic pain couples find themselves facing a major role transition: becoming grandparents. They are also striving to accumulate the financial resources needed for a secure retirement. Other common life stressors in this population include marital problems and job difficulties (with co-workers or supervisors). Interventions at this stage of the life cycle normally focus on these issues or their variants.

The high correlation between illness and significant life changes has been well documented (Achterberg, 1985, p. 172; Engel, 1968). This inherent vulnerability is multiplied when the social climate changes and stressors seem uncontrollable (Feuerstein, et al., 1985; Stern, et al., 1982). Given the complex developmental issues these middle-aged families face, it is no surprise that they have a significant number of chronic pain problems.

The typical middle-aged chronic pain family consists of a couple in their mid-40s with children who are teenage or older; the children are sometimes grown and out of the home. The identified patient may be either male or female, is usually a high school graduate, has had low back pain for several years, and has had one or more surgeries for the pain, with little or no lasting relief. Chronic pain families tend to focus on the patient's physical discomfort and are usually resistant to psychotherapy in any form. However, they are more receptive to educational approaches and to the idea that they can learn how to ease pain and cope with it more effectively.

Chronic pain families usually exhibit several of the following characteristics (Norfleet, et al., 1982, p. 307):
• Interdependence between the primary couple
• Difficulty coping with life changes
• Unclear communication patterns
• Family reinforcement of pain-related behavior
• Drug and/or alcohol abuse
• Pain problems in the "well" spouse
• Unrealistically high expectations
• Sexual problems.

These and other identified problems must be addressed in treatment. Given the at-home context of chronic pain, there are few, if any, contraindications for family intervention with such problems. Indeed, most existing research points to its necessity (Payne and Norfleet, 1985). Many comprehensive pain treatment facilities make family participation a condition of acceptance into the program.

Theoretical frameworks. A learning and systems approach to chronic pain families has proven useful. Briefly, chronic pain is seen as a learned response that is often unwittingly encouraged by well–meaning family members and others in the patient's environment. Family systems theory views the family as a balanced, homeostatic system in which each member influences the others. The symptom of chronic pain can help maintain the family's systemic equilibrium, in which case well members may consciously or unconsciously invest in the patient's dysfunction. Having the symptomatic relative dependent on them makes them feel needed or reassures them that the physically limited spouse won't leave an unhappy marriage. When the symptoms become important to family stability, well family members may resist therapeutic attempts to improve and change the system or the individuals in it, particularly the affected spouse. This occurs even though the entire family may suffer emotionally and view their situation as highly unsatisfactory. When this is the case, newer and more functional states that meet all family members' needs must be substituted; only then will they reach a higher level of homeostasis where the system does not rely on pain or illness to keep it together.

Chronic pain typically places stress on the marriage; the entire family is affected by the patient's frequent depression and unavailability for family activities. Dynamically, chronic pain may serve a variety of functions. Norfleet and colleagues (1982, p. 306) have suggested that chronic pain can:

• Fulfill unconscious dependency needs
• Allow for retribution in a passive-aggressive manner
• Legitimize the failure to complete obligations or live up to high expectations
• Manipulatively control family members
• Avoid existing conflicts.

An understanding of the functions of pain in the family can be important to the nurse planning effective interventions.

Family assessment approaches. Assessment of the chronic pain family is a three-part process: a clinical interview with the couple; observations of their behaviors and interactions during the evaluation; and self-report inventories filled out by each spouse. The pain patient and spouse participate jointly in the family assessment interview. The session is relatively open-ended, with the interviewer directing attention to specific behaviors, as opposed to vague areas of dissatisfaction. It covers the following topics: the family itself, effects of pain on the family, vocational activities, finances, leisure activities, division of labor in the home, psychiatric history, spiritual orientation, sexual relationship, pain behavior, and treatment goals and expectations (Payne, 1982). In addition to providing information about the family's feelings and experiences with pain, this assessment interview furnishes information about how the couple behaves and interacts. It also helps the interviewer form a good working relationship with the patient and spouse.

Preferences for paper and pencil tests vary among clinicians, depending on their training and the particular information they seek. Two tests used by this writer to provide information about the couple's views of their relationship are The Bashford Marital Satisfaction Survey (Bashford, 1977) and The Moos Family Environment Scale (Moos, 1974). The Marital Satisfaction Survey is filled out separately by patient and spouse. Each rates personal satisfaction in 11 areas including family division of labor, success in resolving problems and disagreements, amount and quality of time spent together, and ability to work together as parents. The Family Environment Scale's 10 subscales reflect three larger dimensions: relationship, personal growth, and system maintenance.

Planning

Intervention planning proceeds directly from assessment findings, and must address problems identified at the family level. From the interview and tests, the Martinez family's problem areas were identified as unclear intrafamily communication patterns, family reinforcement of Mrs. Martinez's pain–related behaviors, sexuality, and difficulty coping with the life changes associated with the patient's pain. The specific behaviors targeted in each problem area are shown in Table 21.1.

Family group education serves as the core of effective intervention for chronic pain. Group educational meetings speak to the family on both cognitive and behavioral levels by informing them about chronic pain and teaching them what they can do to help their loved one. Contact with other chronic pain families helps relatives address their affective experience; as members learn new skills and coping techniques, they begin to feel more hopeful. Anger, guilt, depression, and associated feelings decrease.

When emotions are highly charged over given issues, the couple or entire family may require separate therapy sessions directed to their specific problems and responses.

Although chronic pain patients tend to focus on their physical symptoms, family therapy is readily accepted when members see a personal advantage in meeting: for example, an opportunity to master difficult communication skills or resolve conflicts.

Table 21.1 Problem Areas and Behaviors Addressed in Treatment

Problem Areas	Behaviors
• Unclear communication patterns	• Spouse answers questions directed to patient; lack of assertive communication • Poor listening skills; indirect references to financial strain and household chores
• Family reinforcement of pain	• Catering to patient (*e.g.,* fluffing pillows, bringing hot water bottle, family taking over all household duties, leaving patient out of activities)
• Sexual problems	• Cessation of sexual activity
• Difficulty coping with life changes	• Decreased social activities; depression; veiled hostility; avoidance of problem discussion or solution; medication addiction

Intervention

The Martinez family's treatment was directed toward cognitive, affective, and behavioral levels of family functioning (Leahey and Wright, 1985). Although this case intervention took place primarily in an inpatient pain center, it is feasible to treat chronic pain families in an outpatient setting, as long as no urgent drug abuse or other problem makes inpatient medical treatment and supervision mandatory.

Topics pertinent to the Martinez family were emphasized in nursing staff presentations and meetings. These included the relationship between stress and chronic pain, improved communication, family responses to pain, and sexual dysfunction.

Family intervention is a team effort requiring active participation by all staff. Team members contribute to intervention plans, and even information meetings become opportunities to work toward family and patient treatment goals. For example, Mrs. Martinez's physical therapist encouraged her to increase activity and do more for herself. The physician, pharmacist, and nursing staff helped her taper off narcotic analgesics and understand the role of medications and their optimal uses. The nursing staff encouraged her to develop new interests that could be shared with others and helped her focus on becoming self-reliant.

Family group education meetings, held 3 evenings a week, are a formal part of the treatment program; attendance is mandatory for the patient and significant others. These meetings are conducted on a rotating basis by the physician, psychologist, social worker, nurse(s), dietitian, and other member(s) of the treatment team. Staff members conduct sessions in their particular areas of expertise.

The initial meeting is an orientation where family members receive information to help allay their anxiety about the program and to explain the Pain Center's structure and philosophy. Such concepts as self-responsibility, family involvement, and the idea that chronic pain is more than a physical problem are all discussed. The program's rules and mechanics are explained, hospital facilities are shown to the family members, and questions are answered.

This program has been presented in some detail by Norfleet and colleagues (1982); the following discussion illustrates how the program's primary concepts were applied to the Martinez family's first two identified problem areas: unclear communication patterns and family reinforcement of pain.

The family session devoted to communication skills emphasizes clarity. In order to communicate clearly, the sender of a message must first know what information is to be conveyed. A four-step process is taught:

- Knowing what one wants to convey
- Sending a congruent message
- Receiving a message
- Understanding the message.

Step one stresses distinguishing feelings from beliefs and thoughts. One must first know the feeling associated with the message before the message is sent. Step two: the message must be sent clearly if communication is to occur. People who do not know what they want to say may end up sending an incongruent message. For example, a family member might say, "I'm not angry," while body posture and facial expression are saying, "I'm tense and irritable." The receiver does not know which is the real message and is therefore unsure how to respond. Family members practice sending both types of messages—congruent and incongruent—to each other. They experience the difference between the two types and exchange feedback about their reactions to each.

In step three, families learn to listen actively. Some people speak for the entire family, fail to listen, and change the subject when they do not get their way. Family members practice accurately restating what they have heard; sometimes messages are repeated verbatim. Poor listening skills are identified when people require many repetitions to recreate the message sent.

In step four, understanding, a distinction is made between merely hearing the message and interpreting its meaning accurately. Chronic pain patients often misinterpret messages and frequently perceive innocuous comments as criticism. To enhance accurate interpretation, family members may practice an exercise called "Do you mean...?" (Satir, 1972), which is illustrated by the following example:

X. It's a nice day.
Y. Oh, do you mean you want to go outdoors?
X. No.
Y. Do you mean you're mad at me for closing the windows?
X. No.
Y. Do you mean you feel good?
X. Yes.

This exercise teaches people to listen carefully and to clarify ambiguities, rather than to leap to false conclusions based on faulty understanding. It is not uncommon for people to find these exercises very difficult. Indeed, heated arguments can develop during these practice sessions—arguments that may signal someone's need for additional time with a staff member who can help them improve basic skills and clarify communication.

Classroom discussions on family reinforcement of pain usually describe the difference between acute and chronic pain and then teach the family how pain can be a learned response. This class starts with the statement that all pain is real but that there are different types of pain. The family is told that their relative's pain "is chronic (long-lasting), intractable (not responsive to usual treatments), and maladaptive (restricts the life-style)." (Norfleet, et al., 1982, p. 314)

Acute pain is a prompt warning; unlearned, transient, and followed by healing. The chronic pain syndrome, on the other hand, may involve a small amount of acute or respondent pain but consists mostly of learned pain. Typically, the chronic pain patient cannot tell the difference between the two. Learned pain develops through reinforcement. When relatives cater to the patient by waiting on him, massaging painful areas, or taking over household duties, the likelihood that the pain behavior will continue is increased. Indeed, the pleasant consequences reinforce the patient's pain.

The staff must also demonstrate that, however unconscious, unintentional physiologic learning takes place. Family members are asked to sit down and visualize themselves eating a slice of raw lemon. They are asked to imagine the taste of the lemon and the other physical sensations they experience as they eat it. After this fantasized experience, people are asked to report whatever physiologic phenomenon they became aware of. Most of them will report increased salivation and accompanying sensations such as aching jaws and swallowing. Although these responses were based on fantasy, they were both real and unintentional—just as pain can be.

The Martinez family participated actively in treatment and made good progress during the patient's 4-week inpatient stay. Results of the 6 months' follow-up were also good: gains had been maintained and the family had dealt effectively with small crises that in the past might have exacerbated the chronic pain syndrome.

Family involvement is crucial in chronic pain treatment. As noted by Moore and Chaney (1985), such involvement helps family members cope more effectively with their own emotional responses. Family intervention can also help maintain treatment gains. In working with a chronically ill population that includes pain patients, Wooley and colleagues (1978, pp. 399–400) noted that family therapy was one of the factors "associated with short-term success" in an inpatient program and "return to an intact family" was one of the highest predictors of continuing improvement at 1 year after. Wooley and colleagues have suggested that prior to treatment, and when the patient does not return to an intact family after treatment, he might be "using the medical care system as a family substitute" (p. 398).

Intervening with chronic pain families means helping them learn and develop. Haley (1973, pp. 43–44) has expressed this as follows:

"If one thinks of therapy as the introduction of variety and richness into a person's life, the goal is to free the person from the limitations and restrictions of a social network in difficulty. Symptoms usually appear when a person is in an impossible situation and is trying to break out of it... A symptom cannot be cured without producing a basic change in the person's social situation which frees him to grow and develop."

Evaluation

The effectiveness of work with chronic pain families can be evaluated in a number of ways. The problem-oriented assessment identifies specific behaviors as treatment foci. Success in changing these targeted behaviors serves as an important evaluation criterion. Other data that can be useful in program evaluation include pretreatment and posttreatment comparisons of the following: patient and family ratings of satisfaction with their lives, spouse-observed pain behaviors, home/work activity and productivity levels, biopsychosocial dysfunction, and utilization of medical services.

CONCLUSIONS

Intervening with chronic pain families is a critical part of treatment. Successful intervention in such cases requires a team effort; the entire treatment team *must* share common perceptions of the family's problems and of treatment goals. Coordinated, consistent responses from health care professionals can help break restrictive family patterns. Changing the family's response to pain—that is, making the everyday environment less supportive of it—can lead to the discovery of newer and more adaptive ways for the family to be together. Effective treatment of the chronic pain family involves introducing more satisfying ways of interacting in order to help the family achieve a healthier level of functioning.

REFERENCES

Achterberg, J. *Imagery in Healing*. Boston: New Science Library, Shambhala Publications, 1985.

Bashford, M.B. "An Assessment of Direct and Observational Communication Training as Marital Quasi Therapy," Unpublished doctoral dissertation. Columbus, Ohio: Ohio State University, 1977.

Bonica, J. Editorial in *University of Washington Medicine* 7:2, 25, 1980.

Crue, B.L. "Multidisciplinary Pain Treatment Programs: Current Status," *Clinical Journal of Pain* 1(1):31–38, 1985.

Engel, G. "A Life Setting Conducive to Illness: The Giving-up—Given-up Complex," *Annals of Internal Medicine* 69:293–300, 1968.

Feuerstein, M., et al. "Environmental Stressors and Chronic Low Back Pain: Life Events, Family and Work Environment," *Pain* 22:295–307, 1985.

Haley, J. *Uncommon Therapy*. New York: W.W. Norton & Co., 1973.

Leahey, M., and Wright, L.M. "Intervening with Families with Chronic Illness," *Family Systems Medicine* 3(1):60–69, 1985.

Lukensmeyer, W.W. "Management of Patients with Chronic Pain," in *Psychiatry for the Primary Care Physician*. Edited by Freeman, A.M., et al. Baltimore: Williams and Wilkins Co., 1979.

Moore, J.E., and Chaney, E.F. "Outpatient Group Treatment of Chronic Pain. Effects of Spouse Involvement," *Journal of Consulting and Clinical Psychology* 53(3):326–34, 1985.

Moos, R.H. *Family Environment Scale*. Palo Alto, Calif.: Consulting Psychologists Press, 1974.

Norfleet, M.A. "Paradoxical Interventions in the Treatment of Chronic Physical Illness," *Journal of Strategic & Systemic Therapies* 2:63–69, 1983.

Norfleet, M.A., et al. "Helping Families Cope with Chronic Pain: An Integral Part of an Interdisciplinary and Multimodal Treatment Program," in *Group and Family Therapy 1982*. Edited by Wolberg, L., and Aronson, M. New York: Brunner-Mazel, 1982.

Payne, B.A. "A Transpersonal Family Treatment Program for Chronic Pain Patients," Unpublished doctoral dissertation. Menlo Park, Calif.: California Institute of Transpersonal Psychology, 1982.

Payne, B.A., and Norfleet, M.A. "Chronic Pain and the Family: A Review," Unpublished manuscript, 1985.

Satir, V. *Peoplemaking*. Palo Alto, Calif.: Sciences and Behavior Books, 1972.

Stern, G.S., et al. "Stress and Illness: Controllable and Uncontrollable Life Events' Relative Contributions," *Personality and Social Psychology Bulletin* 8(1):140–45, 1982.

Wooley, S.C., et al. "A Learning Theory Model of Chronic Illness Behavior: Theory, Treatment, and Research," *Psychosomatic Medicine* 40(5):379–401, 1978.

22 Intervening with middle-aged families recovering from cardiac surgery

Sally H. Rankin, RN, MSN
Doctoral Candidate
Department of Family Health Care
School of Nursing
University of California
San Francisco, California

Catherine L. Gilliss, RNC, DNSc
Assistant Professor
Department of Family Health Care
School of Nursing
University of California
San Francisco, California

OVERVIEW

This chapter discusses the changes observed in one family whose members participated as a case control in an ongoing study of postcardiac surgery families. Their problems and the nursing care offered to them and other experimental treatment cases are described, and information about evaluating the health of these families presented.

CASE STUDY

Mr. Bartlett was hospitalized for coronary artery bypass graft surgery (CABG), and a family assessment was subsequently completed using the Calgary Family Assessment Model (CFAM). The family is composed of Mr. Bartlett (41 years old), Mrs. Bartlett (also 41), and four young adult children (daughters 24 and 22; sons 20 and 19). All but the youngest son lived outside the home but were available if their parents needed help. Mr. and Mrs. Bartlett were high school sweethearts and married at age 17 following Mrs. Bartlett's pregnancy. Family boundaries and important subsystems are identified in the genogram (Figure 22.1).

Developmentally, the family unit was completing the launching stage (Duvall, 1977) and moving into the middle-aged stage of the family life cycle, with primary tasks of reinvesting in couple identity and developing independent interests. In this case, Mr. and Mrs. Bartlett's own developmental levels were also considered since they affected client recovery.

Figure 22.1 Genogram—The Bartlett Family

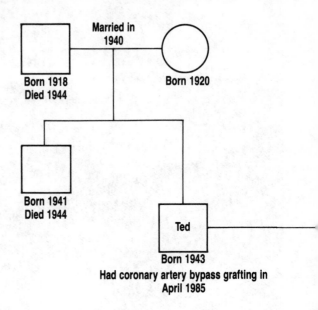

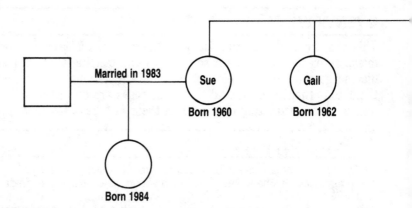

Functionally, this family appeared to communicate thoughts and feelings clearly. The history indicated an ability to solve problems, and members maintained rather traditional roles within a strong parental coalition. The Bartletts seemed to enjoy being together and sharing their experiences.

As a study control case, the family (marital subsystem and one child) was interviewed once during hospitalization, at which time an audiovisual program answering cardiac families' most common questions about exercise, medications, and diet following surgery was viewed and discussed. The family was also contacted by telephone at 3 and 6 months after surgery so that the nurse could evaluate the patient's and the family's physical, social, and emotional recovery.

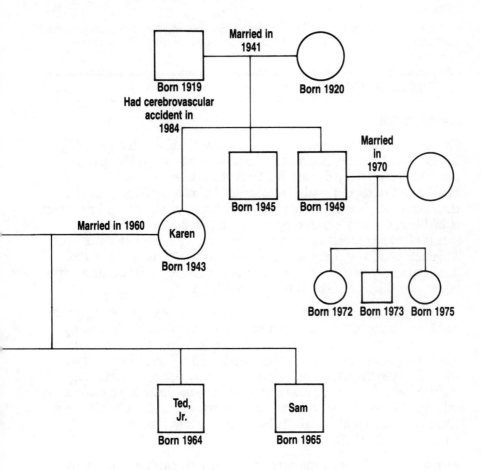

Six months postoperatively, Mr. Bartlett returned to work and resumed most of his normal activities. However, he remained depressed, as evidenced by early-morning awakening, complaints of nonproductivity, and spontaneous crying episodes. Further, he was concerned about the iatrogenic urinary tract infection that had evolved into prostatitis and was resistant to conventional antibiotic therapy. The Bartlett's sexual relationship had not yet resumed. The client had rejected referrals to a counselor from both the nurse and his physician.

Additionally, the couple's interaction pattern had changed since baseline observations were made. Mrs. Bartlett frequently complained that her husband did not exercise enough or eat the right foods. She angrily reminded him to take his medications and call his doctor if he did not feel well. "You've got to do these things for yourself if you want to get better, you know. No one can make you get better," was a common refrain.

His wife's reminders seemed to make Mr. Bartlett irritable, then despondent. "I'm doing everything I can, but it doesn't seem like enough; I'm not sure I'll ever get well. Why, I was better *before* surgery."

NURSING PROCESS

Assessment

The health problem: Coronary artery disease. Morbidity and mortality indices reveal that heart disease takes a high toll on the U.S. population. Coronary artery disease (CAD) is the primary cause of death in the United States and is also responsible for more activity limitation than any other disease (Dracup, 1982; Strauss, et al., 1984). The advent of CABG has been welcomed by many individuals and families as a means of adding precious years to—and improving the quality of—life. Although CABG's efficacy is still debated, it has become one of the most frequently performed surgeries; approximately 200,000 Americans underwent CABG in 1984 (Preston, 1984).

CAD's physiologic risk factors are well-known: age, gender, cigarette smoking, family history, elevated lipid and lipoprotein levels, obesity, and hypertension. The psychosocial profile, however, is less well delineated. Frequently mentioned factors are high-pressure behavior styles, with the Type A personality a prominent descriptor; sociocultural mobility with frequent changes in residence, occupation, or cultural setting; and the presence of anxiety, depression, and sleep disorders (Dracup, 1982; Frank, et al., 1979; Friedman and Rosenman, 1974; Underhill et al., 1982).

Family impact. Though the precise response to cardiac surgery of specific patients and their respective families varies, most families seem to find the experience disorganizing and stressful. Most cardiac families are in mid-life, facing appropriate developmental tasks. These families are at high risk for developmental delay or failure if the nurse or other care provider does not consider their needs.

Some psychosocial characteristics common to families of heart disease patients are beginning to emerge. In a study of patient-spouse recovery from CABG surgery, Gilliss (1984a) found spouses to "hover" and try to control patient behavior, resulting in anger and anxiety for both patient and spouse. In the authors' ongoing (Gortner, et al., in progress) work with families of CABG patients, initial spousal hyper-vigilance, followed by sleeplessness, anxiety, and irritability, has been the pattern. In more stable families, such problems usually resolved naturally with time and improved patient health. Indeed, Penckofer and

Holm (1984) found that within 3 to 8 months postoperatively, most patients reported significant increases in family life satisfaction. Patients and families who cannot re-equilibrate may face issues external to the chronic illness, such as personal or family developmental transitions. Therefore, since developmental tasks can potentiate psychological symptoms, and vice versa, the psychological components of heart disease must be considered interrelated with both the patient's and the family's developmental status. For a discussion of these interrelationships we consider both adult (client) and family developmental level.

Mid-life transitions and heart disease. Whether middle age is a period of turmoil, struggle, and what many refer to as an "identity crisis" (Erikson, 1982; Gould, 1972; Levinson, 1977; Rosenberg and Farrell, 1976; Sheehy, 1976), or whether it is instead a golden period characterized by decreased external pressures and increased security (Deutscher, 1968; Lowenthal and Chiriboga, 1972; Neugarten, 1968), there seems little doubt that middle age is indeed a recognizable life state accompanied by certain developmental tasks and issues.

During the mid-life transition (Levinson, 1977), encompassing roughly the ages of 40 to 45, men are assaulted by tumultuous internal and external struggles. Gould (1972) and Levinson (1977) recognize these years as fraught with discomfort initiated by a personal questioning of values, self-worth, paternal and spousal effectiveness, and achievement of career goals. The process of equilibration requires a great deal of emotional and mental energy even in the healthiest of men. The man who is also assaulted by heart disease and consequent surgery can be expected to experience periods of even greater instability.

During hospitalization, Mr. Bartlett expressed an ambivalence about returning to his demanding position as manager of a food supply distributing business: "I've achieved everything I had hoped for. I make plenty of money and could quit right now and retire. My wife and I could spend all our time travelling or we could move to the country and try farming." Five minutes later he characterized himself as a "workaholic"; he doubted that he could give up his position, and proceeded to call his business office and place immediate orders for increased shipments of foods. Mr. Bartlett's four children were not as dependent on him for financial support as are the children of many men in their 40s. He was painfully aware, however, of his employees' dependence upon him and felt that if he could not continue to direct the business he would be letting them down. Mr. Bartlett returned to work (against advice) on a full-time basis 3 weeks after surgery, but complained that he did not feel that he "had it all together yet" in terms of his ability to think and make decisions. Three months after his surgery he reported, "The rock finally got a crack in it." The analogy is striking: Mr. Bartlett saw himself as the rock that supported his business and to a lesser extent his family, but once the rock cracked he was "no longer in control." Assessing Mr. Bartlett's attempt to deal with mid-life transition reveals an individual trying to behave responsibly within a long-established personal system, one who is coming to terms with significant issues and yet is overwhelmed by major surgery and all of its consequences.

Family developmental stages and heart disease. A great part of Mr. Bartlett's problem during recovery related to the fact that he and his family did not see cardiac surgery as normal for a man of 40. Indeed, the median age of CABG patients has been reported to have increased from 50 years in 1967-70 to 57 years in 1979 (Cosgrove, et al., 1982). With the surgery now proving safe for older patients, many elderly couples are faced with the problems of its recovery. However, for older families both the meaning of surgery and the issues involved in recovery are different from those of their younger counterparts.

What are the consequences of a nonnormative event such as life-threatening illness or surgery on the family unit? If the family is assessed developmentally, it becomes evident that the process might be complicated by the intersection of two competing developmental levels.

In the case of illness timing, it might be proposed that the greater the family's child-related needs and tasks, the greater the upheaval in response to illness. In addition, the greater the adult's developmental tasks, the greater the illness-related family disruption. In the Bartletts' case, the family unit was completing its launching stage and should have been growing comfortable with the tasks of middle-aged families. Wright and Leahey (1984) describe these tasks as:
- Reinvestment in the "couple" identity, with concurrent development of independent interests
- Realignment of the relationship to include in-laws and grandchildren
- Dealing with disabilities and death in the older generation.

Mr. Bartlett's illness timing and surgery were dysynchronous with his family's developmental status, forcing the Bartletts to deal with disability and possible death in their own, rather than the older, generation. This dysynchrony may have been responsible, in part, for Mr. Bartlett's extended recovery period.

Mrs. Bartlett's response to the crisis situation reveals how little is still known about adult developmental phases for women (most normative work has described men). However, available research indicates that for women like Mrs. Bartlett the early child-rearing years are the most stressful. Once the launching stage has been passed, a period of new freedom and growth for women begins (Neugarten, 1979; Heckerman, 1980; Abbott and Brody, 1985). Mrs. Bartlett was developing her own career as a decorator, which may have helped keep her at a healthy distance from her husband's problems. Although both husband and wife characterized her as a supportive, willing listener, Mr. Bartlett noted that "she knows she can whip me now" and worried that he "was too dependent on her, and too much of a liability." Though she was relatively comfortable with her personal developmental phase, the spousal dyad and family unit experienced difficulty in integrating the illness event.

In summary, it was noted that developmental models could be useful in analyzing individual and family responses to cardiac surgery.

Planning

Carter and McGoldrick (1982), subsuming family developmental stage seven under "launching," point out that this is the newest, and now the longest, period of family life. In America, socioeconomic changes have helped mesh the launching and middle-aged stages because grown children are leaving and returning to the family of origin with much greater frequency than was the case even 15 years ago. Longer educational preparation and economic constraints have resulted in extended dependence on parental largesse; additionally, changing marriage/divorce patterns are driving more daughters and sons, and their children, back to the parental home. Another factor that must be considered when discussing this stage is increasing longevity. Many middle-aged families with children of their own and surviving parents find themselves truly "in the middle," responsible for both future and past generations.

When planning care for the middle-aged family experiencing cardiac surgery, it is important to help them fully integrate the event into their existing life patterns and continue to complete their appropriate developmental tasks.

The first task that must be considered when planning for a middle-aged cardiac surgical family is reinvestment in the "couple" identity. Instead of attempting to invest further in parenting roles, the couple must realign the marital relationship. For some couples the home recovery period supports accomplishment of this task, since the spouse may be available to the patient for extended periods of time to assist in activities of daily living and to act as primary caregiver. When planning for the home recovery period, therefore, it is important that the nurses:
• Help the couple understand what is appropriate and helpful caregiving
• Facilitate role flexibility *without* depriving partners of important husband-wife role behaviors
• Help the marital dyad plan creative ways to fill time within the patient's physical limitations.

The second task involves a shifting relationship status among family members outside the marital dyad: children, grandchildren, and in-laws. One of the nurse's most helpful planning activities in this area is rehearsing situations that involve maintenance of the marital dyad boundaries. This is particularly important during the postoperative recovery period, when sleep and rest are an issue. For instance, many families cite as one of their most difficult postoperative tasks controlling the number of visitors and the length of visits. While the couple must be able to ask for help from the children when necessary, they must also be able to refuse requests for help from their children, especially requests to baby-sit for grandchildren or any other activity that will be wearing to the recovering cardiac surgery patient. Wives of patients often find this inability to help their adult children a difficult adjustment. Obviously, preparation of couples for this aspect of the recovery period can be quite helpful.

The third task, dealing with disability and death in the preceding generation, is especially problematic for middle-aged families who must deal with these issues in their own generation. A recovering patient who carries the additional stress of worrying about an aged parent will find recuperation fraught with difficulty. For example, one middle-aged man developed postpericardotomy syndrome 2 months following CABG surgery, during the time his elderly father was hospitalized with a stroke. The involved clinicians believed that the added stress of parental illness caused an increase in this patient's catecholamines and a massive inflammatory pericardial response.

Planning for the middle-aged family that has experienced cardiac surgery involves anticipating potentially problematic family tasks. Another important aspect of planning for these families is building the bridge between inpatient and outpatient care. The authors' work with post-cardiac surgery families indicates that developmental concerns must be balanced with newly abbreviated hospital stays and the introduction of a frequently sicker individual into the home. As part of the protocol for preparing families for discharge, the marital dyad should be mobilized to meet the physical and psychosocial challenges that may arise during postoperative recovery at home. The authors use an audiovisual presentation to help families rehearse some of the emotional facets of the recovery. Cardiac surgery patients, who, thanks to prospective payment plans and DRGs (diagnosis-related groups), are being discharged on the 7th day after surgery, have tremendous educational, physical, and supportive care needs. Establishing a bond with the family during hospitalization and sensitizing them to the issues of recovery can help them cope between the nurse's follow-up telephone calls.

Intervention

Most families can muster the strength and maintain enough flexibility to propel the recovering cardiac surgery patient through postoperative recovery at home. However, *family-focused supportive and educational interventions* during this period can enhance recovery for both patient and family. To this end, the authors' preferred interventions have three components, and are accomplished during both hospitalization and home recovery.

Component I: Individual risk reduction and surgical rehabilitation. Predischarge nursing care includes information aimed at preventing the further development of CAD. Slide/tape programs from the American Heart Association (1976) are shown to the patient and family members. These programs cover exercise, diet, and smoking as well as resumption of sexual and other activity.

Component II: Family risk reduction and surgical rehabilitation. The individual patient—and the family—needs information to prepare for postdischarge experiences. The stress of surgery puts the family at risk for the reemergence of old conflicts and unhealthy behavior patterns; indeed, there is some evidence that discord related to family-generated stressors such as marital separation, divorce, and death of a spouse may help precipitate cardiac illness (Roustad, 1984). Surgical stress can reignite these old problems, so it is not uncommon to see recovering families struggle with increased conflict and fighting, scapegoating of vulnerable members, alcoholism, marital infidelity, or physical illness. While the acting out of stress can provide some relief, it may be costly to the family's overall well-being. The nurse can reduce the risk of these problems and ensure a more tranquil recovery period for the patient through family-focused intervention.

Before discharge, patients and spouses need information about changes in the marital relationship that are common during cardiac surgical recovery. To this end, "Working Together for Recovery," an original (Gilliss, 1984b) slide/tape program that sensitizes patient and family members to the social/ emotional or relationship issues usually confronted during the first 6 weeks of cardiac surgical recovery, is useful. The issues addressed include sleeplessness, anxiety, and depression; the tendencies for families to be overprotective and for patients to overdo; and the need to communicate openly in order to solve the problems created by new diets, schedules, and activities (Gilliss, 1984a).

The nurse can draw on both clinical experience and research data to explain how many couples experience conflict during the recovery period; this conflict is usually related to a number of factors: depression and a feeling of "letdown," sleeplessness, fears about the future, and the numerous adjustments that must be made regarding diet, activity, and medications. The slide/tape viewing is followed by a private counseling session in which the nurse can help personalize the program content to the couple's special needs. Anticipated life-style changes are reviewed and information provided. Couples are encouraged to discuss their fears and to anticipate ways in which their relationship might be at risk during the recovery period.

The nurse can play an essential role in helping couples deal with the conflict that usually revolves around the patient's activity level. For example, wives are frequently accused by their husbands of being over-protective and almost infantilizing in their advocacy of activity limitations. While spousal monitoring of the cardiac surgery patient's activity level usually enhances safe recovery, the marital pair should discuss before discharge how they plan to deal with this issue. Learning that these feelings are experienced by many families helps the couple adjust.

Prior to discharge, the nurse can provide information about supportive community agencies or programs. The Mended Hearts Club, which is sponsored by the American Heart Association and is available in many cities, provides information and an opportunity to share experiences with other couples. Cardiac rehabilitation programs that monitor exercise, explain good nutrition and stress reduction, and offer support groups for patients and spouses can also be helpful. The names of these programs are usually available through the local American Heart Association, as well as through discharge planning nurses and social workers.

Component III: Posthospital recovery. Once patients and their families leave the hospital, the number of contacts they have with the cardiac surgeon or other health care personnel dramatically decreases. The authors consider it very important for nurses to maintain contact with families during this period to assist in early symptom identification and reduce family strain. The authors maintain telephone contact for 8 weeks following surgery and have found this nurse-initiated contact successful in identifying and referring problems to local physicians, reinforcing risk factor modification, and allowing patients and spouses to ventilate personal concerns regarding recovery and their emotional health. Spouses, in particular, usually express great concern regarding the recovery process and often need reassurance that recovery is progressing normally and important milestones are being achieved.

Patients and families are contacted at 3 and 6 months after surgery to ascertain recovery status. At 3 months, most patients who wanted to return to work have done so; almost all have returned to or surpassed their previous activity levels; and families have reorganized to integrate the surgical event into their lives. By 6 months, this integration is even more evident. Most patients say they would repeat the surgery if necessary, and most spouses report that life has returned to normal.

The picture is not uniformly rosy, however. Some patients suffer such postoperative sequelae as iatrogenic infections (*e.g.*, hepatitis), while others display progressive atherosclerotic disease and face further surgery. In some cases, such as Mr. Bartlett's, the patient fails to fully integrate the surgery into everyday life and still suffers postsurgical depression. It is imperative that depression be evaluated, so that it will not be confused with the somatic signs and symptoms of congestive heart failure. Such patients can be referred to cardiologists and family counselors.

Evaluation

Evaluating individual or family recovery from cardiac surgery is a complex process, and very little systematic information about it has been collected. The focus of current research (Gortner, et al., in progress) is to identify the correlates of this recovery; to that end several strategies have proven helpful.

Several pencil and paper questionnaires are available for assessing family functioning as it is seen through the eyes of its members. One such instrument is the Family APGAR (Smilkstein, 1978), a five-item questionnaire that asks about family members' satisfaction with family adaptability, partnership, growth, affection, and resolve. Because one member's perceptions of family functioning may not accurately predict the opinions of others, the authors ask both patient and spouse and/or others in the household, to complete an APGAR during hospitalization and at 3 and 6 months after discharge. This data provides a better understanding of the changes that may occur during the period between surgery and recovery and better identification of discrepancies or agreements between partners.

The Marital Adjustment Scale (Locke and Wallace, 1959) can also help evaluate the impact of cardiac surgery on couples' marital satisfaction. This 16-item pencil and paper questionnaire is administered to both patient and spouse and evaluated for similarities and differences in scores.

Another valuable technique for monitoring recovery outcomes has been the telephone interview. Graduate-prepared nurses specializing in cardiovascular or family nursing who have conducted regular (weekly through 6 weeks) brief (20-minute) interviews with patients and spouses have been able to identify patient and/or family problems. Family members have been asked about their perceptions, their needs, their problems, and how they are addressing the issues raised. Nurses can coach these families by offering information and clarifying expectations and understanding. Table 22.1 presents appropriate topics for such an interview and some sample questions.

Table 22.1 Interview Topics and Questions

Topic	Sample question
Concerns about physical signs and symptoms and pace of recovery	• What have been your concerns since we last talked? How has planned care related to.... (your incision, etc.) worked for you?
Life-style management and risk reduction	• How are you managing to balance your dietary restrictions and your teenager's food preferences?
Couple/spousal concerns	• Have you noticed any of the problems heart surgery patients and their families frequently mention—for instance, feeling "low," fatigued, or irritable? How do you handle these issues with your children and spouse?

CONCLUSIONS

Consistent with existing literature on the family and chronic illness, the authors have found that the families described as "healthy" by expert nurses are those that demonstrate flexibility and inventiveness in meeting such postsurgical demands as dietary changes, new exercise and medication regimens, and pain control. These families can focus on the surgery and recovery when it is most demanding and can also return to their other interests or responsibilities following immediate postoperative recovery—usually after 5 to 8 weeks (Gilliss, 1983). However, because cardiac surgery is a highly stressful and usually unanticipated event in mid-life, nursing care that addresses the family concerns may strengthen the entire unit's health.

REFERENCES

Abbott, D., and Brody G. "The Relation of Child Age, Gender, and Number of Children to the Marital Adjustment of Wives," *Journal of Marriage and the Family* 47(1):77–84, 1985.

American Heart Association and the Santa Clara Heart Association. *An Active Partnership for the Health of Your Heart.* Santa Clara, Calif.: Santa Clara Chapter of the California Heart Association, 1976.

Carter, E., and McGoldrick, M. *The Family Life Cycle: A Framework for Family Therapy.* New York: Gardner Press, 1982.

Cosgrove, D., et al. "Results of Myocardial Revascularization: A 12-Year Experience," *Circulation* 65 (Suppl II):1137–43, 1982.

Deutscher, I. "The Quality of Postparental Life," in *Middle Age and Aging.* Edited by Neugarten, B.L. Chicago: University of Chicago Press, 1968.

Dracup, K. "Psychosocial Aspects of Coronary Heart Disease: Implications for Nursing Research," *Western Journal of Nursing Research* 4(3):257–69, 1982.

Duvall, E. *Marriage and Family Development,* 5th ed. Philadelphia: J.B. Lippincott Co., 1977.

Erikson, E. *The Life Cycle Completed.* New York: W.W. Norton & Co., 1982.

Frank, K., et al. "Psychological Intervention in Coronary Heart Disease," *General Hospital Psychiatry* 1(1):18–23, 1979.

Friedman, M., and Rosenman, R. *Type A Behavior and Your Heart.* New York: Alfred Knopf, 1974.

Gilliss, C. "Identification of Factors Contributing to Family Function Following Coronary Artery Bypass Surgery," Doctoral presentation. San Francisco: University of California, 1983.

Gilliss, C. "Reducing Family Stress During and After Coronary Artery Bypass Surgery," *Nursing Clinics of North America* 19(1):103–12, 1984a.

Gilliss, C. "Working Together for Recovery," An unpublished slide/tape program, 1984b.

Gortner, S., et al. "Improving Recovery from Cardiac Surgery I," Study funded by Division of Nursing, Health Resources Administration, U.S. Public Health Service (in progress).

Gould, R. "The Phases of Adult Life: A Study in Developmental Psychology," *American Journal of Psychiatry* 129(5):521–31, 1972.

Heckerman, C. *The Evolving Female: Women in Psychosocial Context.* New York: Human Sciences Press, 1980.

Levinson, D. "The Mid-Life Transition: A Period in Adult Psychosocial Development," *Psychiatry* 40:99–112, 1977.

Locke, H., and Wallace, K. "Short Marital Adjustment and Prediction Tests: Their Reliability and Validity," *Marriage and Family Living* 21:251–55, 1959.

Lowenthal, M., and Chiriboga, D. "Transition to the Empty Nest: Crisis, Challenge, or Belief?" *Archives of General Psychiatry* 26:8–14, 1972.

Neugarten, B. "The Awareness of Middle Age," in *Middle Age and Aging.* Edited by Neugarten, B.L. Chicago: University of Chicago Press, 1968.

Neugarten, B. "Time, Age and the Life Cycle," *American Journal of Psychiatry* 136(7):887–94, 1979.

Penckofer, S., and Holm, K. "Early Appraisal of Coronary Revascularization of Quality of Life," *Nursing Research* 33(2):60–63, 1984.

Preston, J. "Marketing an Operation," *Atlantic* 254(6):32–40, 1984.

Rosenberg, S., and Farrell, M. "Identity and Crisis in Middle Aged Men," *International Journal of Aging and Human Development* 7(2):153–70, 1976.

Roustad, L. "Adjustment to Chronic Illness and Disability in Mid-Life," in *Chronic Illness and Disability Throughout the Life Span: Effects on Self and Family.* Edited by Eisenberg, M., et al. New York: Springer Publishing Co., 1984.

Sheehy, G. *Passages.* New York: Dutton, 1976.

Smilkstein, G. "The Family APGAR," *Journal of Family Practice* 6(6):1231–39, 1978.

Strauss, I., et al. *Chronic Illness and the Quality of Life,* 2nd ed. St. Louis: C.V. Mosby Co., 1984.

Underhill, S., et al. *Cardiac Nursing.* Philadelphia: J.B. Lippincott Co., 1982.

Wright, L., and Leahey, M. *Nurses and Families: A Guide to Assessment and Intervention.* Philadelphia: F.A. Davis and Co., 1984.

23 Intervening with aging families and Alzheimer's disease

Wendy L. Watson, RN, PhD
Education Coordinator, Family Nursing Unit
Associate Professor, Faculty of Nursing
The University of Calgary
Calgary, Alberta, Canada

OVERVIEW

This chapter presents a systemic-strategic approach to intervening with aging families managing Alzheimer's disease (AD). An AD patient's problems (physical, cognitive, and/or emotional) both affect and are affected by the family. This relationship is demonstrated through a case study. Interventions to interrupt maladaptive interaction patterns, such as devising strategies to modify difficult behavior, using questions as interventions, reframing the situation, offering positive connotations and split opinions, devising rituals, recommending support groups, and facilitating discussion of institutionalization, are described. Iatrogenic double binds are discussed as well as the analogue that exists between the patient-family system and the family-health care professional system.

CASE STUDY

The Simpson family was referred to the Family Nursing Unit, Faculty of Nursing, University of Calgary (Wright, et al., 1985) by the family physician, who recognized their need for assistance in caring for Mrs. Simpson's elderly sister. At the time of referral the household consisted of John, age 75, a retired postal employee; Mary, age 66, a homemaker; and Mary's sister, Margaret, age 74. Margaret had been diagnosed 3 years before as having Alzheimer's disease (AD) and had lived with the family for the past 2 years, since her husband's death. After enjoying "the freedom of retirement" for 8 years, John and Mary now felt trapped and burdened with their caregiving responsibilities. They had even postponed a holiday for the past 2 years. However, the Simpsons insisted that they "knew" that having Margaret with them was the "right and only thing to do."

The family physician reported that Margaret's most recent neuropsychological evaluation suggested that her AD was not as advanced as her problematic and careseeking behaviors would indicate.

Following a thorough family assessment using the Calgary Family Assessment Model (Wright and Leahey, 1984) one major problem was identified: a helping/helplessness cycle in the family system, which appeared to be perpetuating both Margaret's ongoing, debilitating dependence and the couple's perceived entrapment.

Assessment revealed that the couple's main source of information about AD had been the television. Given Margaret's pre-AD history of dependent behavior (i.e., "she's always needed someone to take care of her"), John and Mary assumed that she needed even more help following her diagnosis.

The couple requested that Margaret not be involved in the sessions, and the request itself was seen as providing insight into family functioning. The sister's absence in the sessions was made present through triadic questioning (Tomm, 1984b) and in the delivery of each intervention.

During five family systems nursing sessions over 6 months, the nurse slowly but consistently challenged the family belief that Margaret was incapable of doing anything for herself and had to be "babied" lest she become upset. Also challenged was John and Mary's strong belief that "caring equals 'doing for' and 'helping more.' " Interventions were designed to increase Margaret's performance abilities, reduce the burden on John and Mary, and increase positive feelings in the triadic relationship and between the various dyads.

In the first session, it was determined that much of the talk in the Simpson household centered around Margaret's health. A vicious circle had developed in which the couple inquired about Margaret's health and Margaret complained; the more she complained, the more the couple pursued the topic, and vice versa. In order to interrupt this negative pattern, John and Mary were instructed not to talk of Margaret's health for 2 weeks; they were told, in addition, not to respond to her complaining and to note her reaction. The task was expected to be difficult, and the couple was encouraged to support each other in its completion. In addition, they were asked to stop performing a single task (of their own choosing) that they usually performed for Margaret.

John and Mary arrived for the next session elated. They had decided to stop providing Margaret with a glass of water at breakfast and found that she took the initiative to get it herself. They also noted a marked reduction in her health complaints when they did not discuss her problems with her. During this second session, it was hypothesized that Margaret used her helpless, "out of control" behavior to maintain control within the family. It was also noted that Mary was more reluctant than her husband to believe that Margaret could be more independent. The nurse hypothesized that perhaps Mary's helpfulness represented her *own* attempt to maintain control. To gently challenge family beliefs and interrupt the helping/helplessness cycle a second time, the couple was instructed to perform an "experiment." Twice during each of the next 2 weeks, they were to "pretend helplessness": Mary would declare that she was too tired to finish preparing supper, and John would "pretend confusion and incapability" when trying to make the toaster work for breakfast.

The intervention rippled dramatically through the family system, and by session three the couple began to instigate changes on their own. John had suggested that Margaret, who was incontinent nightly, begin getting her own clean bedsheets and "get more exercise" by going to the bathroom more frequently. Margaret was now getting bedsheets from the closet, making her bed, making toast, dusting the living room furniture, and "apologizing" when she didn't pour her own glass of water at breakfast. In order to maintain these rapid changes, the couple was advised to proceed slowly and to consider what to do with the time that was formerly devoted to worrying about and waiting on Margaret. Three weeks later, the couple reported that Margaret had not been incontinent for 4 consecutive days and was continuing to do more for herself. They stated that her appearance was 100% improved. The couple had gone out 3 afternoons "just to enjoy themselves!" Mary reported that she was finding it "easier to sit back more than I used to."

The nurse attempted to solidify the established changes and further challenge the family through a split-opinion intervention. John and Mary were told that half the team felt there had been just the right amount of change and that the couple should not request any more of Margaret, while the other half were convinced that Margaret could do 10% more and that the couple should continue to seek creative ways of increasing her independence.

The overall effectiveness of family intervention with this AD family became apparent 3 months later when the nurse found it almost impossible to arrange the follow-up session—because the couple was busy making last-minute arrangements for a vacation to Ireland!

THE NURSING PROCESS

Assessment

The health problem: Alzheimer's disease. Alzheimer's disease (AD) has been termed "the silent epidemic" and "the disease of the century"; it now affects the lives of 1.5 million older "victims" and 4.5 million of their families and friends. Who is the AD "patient"? From a family systems perspective, of course, the whole family is the "patient"; however, for purposes of this chapter, the older person with AD will be termed "the patient."

The National Institute of Neurological and Communicative Disorders and Stroke estimates that 15% of people over 65 years of age have varying degrees of dementia or deterioration in intellectual capacity (McKinstry, 1982). Sixty percent of these cases are attributed to Alzheimer's disease.

Alzheimer's disease is a progressively degenerative brain condition with no known cause or cure. It is characterized by neurofibrillary tangles, senile plaques, and granulovascular structures; as these anomalies in the brain increase, cognitive functioning deteriorates. Chronic decline in intellect, memory, judgment, concentration, self-care abilities, and personality all reflect physiologic changes in the brain.

Although the AD's "cause" is not presently known, possible etiologies include viruses, biochemical changes, aluminum intoxication, genetic defects, and immune system malfunction (Schneck, et al., 1982).

Consistent with this elusiveness in cause and cure, accurate diagnosis of AD is difficult; positive confirmation is available only through autopsy. Diagnosis thus revolves around exclusion of other disorders—i.e., drug use, circulatory problems (strokes, cardiac insufficiency), head trauma, tumors, or metabolic disorders (Cohen, 1980)—that might produce similar cognitive symptoms.

Zarit and Zarit (1984) emphasize the need to distinguish dementia from delirium and depression. Depression is the most frequent psychological cause of cognitive impairment in elderly patients and frequently masquerades as dementia (Wells, 1979). A brief mental status examination can be used to differentially diagnose dementia from either depression or delirium (Kahn and Miller, 1978; Zarit, 1980); the history of problematic symptoms will also help establish the diagnosis. Wells (1979) developed a comparative table for differentiating pseudodementia from irreversible dementia, highlighting both family and individual manifestations:

Pseudodementia. Family is aware of dysfunction. Symptoms progress rapidly following a precise, identifiable onset. Patient complains of cognitive loss and communicates strong distress. Nocturnal accentuation of dysfunction is uncommon. "Don't know" answers are typical. Patient's task performance varies widely, even on tasks of similar difficulty.

Dementia. Family is unaware of dysfunction and its severity. Symptoms develop slowly and progress; patient complains very little about cognitive loss and appears unconcerned. Nocturnal accentuation of dysfunction is common. "Near-miss" answers are frequent, and task performance is consistently poor on tasks of similar difficulty.

Although AD is characterized by an insidious onset of symptoms and marked variability in the course of the illness, some guidelines can be presented (Table 23.1). Over a period of years, the patient becomes bedridden, emaciated, and helpless; dementia and physical incoordination increase. Death occurs from infected pressure sores or bronchopneumonia (Dewis, 1982).

Aging families and adult children. Families do not exclude their elderly; indeed, most continue to provide assistance at great personal cost. Twice as many bedridden and housebound elderly patients are being cared for by families as are in institutions (Shanas, 1979), a statistic that holds true for AD patients. Family members care for 90% of America's older, mentally impaired persons (Zarit et al., 1980).

Stimulation, patience, and security have been noted to be three essential ingredients in effective care of the demented (Arie, 1973). Caregivers may understandably be overwhelmed when attempting to operationalize these parameters of care. As AD patients' awareness of their disability decreases, security needs take precedence, further increasing demands on caregivers.

Table 23.1 Stages of Alzheimer's Disease

Stage	Duration (yrs.)	Characteristics
Forgetfulness	2 to 4	• (Possible) First indications: memory loss regarding present events/familiar objects or people (for example, own telephone number, route to office or home) (Dewis, 1982) • Loss of spontaneity, initiative, sense of humor (Hayter, 1974) • Reduced attention span • Withdrawal from activities (first sign of difficulty) (Zarit, 1982)
Confusion	2 to 20	• Progressive memory loss • Aphasia • Agnosia • Apraxia • Wandering • Nocturnal restlessness • Repetitive motion(s) • Temporal disorientation • Mirror sign (inability to recognize self in mirror) (Pinel, 1975)
Dementia*	1	• Complete disorientation • Seizures • Gait disturbances • Pseudoparkinsonism • Forced laughter • Crying • Klüver-Bucy-like syndrome (hyperorality, flat or decreased affect, bulimia, usual agnosia, hypermetamorphosis or compulsively touching everything)

*All symptoms described by Sjogren (1950); Sjogren et al. (1952).

Impact of Alzheimer's disease on the family. AD caregivers (usually a spouse or adult daughter) face time- and energy-consuming responsibilities that must often be discharged at tremendous personal cost in terms of social isolation; lack of time for self, family, and friends; career interruptions; financial drain; and heavy physical labor (Archbold, 1982; Brody and Lang, 1982). The entire experience can produce a variety of conflicting emotions, including sadness, frustration, anger, guilt, discouragement, empathy, rejection, pity, revulsion, and entrapment (Mace and Rabins, 1981). Life narrows, and caregivers may feel very alone. Caregivers, usually women, are caught "in the middle" in three senses: generation, age, and competing demands on their time. The Philadelphia Geriatric Center identifies these "women in the middle" as those most in need of assistance in cases involving aging families (Brody, 1981).

Silverstone (1979) clarifies our understanding of the multiple demands, transitions, and tasks that AD caregivers may face by viewing their situation in terms of their developmental tasks: relinquishing youth, adjusting to the "empty nest" (which Silverstone considers a euphemism for the multitude of feelings this life-cycle stage may generate), facing mortality and age, and assuming a filial role in relation to parents. The interdependence of these tasks can complicate even further the potential conflict between the middle-aged woman's filial, marital, and parental responsibilities, thus placing daughters of aging parents at "the fulcrum of familial stress" (Bloom and Munroe, 1972).

Simos' (1973) seminal study of adult children and their view of the problems of their aging parents concluded that most children can handle their parents' physical problems, even those that may require considerable time and attention. What disturbed them were the psychological, interpersonal, and social problems associated with managing their elderly parents' isolation or ineptness. The adult children studied responded to their perception of these problems by "attempting to console or comfort the parent, struggling with negative feelings aroused by the parent, serving as peacemaker with caretaking personnel and others, dealing with family disruptions set off by the parent, or in rare cases attempting to limit the parent's insatiable demands" (p. 80).

Zarit and colleagues (1980) measured the level of burden experienced by the primary caregivers of impaired elderly; such burdens were evoked by "lack of time for oneself, the excessive dependency of the patient on the caregiver, and (the) caregiver's fears about further deterioration in the patient's behavior" (p. 652).

The results of this investigation indicated that caregivers' burdens were unrelated to behavior problems resulting from the elderly person's impairment. Rather, they seemed associated with the caregiver's degree of social support—specifically the number of visits by other family members to the elderly parent. The correlation was negative; the more support received (as indicated by the number of visits), the less burdened the caregiver felt.

Pratt and colleagues (1985) were among several researchers to examine how Alzheimer's caregivers decreased their perceived burdens. Self-confidence in problem-solving and the ability to reframe (redefine stressful experiences to provide new understanding and facilitate management) were effective internal strategies (McCubbin, et al., 1981). Spiritual and extended-family support were identified as effective external coping mechanisms (McCubbin et al., 1981), as was taking turns providing care ("principle of substitution") (Johnson, 1983; Shanas, 1979).

Spiritual support may provide a basis for assigning meaning to an AD problem, allowing the caregiver "to neutralize a potential stressor by seeking positive attributes in the situation or making positive comparisons to others" (Pratt et al, 1985, p. 31). Because of the numerous losses accompanying Alzheimer's and the need for caregivers to continually modify their reactions to the patient in order to maintain a calm environment, many find spiritual support particularly helpful.

Pratt and coworkers (1985) associated an internal strategy of "passivity," employing avoidance responses, with higher levels of caregiver burden. This association may be understood by hypothesizing that high levels of perceived burden evoke passivity. The more passive and nonconfident one is, the more burdened one becomes.

Perceptions of burden were found to be related to the caregiver's health status. Those in excellent or good health felt lower burden levels than those in fair or poor health. Seventy-nine percent of caregivers studied indicated that caregiving had negatively affected their health status; 35% indicated a great negative effect on health, while 44% cited moderate impact.

Family impact on Alzheimer's disease. So far, this chapter has emphasized the impact of AD on the family. But what of the impact of the family on AD? Roth (1977) and Tomlinson and colleagues (1970) found that up to half of all behavioral problems in Alzheimer's and vascular dementia patients arise from factors other than brain cell loss. These additional factors included the patient's personality, personal history, and current life situation.

Interaction patterns in aging families can stimulate, exacerbate, or ameliorate AD deficits. Herr and Weakland (1979b), operating from a brief strategic therapy model, have broadened their perception of age-related problems from "seeing these problems as arising only from individual, age-related and usually irreversible or progressive deficits, to seeing that at least part of the difficulties involved may be related to family communication" (p. 144). They define communication as the "patterns of interactions which have the potential for pathogenesis" (p. 145).

Herr and Weakland also assert that elements of the traditional double bind can be present in the adult child–aging parent relationship and may promote diagnosis of senile dementia. For example:
• An *intense relationship* exists due to the increased dependency needs of the elder and/or the social pressures on the adult child.
• Advancing age prompts emergence of sensitive topics that may involve *contradictory levels of messages* to the elder. For example, the following

contradictory message may be given to a recent widow by her children: "We will help you to remain independent. If you refuse our help (by not following all our advice and directives) this will be a sign to us that you are unable to continue living independently" (p. 147). The message is paradoxical. The only way the mother can remain independent is to be dependent (follow orders).

• The *opportunity* to leave the field is minimal for the elder because of physical, social, and economic restrictions.

• "Elders may have *difficulty commenting on the contradiction* because of minor cognitive impairments which would not be of much significance in other respects" (p. 147).

Therefore, it is useful to look beyond the question of "Why did this problem first appear?" to that of "What is the cycle of interaction in the family system that maintains or escalates the problems of the family coping with Alzheimer's?" (Weakland et al., 1974).

Attention to the cybernetic aspects of family interaction can also provide vital information about the elderly, their problems, and potentials (Watson and Wright, 1984). Circular epistemology looks for recurrent negative patterns—that is, vicious cycles of interactions. It prompts a shift from evaluating family members' intentions to evaluating the effect(s) of their behavior...and the effect of the effect(s) (Tomm, 1984a). Circular causality perspectives can provide new pieces to the Alzheimer's family puzzle.

As AD progresses, family members frequently report that their loved one (the patient) becomes a virtual stranger, doing things that are uncharacteristic of the former self. This "strange" behavior elicits uncharacteristic responses from the family members, which can lead to a house full of "strangers," all of them trying to make sense out of each other's behavior. As a result, the AD caregiver may become preoccupied with the physical aspects of care and begin to "talk over" the patient as if he were not present. "When this happens the patient's world begins to die around him, and his motivation to remain connected to reality diminishes" (Dewis, 1982, p. 34), which verifies to the caregiver that the patient is "not really there." The cycle perpetuates itself, aggravating Alzheimer's symptoms.

AD, particularly in its early stages, has few physical symptoms; that can make it difficult for the family to lower their expectations of the patient. One person said, "If I wore a bandage or used a crutch I would get more understanding" (Dewis, 1982, p. 33). Families may respond instead by exhorting the patient to change, thus increasing his frustration and discouragement. Family members may then conclude that "if only he wouldn't get discouraged and (would) just try harder he could do more."

Even when the disease is finally acknowledged and becomes "visible," either through patient behavioral/personality changes or through family education, the family may render the patient "invisible" by not expecting anything of him because he is "not there." The more they think of the patient as "not there," the less connected he will be to them or to reality, once again perpetuating a counterproductive cycle.

Family assessment model. The Calgary Family Assessment Model (CFAM) (Wright and Leahey, 1984) can be used to assess aging families coping with Alzheimer's disease. The visual impact of the two tools for *structural* assessment—that is, the genogram and the ecomap—make them immediately useful to the nurse. Diagramming three generations of family members, their ages, occupations, and living arrangements facilitates identification of potential family resources.

The ecomap diagrams each family member's contacts with "outside" systems, for example, work, church, community, and friends. A "before" and "after" AD ecomap is especially revealing, since family members typically become isolated from former social contacts as the illness progresses. The nurse may uncover through ecomap questions a pattern of diminishing personal and increasing professional contacts. Sample questions include:
• "How have your friends responded to your husband's AD diagnosis?"
• "With what other health care professionals is your family presently involved?"

Developmental assessment focuses on the three major tasks of aging families:
• Shifting from the work role to leisure and/or retirement.
• Maintaining both systemic and individual functioning while adapting to increased age.
• Preparing for one's own death and dealing with loss of spouse, siblings, and/or parents (Wright and Leahey, 1984).

The developmental impact of AD can be assessed through such questions as:
• "What did [the patient's] forgetfulness affect first: his work or leisure?"
• "What do you and [the spouse/patient] still do together, in spite of the illness, to make you feel like a couple?"
• (To adult child) "Of your mother and father, whom do you think was more satisfied with his or her life's accomplishments before [the patient's] AD was diagnosed?"

Instrumental functioning is a particularly critical area in AD families. The caregiver's burden and the family's abilities to assist the primary caregiver and utilize community resources effectively can be assessed through direct questioning about the routine activities of daily living.

The CFAM's nine *expressive functioning* areas help nurses assess the AD family's underlying dynamics; one area, beliefs, is especially useful. A nurse must understand each family member's beliefs about AD. Such information can be obtained by asking, "What is your understanding of Alzheimer's disease?" or, "What do you think causes Alzheimer's disease?" or, "How do you think your family is coping with Alzheimer's at this time?"

AD myths and misconceptions abound, and nurses can play a vital role in providing and clarifying information. Several points should receive particular emphasis:
• Senility is not a normal part of growing old.
• The patient may be the first to know that something is wrong; one cannot assume that AD patients do not suffer because they do not know that anything is wrong.
• AD is not contagious.
• AD does not result from excessive strain or emotional stress.
• AD-related mental declines are not from laziness.

Assessment of the presenting problem. Since AD's stages may vary from person to person, and therefore from family to family, the caregivers cannot foresee the duration, type, or severity of symptoms. A nurse must therefore obtain or record specific descriptions of the patient's behavior, cognition, and affect at the time of initial assessment. The nurse must find out what behavioral, cognitive, and emotional changes the family has weathered, and how they weathered them.

To intervene effectively and efficiently with AD families, nurses need to obtain a clear picture of the disease problem in the family context. This requires asking each family member, "What is the problem that is concerning your family the most at this time?" This process is vital, since a problem without a definition is a problem without a solution (Herr and Weakland, 1979a).

In defining the problem, it is important to be specific:
• Ask the patient and family about specific instances of forgetfulness and behavioral problems.
• Avoid accepting such vague descriptions as "he had poor judgment."
• Obtain a specific history of the problem, and the situation(s) in which it arises, in order to place complaints in a broader context. For example, a person who has always had a poor memory for names should not be labelled demented if that trait continues into old age.

Memory problems may arise only in specific contexts, "either antecedent to some event or when the problem results in positive consequences or reinforcements for the individual" (Zarit, 1979, p. 242). It is always important to look for a functional basis for the difficulty.

When an individual problem has been specifically outlined and illustrated with examples, a nurse may steer discussions to a more systemic level by asking how the situation concerns family members. She might ask an adult daughter, for instance, "How is your father's forgetfulness and confusion a problem for you?"

Exploring each family's attempts to resolve its problems can also reveal any vicious interactional cycles that might maintain or escalate the AD problem. Questions such as, "When your husband forgets his words, what do you do?" or, "What has worked the best/the worst?" can be helpful.

Finally, assessing the presenting problem involves goal setting. Herr and Weakland (1979a) offer a useful question: "What is the smallest amount of change that would indicate to you that you are making progress in solving the problem?"

Planning

The information derived through assessment allows the nurse to formulate hypotheses about the interaction between family dynamics and the problematic AD symptom(s)—hypotheses that will guide intervention.

Zarit (1979) specifies several intervention goals for families coping with progressive cognitive deterioration of an elderly member (Table 23.2). Working from a systemic (Tomm, 1984a) and a strategic (Fisch, et al., 1982) perspective of family dynamics, the intervention goal(s) is (are) to introduce greater complexity into the family system and to build upon existent but formerly untapped family competencies and resources.

Table 23.2   Intervention Goals for AD Families

- Maintain maximum patient independence/function.
- Strengthen family caregiving capacity through emotional and informational support.
- Correct misconceptions about AD.
- Encourage/permit caregiver(s) to meet personal needs.
- Respond to patient's major behavioral problems.
- Arrange for appropriate outside support/care services.

Intervention

The systemic-strategic approach directs therapeutic efforts toward changing interactional patterns between people rather than toward changing a particular individual.

Provide information. Simply introducing new information about AD into
a family system can interrupt vicious cycles of family interaction,
because family members characteristically act according to their beliefs/
perceptions of "reality." New information may change not only the
existing beliefs/perceptions of the illness, but also perceptions of family
members' behaviors and motives, resulting in a "new family reality."
AD families need information about the causes, cures, and consequences
of cognitive decline (Zarit and Zarit, 1984) and about the course of
the illness (Gwyther and Matteson, 1983).

Causes of AD. The nurse should explain that the causes of AD are not
currently well understood. Genetic inheritance has been considered
but not confirmed; the slow-acting virus hypothesis has not been substantiated. Inactivity is considered not a cause but a result of AD (Zarit
and Zarit, 1984).

Cures. Zarit and Zarit (p. 240) also point out that "one of the most
crucial parts of an intervention is to dissuade (the family) from seeking
out quack or ineffective cures while still maintaining hope that something can be done."

Consequences of cognitive decline. The nurse can help the AD family
understand memory loss by explaining that the patient cannot remember
that he/she forgets and that forgetfulness does not result from lack of
effort, and by elucidating its behavioral impact.

Disease course. Gwyther and Matteson (1983) indicate that most families
who have received basic AD information want to know how the disease
will progress. This is especially true of families who have coped effectively in the past by gathering information and making plans. However,
three issues can complicate this process:
• family ambivalence about how much they want to know about the
disease (Gwyther and Matteson, 1983)
• highly idiosyncratic disease processes, which make it difficult to
predict specific functional changes over time (Berman and Rappaport,
1984)
• variation in family members' knowledge about AD, their misconceptions, and their desire for more information.

The nurse should verbally ascertain each family member's present
understanding of AD and perceived knowledge deficit, and then provide
specific information *in writing.* Two communication skills are better
than one, especially when a family is confused and in crisis.

Zarit (1982) does not consider the concept of AD stages useful since
patient deficits and the symptoms that families find distressing vary
widely. Gwyther and Matteson (1983, p. 94) however, determined that
"the stages of the illness offer some structure for the family caregiving
efforts."

Given the debatable usefulness of guidelines for patient decline, it is beneficial to inform family members about *their own* changes relative to the patient. Relatives need to recognize and prepare for the progressive loss of the family member they know. They must acknowledge that the patient's ability to fulfill established family roles (e.g., "Mr. Fix It," "peacemaker," "news agency") will decline or disappear. As the patient deteriorates, family members will be required to "assume the role of 'protective kin,' 'pocket brain,' or 'interpreter' for their disabled relative" (Gwyther and Matteson, 1983, p. 94). They will be forced to make decisions for their relative without his concurrence or approval.

Modify difficult behavior. Specific strategies for managing the emotional and behavioral problems common to Alzheimer's patients should be explained to the aging family. A compilation of suggestions offered is found in Table 23.3.

Use questions as interventions. The interview process—specifically circular questioning—can be used to release new information into a "stuck" family system. By encouraging family members to explore differences and acknowledge connections between their behaviors and their beliefs, implicit information can become explicit and "new" (Tomm, 1984b). Tomm explains that productive interview questions are based on two fundamental assumptions: that information lies in differences and that a behavior's meaning is derived from its context.

Circular questions—for instance, difference, behavioral effect, hypothetical, and triadic—probe the family system and mobilize existing but previously inaccessible internal resources. For example, when instrumental tasks change as a result of the patient's decreasing abilities, it becomes important to ask, "Which of the tasks that your husband used to perform will be most difficult for you to assume? Who can help you the most with this? Who in the family would be most helpful?"

The nurse's questions can help the family support its caregivers and recognize caregiving efforts. For instance, in a meeting with family members, the nurse might ask an adult child, "What do you think your father might be most grateful to your mother for these days?"

As AD shatters family members' dreams and life expectations, other family supports are needed and can be stimulated. In a family interview an adult child may be asked, "How different do you think life is for your mother now that your father has AD? What dreams and expectations did she have that she feels cannot be fulfilled? Which dreams can still be realized? Which need modification or letting go?"

Questions useful for prompting the family to examine its beliefs about the patient's abilities are:
• "Was there something that [the patient] did in the last month that surprised you?"

Table 23.3 Caregiving Strategies for Alzheimer's Patients

Patient Problems	Initial Family Reaction	Family Members' Interventions
Sleep disturbance	Sleep disturbance, irritability	• Keep patient awake during day. • Adjust time of patient's tranquilizer. • Provide exercise for patient. • Provide soothing stimulation (massage).
Exacerbation of symptoms in the evening (i.e., increased confusion)	Decreased patience	• Identify patient's "worst" time period. • Identify events/activities contributing to stimulus overload. • Decrease stimulation in environment around that time. • Get more rest. • Use diverting tasks.
Repetitive questions	"Last straw" effect	• Recognize that repetitive questions derive from fear and uncertainty. • State "I will take care of you." • Ignore questions. • Give attention to patient.
Repetitive acts	Annoyance	• Give patient a task to do or a soft toy. • Use gentle but firm touch to curtail activity.
Clinging/following	Distress, irritation, lack of privacy	• Recognize that the world is a strange place to someone who cannot remember. • Reframe patient behaviors from "irritants" to "compliments." • Remember that a patient is confident that you know the world. • Give patient something to do. • Find someone to be with patient. • Take time for self periodically.
Complaints, insults, accusations	Insulted, angry; fear that patient will insult/alienate outside help, therefore reluctant to ask for assistance	• Be empathetic; consider patient's point of view. • Look for underlying meaning and respond sympathetically. • Interpret malevolent remarks in a benevolent way; e.g., "You are cruel" may be a way of saying "life is cruel."
Misinterpretation of sounds and sights	Fear regarding personal safety (i.e., is there *really* someone in the house?), patient's stability (i.e., is patient *really* crazy?)	• Keep environment well lighted. • Explain what things are, but do not disagree directly. • Address patient directly by name. • Do not talk about patient in third person in patient's presence.
Demanding behavior	Feel manipulated, attributing demands to patient's pre-AD style of relating.	• Recognize that manipulation takes planning. • Relabel "demanding" behavior as patient's "need to be connected." • Look for something that is making patient feel lonely, abandoned, frightened.

(continued)

Patient Problems	Initial Family Reaction	Family Members' Interventions
Demanding behavior *(continued)*		• Be specific and direct: "I will see you (when)." • Set limits on what you can do. • Determine extent of patient disabilities.
Apathy/listlessness	Hopelessness, exhaustion	• Keep patient active. • Do simple tasks that patient can perform successfully. • Go for a walk. • Play music.
Anger	Defensiveness, anger	• Respond calmly. Do not respond with anger. • Remove patient from the stimuli that prompted outburst or remove stimuli.
Difficulty understanding directives/communicating	Impatience	• Keep assuming that patient can understand. • Supply word(s) if patient appears to be fumbling. • Look for meaning in patient behaviors. • Recognize that hearing loss often accompanies cognitive decline. • Recognize that patient may be able to read, even if unable to talk. • Keep voice low; remember that a male voice is easier to hear. • Repeat directives using same gestures and words. • Allow patient 2 minutes to respond.
Frustration related to not being able to succeed at former tasks.	Desire to take over and "do for"	• Break tasks into sequential steps or pieces.
Losing weight Not eating	Worry, frustration, impatience	• Offer one food at a time. • Offer six small daily meals. • Decrease external stimulation at meal time. • Allow patient 40 minutes per meal. • Relax.
Depression about declining cognitive abilities	Helplessness, protectiveness, withdrawal	• Ask patient what having AD means to him/her. • Be honest about diagnosis. • Involve patient in pleasant activity.
Aggressive behavior	Anxiety	• Recognize patient's sensitivity to nonverbal behavior. • Look for what might have provoked aggression (rushing, etc.). • Keep track of situations triggering adverse reactions. • Remove patient from situation.

(continued)

Table 23.3   Caregiving Strategies for Alzheimer's Patients
(continued)

Patient Problems	Initial Family Reaction	Family Members' Interventions
Nocturnal wandering	Worry, sleep disturbance	• Recognize that much wandering is goal-directed even if patient cannot express goal. • Provide rocking chair, music. • Walk patient during day. • Keep patient active during day. • Secure name tag on patient. • Dead-bolt doors. • Provide stuffed animal (has been found to decrease wandering and repetitive behaviors).

Sources: Mace and Rabins, 1981; Hirst and Metcalf, 1985.

• "What circumstances surrounded this event?"
• "How did the family members respond?"
• "Who was the most surprised?"
• "What was the last thing [the patient] did that seemed like his old self?"
• "What sense do you make out of this change in behavior?"

The nursing interview can also be used to facilitate resolution of problems associated with such AD behaviors as wandering. Useful questions include:
• "When [the patient] wanders, what does [the caregiver] do?"
• "Is [the patient] wandering more now than last month?"
• "What do you think is most upsetting to the [the caregiver] about (the patient's) wandering behavior?"

Reframing. Reframing provides a new way of looking at a situation or problem (Herr and Weakland, 1979a) for the purpose of generating new solutions. When family caregivers are encouraged to look for underlying, benevolent meanings to the AD patient's malevolent or noxious behavior, they are being encouraged to "reframe" (see Table 23.3 for examples). Families of AD patients must be reminded that the patient has no memory of the moments that went before (Mace and Rabins, 1981); they need to understand that the behavior is not willful or intended to irritate, but is instead beyond the patient's control. This relabeling can break a vicious cycle of argument between patient and family members.

Although all family caregivers require periodic respite, many reject such suggestions for fear of neglecting their perceived responsibility to the patient. They may feel guilty about taking time for themselves or frustrated by the conflicting desire to "take time off" and the desire to "take care of" the loved one. "Do not tell me to take time for myself.

If more than one person tells me to take time for myself, I am going to scream" is a commonly expressed sentiment and a definite indication that the caretaker *needs* some personal time.

By reframing, "taking time off" for oneself as another way of "taking care of" the patient, caretakers can often balance AD care and their own needs more effectively. In a particularly work-oriented family, the nurse might even prescribe relaxation as a family task—so that it seems like work!

Provide an opinion. The nurse might deliberately offer a summary statement, explanation, or opinion that differs from prevailing family beliefs.

Positive connotation. With positive connotation, the symptom is reframed and connected to other behaviors in the family system, and vice versa. "The presenting problem is construed as a solution (albeit a temporary one) to some other hypothetical or implied problem that could or would occur should the symptom not be present" (Tomm, 1984b, p. 264). The nurse must identify connections carefully and select issues relevant to the family's current life situation; in short, the opinion must be plausible, based on information that the family itself provided in response to circular questions (Tomm, 1984). For example, a wife refused to take her cognitively-impaired husband home after hospitalization, which incited her children to anger and action. Her behavior was positively connoted as a demonstration that she needed her family's help with the caretaking responsibilities and allowed a positive opportunity for the children to demonstrate their concern. Because the mother had previously done everything for herself, her behavior was positively connoted as being sensitive to her children's awkwardness in offering unsolicited help. The children's behavior was positively connoted as sensitivity to their mother's "little red hen" approach to life and concern about undermining her independence.

Split-Opinion. Split-opinion can be a useful intervention if intrafamily conflict hinders decision making. For example, family members may argue *ad nauseum* about the AD patient's functional abilities and about the need for institutionalization. During a family interview, the nurse can maintain engagement with the various family factions and stimulate decision making by mirroring their positions and/or by adding another perspective. The important thing is to avoid showing a preference for any particular point of view.

A nurse delivered the following split-opinion to an AD family at the end of a family interview: "Part of me feels that your husband/father can do a little more than what he is presently doing. That part of me would like you to do a little less for him next week. However, another part of me thinks that your husband/father is doing all he can do; in fact, that part of me is concerned about what might happen to you and your relationship with him and others if he did any more. That part of me would like you to think about and write down the consequences of your husband/father doing more and of you doing less."

Devise rituals. A therapeutic ritual is a specific task to be carried out by family members. This task is not intended to become part of the daily activity pattern; rather, it is to be used as an experimental change in usual family interaction patterns.

A caregiver reluctant to take respite despite persistent recommendations by the family and nurse was advised by the author to "make a list of things you used to enjoy doing that would consume no more than one hour of your time. Write each of these activities on a separate piece of paper. Place the pieces of paper in a bowl. Every Sunday night select one piece of paper from the bowl and see what your task for the week is. Schedule this duty into your week's labors." This ritual employed the client's language of hard work whenever possible. Leaving the choice of activity up to chance reduced the guilt that might be associated with "choosing" to take time off.

Rituals introduce clarity where there is too much confusion within the family. An odd day/even day ritual (Selvini, et al., 1978) can help sort out contradictory double-binding behaviors by prescribing sequence (Tomm, 1984b).

Eliminate double binds. While a planned double bind can sometimes be useful, the intervening nurse must be careful not to unintentionally "double bind" the caregiving family. Instructions given to family members often appear to send conflicting messages (for example, Mace and Rabins, 1981; Gwyther and Matteson, 1983). Gwyther and Matteson (1983) say that the AD patient cannot show appreciation because of cognitive deficits, yet they also assert that the patient may feel robbed of independence and resent caregiver intrusion. In other words, the instructions assert that the AD patient is at once aware and unaware, on different cognitive levels. Caregivers are told that patients do not understand but are also told to speak directly to them.

Another contradiction occurs when family members are cautioned not to respond to an AD patient as they would to a well-functioning person because this might *provoke catastrophic reactions* in the cognitively-impaired person. At the same time, caregivers are told that they are *not responsible for the reactions* and declining abilities of the patient. If there is a catastrophic reaction, the caregivers are told, "Don't worry, the patient will forget" (Mace and Rabins, 1981).

The caregiving family is thus in a paradoxical situation. The AD patient looks well and yet behaves "inappropriately." The relationship is intense; the patient gives conflicting messages, as do helping professionals; the caregiver can neither comment on the situation nor "leave the field." All the elements of a classic double bind (Watzlawick et al., 1967) are present.

Recommend a support group. Faced with the confusion and burdens of caring for an AD-afflicted relative, many families find consolation in talking with others who have "been there." Support groups offer both an emotional outlet and a source of management techniques. Support from family and friends reduces stress and vulnerability to illness (Caplan, 1981) and may reduce the caretaking family's sense of burden (Zarit et al., 1980). Group support may allow family members to delay the AD patient's institutionalization and enhance the family's ability to cope with the dementing illness.

Lazarus and colleagues (1981) studied changes in the psychological well-being of participants in a discussion group for relatives of Alzheimer's patients. Compared to nonparticipating AD relatives, group members felt more in control of their own lives and less at the mercy of fate.

By analyzing the most effective parameters of AD support groups, Kapust and Weintraub (1984) devised a flexible group approach that suits the constantly changing nature of AD management. They recommend that group sessions be scheduled realistically—in light of the special problems of AD caregiving—and that outside help with the patient during meetings be facilitated. The researchers also suggest that groups be heterogeneous and contain only 5 to 10 people, most or all of whom should be family members (spouse or adult children) caring for patients with varying degrees of AD-related impairment and living in diverse locations (i.e., home, institution). "Those with relatives still at home can become prepared for what lies ahead. Those with relatives in a nursing home can recall what it was like to have the patient at home. These comparisons are critical in coping with the gradual loss they are experiencing" (p. 460).

Through education and emotional ventilation/validation, support groups can deal with the following issues: the patient's medical work-ups, management problems, emotional reactions to having family roles changed by AD, utilization of community resources, and thoughts about the future.

Address the issue of institutionalization. Using the interventions just described, nurses can help family members cope more effectively with the problems presented by AD, perhaps delaying or even preventing institutionalization. However, when the patient's psychological and physical needs outweigh family and community resources, institutionalization becomes necessary.

Geiger and Berman (1983) identified five reasons for institutionalizing patients with a dementing illness:
• physically assaultive behaviors
• major physical/medical care needs
• incontinence
• physical/emotional illness in the caregiver
• financial inability to maintain patient at home.

If institutionalization is not discussed until the decision *must* be made, family members are usually too emotionally, physically, and financially exhausted to think clearly. Advance planning will allow more—and more productive—family involvement. To stimulate family discussion of this difficult decision while energy and time are still available, the nurse might ask family members, "How bad would things have to get for you to think about alternative living arrangements for [the AD patient]?" or "What would you observe in [the primary caregiver] that would indicate that it is time to place [the patient] in a nursing home?"

The family coping with AD will have many opportunities to discuss difficult topics during the course of their loved one's illness; those topics include management of property and financial affairs, mental incompetence, and power of attorney, just to name a few. The nurse can prepare the family for these highly sensitive discussions by involving as many family members as possible in early assessment sessions. Family members who feel that their perceptions of the problem are valued will be more likely to continue their support through difficult decision-making processes.

Evaluation

Evaluation is an ongoing process—not a terminal objective. The nurse working with the AD family must evaluate family responses to interventions continually; nursing interventions are like trial balloons that may either fly or fall but will always provide information helpful in generating other interventions.

Wasson and co-workers (1984) evaluated their outreach treatment to psychiatrically impaired elderly by defining "improvement" as:
• decreased symptoms
• increased sense of well-being (patient); and/or
• significantly reduced tension in relationships between the patient and significant others.

Patients with dementing illnesses demonstrated more improvement than those diagnosed with depressive or paranoid disorders.

From the family systems perspective, it is important for nurses to analyze how the interventions impact not only on the AD patient, but also on family members. It is important to note that family improvement will manifest itself in reduced caregiver symptoms, increased well-being in family members, a decreased sense of burden, and more positive perceptions of family relationships.

CONCLUSIONS

Effective intervention with aging families with AD must consider analogous patient and family experiences. The helplessness, suspicion, and confusion every patient feels are mirrored in family member interactions with the patient and with helping professionals.

This chapter has presented interventions to help AD families overcome their caregiving problems. As the AD patient becomes increasingly dependent on the family, so too may the family become dependent on the nurse's interventions. Unwittingly, the nurse may foster dependence and decreased functioning in the family, just as the family may foster the patient's debilitation. Therefore, the most important interventions are those that expose and interrupt the dependence and helplessness that exists between patients and families, and between families and nurses.

REFERENCES

Archbold, P.G. "All-Consuming Activity: The Family as Caregiver," *Generations* 7:12–13, 40, 1982.

Arie, T. "Dementia in the Elderly: Diagnosis and Assessment," *British Medical Journal* 4:540–43, 1973.

Berman, S., and Rappaport, L. "Social Work and Alzheimer's Disease: Psychosocial Management in the Absence of Medical Cure," *Social Work in Health Care* 10(2):53–70, 1984.

Bloom, M., and Munroe, A. "Social Work and the Aging Family," *The Family Coordinator* 21:103–115, 1972.

Brody, E.M. " 'Women in the Middle' and Family Help to Older People," *Gerontologist* 21(5):471–80, 1981.

Brody, E.M., and Lang, A. "They Can't Do It All: Aging Daughters with Aging Mothers," *Generations* 7:18–20, 37, 1982.

Caplan, G. "Mastery of Stress: Psychosocial Aspects," *American Journal of Psychiatry* 138:413–20, 1981.

Cohen, G. *Fact Sheet: Senile Dementia.* Washington, D.C.: Mental Institute of Mental Health, U.S. Department of Health, Education & Welfare, 1980.

Dewis, M.E. "Alzheimer's Disease: The Silent Epidemic," *Canadian Nurse* 78(7):32–35, 1982.

Fisch, R., et al. *The Factors of Change: Doing Therapy Briefly.* San Francisco: Jossey-Bass, 1982.

Geiger, D., and Berman S. Personal interviews with spouses of Alzheimer's disease patients at Veterans Administration Medical Center, Palo Alto, Calif., 1983.

Gwyther, L.P., and Matteson, G. "Care for the Caregivers," *Journal of Gerontological Nursing* 9(2):93–95, 110, 116, 1983.

Hayter, J. "Patients Who Have Alzheimer's Disease," *American Journal of Nursing* 74:1460–63, 1974.

Herr, J.J., and Weakland, J.H. *Counseling Elders and Their Families.* New York: Springer Publishing Co., 1979a.

Herr, J.J., and Weakland, J.H. "Communications Within Family Systems: Growing Older Within and With the Double Bind," in *Aging Parents.* Edited by Ragan, P.K. Los Angeles: University of Southern California, 1979b.

Hirst, S.P., and Metcalf, B.J. "Alzheimer's Disease: A Nursing Perspective," Workshop conducted at the University of Calgary, Calgary, Alberta, 1985.

Johnson, L.C. "Dyadic Family Relations and Social Support," *Gerontologist* 23:377–83, 1983.

Kahn, R.L., and Miller, N.E. "Assessment of Altered Brain Function in the Aged," in *The Clinical Psychology of Aging.* Edited by Storandt, M., et al. New York: Plenum Press, 1978.

Kapust, L.R., and Weintraub, S. "Living with a Family Member Suffering from Alzheimer's Disease," in *Helping Patients and Their Families Cope with Medical Problems: A Guide to Therapeutic Group Work in Clinical Settings.* Edited by Roback, H.B. San Francisco: Jossey-Bass, 1984.

Lazarus, L.W., et al. "A Pilot Study of Alzheimer Patients' Relatives Discussion Group," *Gerontologist* 21(4):353–58, 1981.

Mace, N.L., and Rabins, P.V. *The 36-Hour Day.* Baltimore: Johns Hopkins University Press, 1981.

McCubbin, H., et al. F-COPES (Family Crisis-Oriented Personal Evaluation Scales) Measuring Instrument. St. Paul: Family Social Science, University of Minnesota, 1981.

McKinstry, D.W. "Diagnosis, Cause and Treatment of Alzheimer's Disease," *Research Resource Reporter.* (U.S. Department of Health & Human Services) 6(6), 1982.

Pinel, C. "Alzheimer's Disease," *Nursing Times* 71(3):105–06, 1975.

Pratt, C.C., et al. "Burden and Coping Strategies of Caregivers to Alzheimer's Patients," *Family Relations* 34:27–33, 1985.

Ragan, P.K., ed. *Aging Parents.* Los Angeles: Ethel Percy Andrews Gerontology Center, University of Southern California, 1979.

Rosin, A.J. "The Physical and Behavioral Complex of Dementia," *Gerontologist* 23:37–46, 1977.

Roth, M. "Recent Progress in the Psychiatry of Old Age and Its Bearing on Certain Problems of Psychiatry in Earlier Life," *Biological Psychiatry* 5:102–05, 1977.

Schneck, M.K., et al. "An Overview of Current Concepts of Alzheimer's Disease," *American Journal of Psychiatry* 139(2):165–73, 1982.

Selvini Palazzoli, M., et al. "A Ritualized Prescription in Family Therapy: Odd Days and Even Days," *Journal of Marriage & Family Counseling* 4(3):3–9, 1978.

Shanas, E. "The Family as a Social Support System in Old Age," *Gerontologist* 19:169–74, 1979.

Silverstone, B. "Issue for the Middle Generation: Responsibility, Adjustment, and Growth," in *Aging Parents.* Edited by Ragan, P.K. Los Angeles: University of Southern California Press, 1979.

Simos, B.G. "Adult Children and Their Aging Parents," *Social Work* 18:78–85, 1973.

Sjogren, T., et al. "Morbus Alzheimer's and Morbus Pick: Genetic, Clinical & Pathoanatomical Study," *ACTA Scand* 82:1–152, 1952.

Sjogren, H. "Twenty-four Cases of Alzheimer's Disease: A Clinical Analysis," *ACTA Med. Scand.* (Supp), 246:225–33, 1950.

Tomlinson, B.E., et al. "Observations on the Brains of Demented Old People," *Journal of Neurological Science* 11:205–42, 1970.

Tomm, K. "One Perspective on the Milan Systemic Approach. Part I: Overview of Development, Theory and Practice," *Journal of Marital and Family Therapy* 10(2):113–25, 1984a.

Tomm, K. "One Perspective on the Milan Systemic Approach. Part II: Description of Session Format, Intervening Style and Interventions," *Journal of Marital and Family Therapy* 10(3):253–71, 1984b.

Wasson, W., et al., "Home Evaluation of Psychiatrically Impaired Elderly: Process and Outcome," *Gerontologist* 24(3):238–42, 1984.

Watson, W.L., and Wright, L.M. "The Elderly and Their Families: An Interactional View," in *Families with Handicapped Members.* Edited by Hansen, J.C., and Coppersmith, E.I., Rockville, Md.: Aspen Systems Corp., 1984.

Watzlawick, P., et al. *Pragmatics of Human Communication.* New York: W.W. Norton & Co., 1967.

Weakland, J.H., et al. "Brief Therapy: Focused Problem Resolution," *Family Process* 13:141–68, 1974.

Wells, C.E. "Pseudodementia," *American Journal of Psychiatry* 136:7, 896, 1979.

Wright, L.M., et al. "The Family Nursing Unit: Clinical Preparations at the Master's Level," *The Canadian Nurse* 81:26–29, 1985.

Wright, L.M., and Leahey, M. *Nurses and Families: A Guide to Family Assessment and Intervention.* Philadelphia: F.A. Davis Co., 1984.

Zarit, J.M. "Predictors of Burden and Distress for Caregivers of Senile Dementia Patients," Unpublished doctoral dissertation. Los Angeles: University of Southern California, 1982.

Zarit, S.H. *Aging and Mental Disorders: Psychological Approaches to Assessment and Treatment.* New York: The Free Press, 1980.

Zarit, S.H. "The Organic Brain Syndrome and Family Relationships, "in *Aging Parents.* Edited by Ragan, P.K. Los Angeles: Ethel Percy Andrews Gerontology Center, University of Southern California, 1979.

Zarit, S.H., and Zarit, J.M. "Psychological Approaches to Families of the Elderly," in *Chronic Illness and Disability Through the Life Span: Effects on the Family.* Edited by Eisenberg, M.G., et al. New York: Springer Publishing Co., 1984.

Zarit, S.H., et al."Relatives of the Impaired Elderly: Correlates of Feelings of Burden," *Gerontologist* 20(6):649–55, 1980.

INDEX

A

ABCX Model, 104
Absence seizure, 278
Adaptation model, 10
Adolescents
  with Crohn's disease, 168-185
  with diabetes, 308-318
  normal development of, 170
  obesity and, 319-341
Affective level of family functioning,
  70, 72, 362
Aging families, 200-215, 381-404
Alzheimer's disease, 381-404
  characteristics of, 383
  family assessment models for, 389
  impact on family, 385
  institutionalization and, 399-400
  stages of, 385, 392
  strategies for caregiver, 394-396
  support groups, 399

B

Behavioral level of family functioning,
  72-73, 362
Birth defects. *See* Congenital defects.

C

Calgary Family Assessment Model, 11,
  59, 108, 110, 114-116, 123, 124-
  125, 172, 234, 243, 268, 298,
  319, 349, 389
Cerebral palsy, prevalence of, 121
Child Health Assessment Intervention
  Model, 124, 125

Chronic illness
  assessment and, 58-66
  assumptions about, 56-58
  definition of, 12
  and the elderly, 13, 186-199, 381-
    404
  ethnicity and, 77-100
  family interventions in, 66-67
  family reactions to, 56-58, 70, 72,
    179, 266-268
  family tasks in, 16, 137-138
  nursing interventions in, 68-73
  patient reactions to, 20
  psychosocial factors in, 33-36
Circumplex Family Assessment Model,
  109, 111, 112, 189, 191
Cleft lip and cleft palate, 243-256
  family reactions to, 248-250
  nursing interventions in, 251-254
Cognitive level of family functioning,
  69-70, 362
Communication, dysfunctional, 319-
  321, 333, 336
Community health nursing, 4
Congenital defects, 102-119, 243-256,
  257-274
  parental reactions to, 103
  sibling reactions to, 107
Continuous ambulatory peritoneal
  dialysis, 231
Coping Health Inventory for Parents,
  111, 112, 143
Coronary artery bypass grafting, 370
Coronary artery disease, 370
Crisis management, 16-17
Crisis research, 103-107
Crohn's disease, 168-185
  body image and, 176
  family assessment model for, 172
  incidence of, 169
  sexual maturation and, 176
  sibling reactions to, 171
  symptoms of, 168-169